T0356660

An Introduction to Community and Primary Health Care

Fourth edition

Nurses and other health care professionals play a vital role in providing equitable, collaborative health care in the community. A primary health care approach is underpinned by the social model of health care and examines how social, environmental, economic and political factors affect the health of individuals, families and communities. *An Introduction to Community and Primary Health Care* provides a comprehensive and practical explanation of the fundamentals of this approach, preparing learners for professional practice in Australia and Aotearoa New Zealand.

The fourth edition has been restructured into four parts covering theory, working with diverse communities, key skills for practice, and the professional roles that nurses and other health care practitioners can play in primary care and community health practice. Each chapter has been thoroughly revised to reflect the latest research and includes up-to-date case studies, reflection questions and critical thinking activities to strengthen students' knowledge and analytical skills. A new postface reflects on the future directions of primary health care.

Written by an expert team of nurse authors with experience across a broad spectrum of professional roles, *An Introduction to Community and Primary Health Care* remains an indispensable resource for students of nursing and other health care professions.

Diana Guzys is Lecturer in Nursing in the School of Nursing, College of Health and Medicine at the University of Tasmania.

Elizabeth Halcomb is Professor of Primary Health Care Nursing in the School of Nursing at the University of Wollongong.

Cambridge University Press acknowledges the Australian Aboriginal and Torres Strait Islander peoples of this nation. We acknowledge the traditional custodians of the lands on which our company is located and where we conduct our business. We pay our respects to ancestors and Elders, past and present. Cambridge University Press is committed to honouring Australian Aboriginal and Torres Strait Islander peoples' unique cultural and spiritual relationships to the land, waters and seas and their rich contribution to society.

Cambridge University Press acknowledges the Māori people as tangata whenua of Aotearoa New Zealand. We pay our respects to the First Nation Elders of New Zealand, past, present and emerging.

Edited by
Diana Guzys and Elizabeth Halcomb

An Introduction to Community and Primary Health Care

Fourth edition

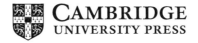

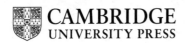

Shaftesbury Road, Cambridge CB2 8EA, United Kingdom

One Liberty Plaza, 20th Floor, New York, NY 10006, USA

477 Williamstown Road, Port Melbourne, VIC 3207, Australia

314–321, 3rd Floor, Plot 3, Splendor Forum, Jasola District Centre, New Delhi – 110025, India

103 Penang Road, #05–06/07, Visioncrest Commercial, Singapore 238467

Cambridge University Press is part of Cambridge University Press & Assessment,
a department of the University of Cambridge.

We share the University's mission to contribute to society through the pursuit of
education, learning and research at the highest international levels of excellence.

www.cambridge.org
Information on this title: www.cambridge.org/highereducation/isbn/9781009464659

First published 2014
Second edition 2017
Third edition 2021
Fourth edition 2025

Cover designed by Bec Yule, Red Chilli Design
Typeset by Lumina Datamatics Ltd

A catalogue record for this publication is available from the British Library

A catalogue record for this book is available from the National Library of Australia

ISBN 978-1-009-46465-9 Paperback

Additional resources for this publication at www.cambridge.org/highereducation/isbn/9781009464659/resources

Contents

Part II   Diverse communities

Chapter 13   Digital health   208
Isabelle Skinner

Chapter 14   Managing chronic health conditions   224
Catherine Stephen, Wa'ed Shiyab and Elizabeth Halcomb

Part IV   Community and primary health care roles

Chapter 15   Community health nursing   242
Amanda Moses, Judith Anderson and Melissa Hanson

About the authors

Editors

Diana Guzys RN, MN, Grad Dip Ed, Grad Dip Adolescent Health & Welfare, B Pub Hlth is Lecturer in Nursing in the School of Nursing, College of Health and Medicine at the University of Tasmania. After relocating to a rural environment and taking up a community health nursing role, Diana embraced a change in her professional practice and career direction. Health education and health promotion was the mainstay of her practice for over two decades, first as a generalist community health nurse and later as a secondary school nurse. Her current research demonstrates a return to seeking ways to improve and optimise the health of rural communities, and professionalism and practice of student nurses in rural and regional Australia.

Elizabeth Halcomb RN, BN(Hons), Grad Cert IC Nurs, Grad Cert Higher Ed, FACN, PhD is Professor of Primary Health Care Nursing in the School of Nursing at the University of Wollongong. She leads a strong research program in primary care nursing, with an emphasis on nursing in general practice, chronic conditions, preventive health and nursing workforce issues. In 2018, she was inducted into the Sigma Theta Tau International Nurse Researcher Hall of Fame for her work in primary care nursing. In 2019, she was the first nurse awarded the Charles Bridges-Webb Medal by the Australasian Association for Academic Primary Care for her significant contribution to academic primary care teaching and research. Her research program has provided new insights into the primary care nursing workforce and team-based models of care, particularly for disease prevention and chronic condition management.

Contributors

Catina Adams BA(Hons), GDipEd, RN, RM, MClinNursing, PhD, MACN, FHEA, CF is an academic midwife and nurse who coordinates the Child, Family, and Community Nursing course and is the Postgraduate Nursing Discipline Lead at La Trobe University. She was awarded her PhD in 2022, asking how the Enhanced Maternal and Child Health program supports women experiencing family violence. Her research interests include neurodivergence; family violence; perinatal anxiety; child, family and community nursing practice; the scholarship of teaching and learning; telehealth and clinical governance.

Judith Anderson RN, PhD, MN, MHSM, BN is adjunct Associate Professor at Charles Sturt University. Her career has been based in rural and regional Australia, working in community health, aged care, acute care and mental health. Judith has held various positions, including clinical nurse educator and nurse manager. In academia, she has taught and researched nursing, paramedicine and health care management and has published in these areas. Her current research focuses on marginalised groups, their access to health care and how to support them within the health care workforce.

Jessica Biles PhD, M(Ed), BN is Associate Professor in Nursing in the School of Nursing, Paramedicine and Healthcare Sciences at Charles Sturt University. Her PhD was a phenomenological study that focused on Indigenous cultural competence development across a cohort of bachelor of nursing degree students. Jessica works with regional communities and local health districts supporting the development and growth of ground-up community driven research initiatives and projects. Her current work focuses on ways to improve workforce and cultural capability for regional people. Jessica is the co-editor of *Aboriginal and Torres Strait Islander Health and Wellness* and is currently an international representative for the European Transcultural Nursing Society.

Bronwen Blake RN, Dip App Sc(Nurs), MIPH, MN(NP), Grad Dip Nurse (Immigration Health) is Clinical Nurse Consultant of the NSW Refugee Health Service. Bronwen's nursing career has been vast and varied, and she has qualifications in ICU and tropical nursing. She has worked with refugees and asylum seekers for most of her nursing career in Australia and internationally. Bronwen is currently on advisory committees for female genital mutilation and tuberculosis and is a member of the executive committee for the Refugee Nurses of Australia.

Rebecca Bosworth RN, BN Hons, PhD is Lecturer and Career Development Fellow in the School of Nursing at the University of Wollongong and an adjunct Lecturer at the National Drug and Alcohol Research Centre, University of New South Wales. Rebecca's PhD was in public health related to men living with HIV with an opioid use disorder seeking methadone maintenance treatment pre-release in a Malaysian prison. Rebecca has collaborated with the United Nations Office on Drugs and Crime (UNODC) about the prevalence of HIV, tuberculosis and viral hepatitis, and HIV-related mortality among people in prison, as well as the availability of interventions to prevent HIV transmission in prisons globally. Rebecca has a keen interest in improving the health and well-being of people who experience incarceration, specifically on topics such as their oral health, suicide prevention, illicit drug use, drug-related risk behaviours and harm reduction. Rebecca is a member of the International Corrections and Prisons Association (ICPA) health care network.

Donna Burt RN, Dip Health Sci, Grad Dip (Business Studies) is an experienced registered nurse who has worked as a health and safety professional for more than 20 years in a variety of industries including government, construction, agriculture, manufacturing and health care.

Kaara Ray B. Calma RN, BN(Hons), PhD is Lecturer in the School of Nursing and Midwifery at Griffith University. In 2018 she was appointed as one of the 21 World Health Organization's (WHO) Primary Health Care Young Leaders. She currently works with WHO leaders and international PHC professionals advocating for PHC as the vehicle to achieve universal health coverage on a local, national and global scale. In 2019, Kaara was awarded 'Recently Graduated Nurse of the Year' by the Australian Primary Health Care Nurses Association. As an academic, Kaara is the primary convenor for the Chronic Condition Management unit and teaches the undergraduate and postgraduate programs.

Lisa Chalmers MPH, BN, Cert(NIC) is Director of Health and Wellbeing at Barker College in Sydney and Board Director at the Australian Primary Health Care Nurses Association. She has over 30 years' nursing experience in a range of primary and tertiary health care settings. Lisa is strongly committed to championing the work of school nurses across Australia so that they are recognised for the incredible work they do and are supported as they seek to care for, educate and promote positive health behaviours for the future generation.

Sandy Eagar BAdvN, MRes(Hons), FACN, RN is Nurse Manager of the NSW Refugee Health Service with experience in refugee health, emergency nursing, education and management. Sandy has represented the Australian College of Nursing on the Detention and Immigration Health Advisory Groups, providing expert advice to the Department of Immigration and the Department of Home Affairs. She was recently the chairperson of the Refugee Nurses of Australia.

Leah East RN, BN(Hons), PhD, GradCertAP, Cert Reproductive and Sexual Health (Nursing) is Professor in Nursing at the University of Southern Queensland. Leah is passionate about primary health care, particularly women's health. She has held multiple positions associated with community, women's health and primary health practice, and is an active researcher.

Melanie Eslick RN, BA, BN, MNurs(ClinEd) is Lecturer in Nursing in the School of Nursing at the University of Tasmania. Prior to nursing, Mel spent many years as a clinical nutritionist in primary care. As a registered nurse and clinical trials coordinator, she specialised in cancer care in outpatient and cancer clinics. Her current research relates to health professionals' responsiveness to patients' health literacy, and student nurses' perceptions of professionalism.

Fiona Groome RN, GradDip(Occ Health) is Nurse Manager for Air New Zealand's Aviation and Occupational Health Unit. In 2013 she was awarded New Zealand Occupational Health Nurses Association New Member Award 2013. Fiona was previously president of the Auckland branch of the New Zealand Occupational Health Nurses Association. She has worked in settings across Australia and New Zealand including occupational health industries and contributed to a number of projects, including research on smoking culture and the proposal for smoke-free New Zealand Defence Forces.

Melissa Hanson BN, BSc(Hons) Nursing, GCertEmergNur, MN is Lecturer in Nursing at Charles Sturt University and a nurse practitioner specialising in emergency and critical care, and palliative care. She has been nursing since 2006 and has worked in metropolitan Sydney and rural and remote New South Wales. She is an active proponent for the *Voluntary Assisted Dying Act in New South Wales*.

Leesa Hooker RN, RM, GradCert CritCare, GradDipPH (Child and Family Health Nur), MHlth Sci, PhD is Professor of Maternal and Child Health Nursing and Associate Dean Research and Industry Engagement at the La Trobe Rural Health School, La Trobe University. She is a principal research fellow, leading two streams of research on reducing sexual and gender-based violence and child, family and community health. She has expertise in the epidemiology of family violence, women's mental health, sexual and reproductive health and parenting.

Sharon James RN, BN, Grad Dip(OHSN), MPH, PhD is a research fellow and project manager at the Sexual and Reproductive Health for Women in Primary Care (SPHERE)

Centre of Research Excellence (CRE) on the Australian Contraception and Abortion Primary Care Practitioner Support (AusCAPPS) Network. She has 25 years' experience in primary health care nursing and is a board director of the Australian Primary Health Care Nurses Association. Her experience in primary health care includes occupational health, general practice, undergraduate education and research. Sharon is a qualitative and mixed methods researcher with interests in women's health, abortion, long-acting reversible contraception, lifestyle risk, preventive care, interconception health and nursing roles in primary health care.

Natasha Jojo PhD, MSc(Nsg), BSc(N), Grad Cert(N), RN is Assistant Professor in the Faculty of Health at the University of Canberra. With a background in mental health, Natasha's research focuses on developing and evaluating programs for children with intellectual disabilities and supporting their parents, teachers and carers. She is a member of the Australian College of Mental Health Nurses, ASID (Australasian Society for Intellectual Disability), IASSIDD (International Association for the Scientific Study of Intellectual and Developmental Disabilities) and the Professional Association of Nurses in Developmental Disability Australia (PANDDA).

Sally Kane RN, Grad Dip OHN is Environment Health and Safety Manager at Agilent Technologies, a multinational high-tech company in the analytical chemical instrumentation business, a position she has held for 32 years. She is passionate about occupational health and safety and has overseen many changes in the way that people work. Sally has been involved in the Australian College of Occupational Health Nurses and the Australian and New Zealand Society of Occupational Medicine (ANZSOM) after it merged 16 years' ago. She was instrumental in developing the ANZSOM Occupational Health Nurse, Nurse Competency Standards and Nurse Recognition Program.

Grant Kinghorn RN, BN, MN(Mntl Hlth), PhD is Lecturer in the School of Nursing at the University of Wollongong. He has worked in correctional and forensic mental health environments for over 10 years. Grant has recently completed his PhD at the University of Wollongong, undertaking a study about nurses' transition into forensic mental health employment.

Fiona Landgren BPharm, GradDip(HospPharm) is Secretariat Manager at the Australian and New Zealand Society of Occupational Medicine and Director of Project Health Pty Ltd.

Lauretta Luck RN, BA, MA, MACN, PhD is Director of the Centre for Nursing and Midwifery Research, a conjoint position of the School of Nursing and Midwifery, Western Sydney University and Nepean Blue Mountains Local Health District. Lauretta has extensive experience researching nursing education and the nursing workforce and has expertise on the challenge of workplace violence towards nurses.

Susan Mlcek PhD, M Comm, MA(Comm & Cultural Studies), GCULM, BA Ed, BSW is Māori from Tauranga, New Zealand. She is a member of the Ngāi Te Rangi Iwi (tribe) and Ngāi Tukairangi Hapū (sub-tribe). Susan has a PhD in community development and management and is an associate professor in human services and social work. Her research areas include decolonising methodologies, Whiteness studies, cross-cultural competencies and culturally responsive practice, Indigenous approaches to research, and rural and regional social services delivery.

Amanda Moses BN, Grad Cert(OncNur), MN(NP), Grad Cert(L&T HE) is Lecturer at Charles Sturt University, primarily teaching undergraduate students with a focus on chronic disease management. She is a nurse practitioner and has over 40 years of nursing experience working in metropolitan, rural and remote locations. Amanda has a passion for improving the quality of life for people with chronic and complex conditions.

Ruth Mursa RN, DipAppSc(Nurs), MN(NursPrac), MN(AdvPrac Child, Youth and Family Nurs), Grad Cert Med & Forensic Management of Adult Sexual Assault, GradDipNg(ConNurseAdvis), Cert Sexual and Reproductive Health(Nurs) is an endorsed nurse practitioner and a PhD candidate at the University of Wollongong exploring men's engagement with general practice. Ruth has extensive clinical nursing experience within primary health care settings, including general practice and reproductive and sexual health.

Christopher Patterson RN, BN(Hons), MN(Mental Health), PhD is Associate Professor within the School of Nursing at the University of Wollongong. He is an active researcher with interests including pre-registration nursing education, mental health stigma and improving the health of people with the lived experience of mental illness. Christopher is also the co-founder and co-director of Recovery Camp, an award-winning program that provides immersive, experiential learning opportunities for nursing students and professionals focusing on mental health recovery and reducing stigma.

Kath Peters RN, BN(Hons), Grad Cert HE, PhD is Professor and Associate Dean (International and Engagement) in the School of Nursing and Midwifery at Western Sydney University. She has extensive clinical nursing and research experience with a strong background in health research and qualitative methodologies. Her areas of research expertise include women's health, underserved and marginalised populations and the health workforce.

Caroline Picton RN, BN(Hons), PhD is a clinical nurse specialist in mental health with an emphasis on delivering sensory modulation strategies to enhance psychosocial recovery and well-being. Caroline has extensive experience using recovery-oriented and trauma-informed practice with people living with a mental illness. She is a facilitator trainer of several models of care that are working towards zero suicides and reducing the use of seclusion and restraint in mental health units. The focus of her research is on using therapeutic recreation in outdoor nature-based settings to enhance mental health.

Maryanne Podham RN, BSci(Hons), GradCert(Clin Ed), MN(Clin Educ) is Lecturer in Nursing at Charles Sturt University. She has extensive clinical and teaching experience. Her research interests include advance care planning, end-of-life care and rural health.

Ravina Raidu RN, MN, BN(Hons), GradCert(Clin Nurs &Teach), GradCert(Clin Redesign), GradCert(Addiction Studies), Dip Project Mgmt, Dip Leadership & Mgmt is a tutor and project coordinator in the School of Nursing at the University of Wollongong. With over 25 years of experience as a clinician and educator, she has an extensive background in drug health and mental health nursing. Ravina's research interests are in clinical supervision, emotional intelligence in leadership, vicarious trauma and trauma nursing awareness within the drug and alcohol sector.

Wa'ed Shiyab RN, MSN is a PhD candidate in the School of Nursing, University of Wollongong. Her doctoral research explores nurses' use of mHealth apps in the management of chronic conditions.

Isabelle Skinner RN, RM, PhD, MPH&TM, MBA, GradDip Prof Comm(multimedia) is Conjoint Professor in the School of Nursing, University of Tasmania and the Tasmanian Health Service North West as well as the Nursing Director Education and Research. Isabelle has been researching, consulting about and implementing digital health innovations for over 20 years. She is currently researching the integration of wearable technologies into clinical management systems.

Catherine Stephen RN, BN, BN(Hons), PhD is Lecturer at the School of Nursing, University of Wollongong. Her doctoral project is a randomised control trial of a nurse-led intervention to improve hypertension management in primary care. Catherine is an early career researcher with a keen interest in primary health care, nurse-led intervention, chronic disease and hypertension management.

Michelle Stirrup RN, GradDip(Occupational Health and Safety), BPhEd has a decade of experience in occupational health. She has worked in food, manufacturing and aviation industries in New Zealand and within food processing in Australia. After completing a degree in physical education, her passion for physical rehabilitation and using exercise to manage medical conditions led her to a career in nursing.

Cristina Thompson RN, RM, BA, MBA is an Honorary Senior Fellow and PhD candidate at the University of Wollongong and an experienced health service researcher. Cristina has worked as a clinician and senior manager in rural and metropolitan health settings. She has expertise in health promotion, health service development, planning and evaluation. Her PhD is about investigating loneliness and social isolation in older people and the contribution of primary care in addressing this issue.

Kathleen Tori ENP, MN(NP), MHlthSci, BHlthSci, CCRN, GradDip VET, MACN, FACNP is a nurse practitioner and Professor of Nursing for the School of Nursing at Charles Sturt University. Her clinical, academic and research interests include all facets of nursing models of health care delivery: transitional processes of advanced nursing roles, barriers and enablers that challenge the successful implementation of alternate health service delivery, economic impact, digital health and sustainability of emerging nurse-led health care, particularly in rural areas.

Henrietta Trip DipNS, CertAdultTchg, BN, MHealSc(Dist), PhD is Senior Lecturer and Academic Lead with the Department of Nursing – Te Tari Tapuhi, University of Otago. Henrietta's nursing, teaching and research is focused on the self-management of long-term conditions across the lifespan for people with learning (intellectual) and developmental disability. This includes social models and accessibility for health care outcomes and workforce development.

Dean Whitehead RN, PhD, MSc, MPH, BEd, FACN is Senior Lecturer in the Institute of Health and Wellbeing at Federation University Australia. He has published widely in the fields of health promotion, health education, public health, primary health care, health policy and research methodology within and outside the nursing disciplines.

Anna Williams BHlthSci(Nur), MPH, PhD, RN is Deputy Head of School (Research) in the School of Nursing & Midwifery at the University of Technology, Sydney. Anna has expertise in primary health care research and evaluation, with specific research interests in the implementation and evaluation of complex interventions in primary health care, chronic illness management and aged care, especially the care of people experiencing dementia.

Nathan J. Wilson RN, BSocSC, MSc, GradCert App Stats, PhD is Professor in the School of Nursing & Midwifery at Western Sydney University. He has research interests in applied research that enhances the health, well-being and social participation of people with long-term disabilities, in particular people with intellectual and developmental disability. Nathan has expertise on the intersection of intellectual disability, social inclusion, the nursing workforce, men's health and sexual health. Professor Wilson was recently the president of the Professional Association of Nurses in Developmental Disabilities, Australia (PANDDA) and has led many campaigns to promote the specialty role of nurses who work with people with intellectual disability.

Rhonda Wilson RN, CMHN, PhD is an internationally recognised mental health nursing scientist with a research focus on digital health interventions. She is Professor of Mental Health Nursing at RMIT University. Over the past 36 years, she has worked in various roles as a clinical nurse, researcher and academic in Australia, Denmark and New Zealand. As a Wiradjuri (First Nation) descendent, she is a vigorous advocate and activist for the promotion of cultural safety and decolonisation in our education and health institutions. She is the current President of the Australian College of Mental Health Nurses.

Preface

This book provides an easy-to-read foundation for nursing students and nurses to introduce working in community and primary health care.

Part I introduces the key concepts that underpin primary health care nursing practice and explores how a nursing career can be developed in primary health care. The chapters provide a basic overview of these concepts to enable students to explore the associated theory and build a fundamental understanding that is so often assumed but not taught.

Part II provides insight into working with diverse communities, including priority groups such as those living with disability, rural communities and Indigenous peoples. Also, within this section, the issues of gendered health and mental health promotion are discussed. The focus on understanding the needs of diverse communities and the impacts of diversity on health care access are vital to ensuring 'health care for all'.

Part III provides information about specific community and primary health care skills. This information is discussed at a beginning practitioner level to be used as a launch pad for future clinical practice.

Part IV presents various community and primary health care nursing roles to enable students to explore the numerous career opportunities available in the sector. These chapters also demonstrate how the concepts discussed in the earlier sections of the text are implemented in practice. While these nursing roles cover a range of areas in which registered nurses contribute to the community's health and well-being, they are not an exhaustive list. Different jurisdictions and regions may have a range of roles in which nurses practice outside of the hospital. The opportunities are endless! One of the most exciting aspects of working in community and primary health care settings is that it offers many unique and eclectic practice possibilities to meet the diverse health needs of individuals, their families and communities.

Acknowledgements

We would like to acknowledge the work of Eileen Petrie, a co-editor of the first edition of this text, and Rhonda Brown and Dean Whitehead for their contributions to co-editing previous editions.

We also wish to acknowledge all those who contributed to the first and second editions: Jacqueline Allen, Nick Arnott, Christine Ashley, Stéphane Bouchoucha, Kerryn Butler-Henderson, Gabrielle Canfield, Leona Evans, Sandi Grieve, Barbara Hanna, Anne Hepner, Gylo Hercelinksjy, Kath Hoare, Kim Hyde, Dean Hyland, Lynda Jarvis, Basseer Jeeawody, Denise Johnston, Joanne Joyce-McCoach, Gail MacVean, Susan McInnes, Maree Meredith, Marisa Monagle, Rebecca O'Reilly, Susan Reid, Wayne Rigby, Vanessa Robertson, Andrea Scott and Kerry Taylor.

Cambridge University Press and the authors would like to acknowledge the feedback provided by peer reviewers of the draft manuscript, including Shazia Shehzad Abbas, Holly Clegg, Danijela Gasevic, Renju Joseph, Kerry Hampton, Navneeta Reddy, Loma-Linda Tasi, Colleen Van Lochem and Claire Verrall. Their feedback and comments were invaluable to the development of this edition.

The editors and Cambridge University Press would like to thank the following for permission to reproduce material in this book.

Cover image: © Getty Images/marumaru. **Figure 1.2**: reprinted from *Ottawa Charter for Health Promotion, WHO*, © (1986). **Figure 1.3**: reproduced with permission from the United Nations. The content of this publication has not been approved by the United Nations and does not reflect the views of the United Nations or its officials or Member States. **Figure 4.1**: reprinted from International Classification of Functioning, Disability, and Health (ICF), WHO, © (2001). **Figure 5.1**: © 2013, Springer Nature. Reproduced from Levesque et al.; licensee BioMed Central Ltd. Reproduced under Creative Commons Attribution License 2.0, http://creativecommons.org/licenses/by/2.0. **Figure 6.1**: reproduced with permission from Australian Human Rights Commission (2018). Face the facts: Gender equality. Retrieved from www.humanrights.gov.au/our-work/education/face-facts-gender-equality-2018 © Australian Human Rights Commission 2018. **Figure 6.2**: © 2022, AIHW. Reproduced under Creative Commons Attribution License 4.0, https://creativecommons.org/licenses/by/4.0/. **Figure 6.3**: reproduced by permission, NSW Health © 2024. **Figure 6.4**: © 2019, AIHW. Reproduced under Creative Commons Attribution License 4.0, https://creativecommons.org/licenses/by/4.0/. **Figure 7.1**: reproduced from Whitehead, D. (2011). Before the cradle and beyond the grave: A lifespan/settings-based framework for health promotion. *Journal of Clinical Nursing, 20*(15–16), 2183–94. © 2011 Blackwell Publishing Ltd. Reproduced with permission of John Wiley & Sons Ltd. **Figure 9.1**: reprinted from Framework for Action on Interprofessional Education and Collaborative Practice, WHO, p. 29, Copyright (2010). **Figure 9.2**: was supported by Healthcare Excellence Canada (HEC). Those preparing and/or contributing to this figure disclaim all liability or warranty of any kind, whether express or implied. From Oandasan,

I., Baker, G., Barker, K., Bosco, C., D'Amour, D., Jones, L., et al. (2006). Teamwork in healthcare: promoting effective teamwork in healthcare in Canada. Canadian Health Services Research Foundation. **Figure 10.1**: © Nursing Council New Zealand. Adapted and reproduced with permission of the Nursing Council of New Zealand. **Figure 12.1**: © 2001 Blackwell Science Ltd, Journal of Advanced Nursing. Reproduced with permission. **Figure 12.2**: © 2001 Blackwell Science Ltd, *Journal of Advanced Nursing.* Reproduced with permission. **Figure 12.3**: © 2003 Blackwell Publishing Ltd. Reproduced with permission. **Figure 12.4**: © The authors, 2005. Reproduced with permission of Lawrence W. Green. **Figure 12.5**: © 2003 Blackwell Publishing Ltd, *Journal of Advanced Nursing.* Reproduced with permission. **Figure 14.1**: reproduced with permission from Glasgow, R.E., Davis, C.L., Funnell, M.M. & Beck, A. (2003). Implementing practical interventions to support chronic illness self-management. *The Joint Commission Journal on Quality and Patient Safety*, 29(11), 563–74, Copyright © 2003 Joint Commission on Accreditation of Healthcare Organizations. Published by Elsevier Inc. All rights reserved. **Figure 21.4**: © 2023 Turning Point. Reproduced with permission. **Figure 22.1**: © 2023 UNHCR. Reproduced with permission. **Figure 23.1**: © The Australian and New Zealand Society of Occupational Medicine Inc. Reproduced with permission.

Table 17.1: © Commonwealth of Australia 2013. Reproduced with permission.

Some material in Chapter 7 has been adapted from Whitehead, D. (2011). Before the cradle and beyond the grave: A lifespan/settings-based framework for health promotion. *Journal of Clinical Nursing*, 20(15–16), 2183–94. © 2011 Blackwell Publishing Ltd. Reproduced with permission of John Wiley & Sons Ltd.

Some material in Chapter 12 has been adapted from Whitehead, D. (2003). Evaluating health promotion: A model for nursing practice. *Journal of Advanced Nursing*, 41, 490–8. © 2003 Blackwell Publishing Ltd, Journal of Advanced Nursing. Reproduced with permission of John Wiley & Sons Ltd.

Every effort has been made to trace and acknowledge copyright. The publisher apologises for any accidental infringement and welcomes information that would redress this situation.

PART I

Theory

1 Community and primary health care

Diana Guzys and Melanie Eslick

LEARNING OBJECTIVES

At the completion of this chapter, you should be able to:

- describe the principles of primary health care (PHC) and how these are linked to adopting the social model of health.
- recognise social determinants of health and how they relate to social justice and health equity.
- identify health promotion principles and strategies.
- explain the intersection of PHC, public health, primary care and communities.

Introduction

Holistic – consideration of the physical, mental, social and spiritual aspects of a person.

Social justice – an ethical principle that requires the outcome of an action to result in equality for all.

Health equity – recognition of differing circumstances requiring differing resource allocation or opportunities to achieve equality in health outcomes (WHO, 2021).

Empowerment – facilitating individuals, groups or communities to assume greater control over factors that influence their quality of life and health outcomes (WHO, 2021).

PHC is a philosophy or approach to health care where health is acknowledged as a fundamental right, as well as an individual and collective responsibility. A PHC approach to health and health care engages multisectoral policy and action which aims to address the broader determinants of health; the empowerment of individuals, families and communities in health decision making; and meeting people's essential health needs throughout their life course (World Health Organization (WHO), 2021). A key goal of PHC is universal health coverage, which means that all people have access to the full range of quality health services that they need, when and where they need them, without financial hardship (United Nations General Assembly (UNGA), 2019).

The PHC approach is **holistic**. It is founded on the social model of health, recognising that a person's health is shaped by their biology, social group and family influences; community factors; economic and environmental effects; as well as public policy. **Social justice**, **health equity**, **empowerment** and participation, **health promotion** and **prevention** are key principles of PHC. In a just society, everyone is supported to achieve and maintain optimal health and well-being. Improvements in health and **well-being** are achieved by addressing the social and environmental determinants of health and reducing the burden of preventable and non-communicable disease.

In this chapter, the social model of health and social determinants of health are explained, as well as the key frameworks underpinning PHC. The concept of health promotion – a fundamental component of PHC – is introduced.

PHC, primary care and community practice

Some people mistakenly believe that any health service delivery that occurs within a community setting constitutes PHC. However, PHC is a philosophy or approach to health care that aims to address the broader determinants of health, emphasising social justice, not simply providing treatment outside hospital settings. At the heart of PHC is the recognition of the impact of social determinants of health and working to address these through health promotion action. The term 'primary health care' is commonly misunderstood and erroneously used interchangeably with the term 'primary care'. Primary care is only a subset of PHC. Primary care is usually the first contact individuals have when they seek health care and typically occurs outside of hospitals. Intervention is the core activity of primary care provision, the focus of care being early diagnosis, effective treatment and disease management of an individual. Primary care services include general practices, community pharmacies, various allied health services, community nursing services, maternal and child health services, mental health services, drug and alcohol services, sexual health services and oral health and dental services (Department of Health, 2022). Fundamental to working from a PHC approach, whatever the health care setting, is acknowledging the significance of the social model of health and seeking to mitigate the influence of social determinants of health that negatively affect individuals, communities or specific population groups.

The social model of health

Health care systems have traditionally developed to respond to illness and disease, rather than to create and support wellness. Advances in science entrenched the biomedical model of health, which considers illness as a matter of cause and cure (Rocca & Anjum, 2020). However, this view has been challenged in the face of mounting evidence, which demonstrates that achieving health and well-being is far more complex. The social model of health takes a broader view of the complex interactions occurring within a society that influence individual and community health and well-being. Various factors that can positively or negatively influence achieving and maintaining good health and well-being are now recognised and are collectively referred to as the **social determinants of health**.

A key principle underpinning the social model of health is social justice. In health, as in many other areas, equality is achieved by adopting an equitable approach. It is essential not to confuse equity with equality. Health equality refers to all people having the same health outcome – ideally, this is to achieve their full health potential – while health equity refers to providing resources and services in response to people's needs to achieve health equality. As Nutbeam and Kickbusch (1998, p. 355) explain, 'Equity in health means that people's needs guide the distribution of opportunities for well-being'. The social determinants of health influence **health inequities**.

To achieve social justice, we must act to reduce social inequity (Taylor et al., 2021). Nurses have a professional duty to advocate for equity and social justice in health, addressing health inequities by providing non-discriminatory, person-centred appropriate and accessible care (International Council of Nurses (ICN), 2023). Inequities can be reduced by addressing the broader determinants of health, by empowering individuals and communities, and by facilitating access to appropriate and sustainable health care (Taylor et al., 2021). Health outcomes are influenced by economic, social, political and environmental conditions. The health care

---

Health promotion – strategic action engaging social and political processes enabling people, individually and collectively, to increase control over the determinants of health and thereby improve their health (WHO, 2021).

Prevention – measures to reduce the occurrence of risk factors, prevent the occurrence of disease, arrest its progress and reduce its consequences once established (WHO, 2021).

Well-being – a positive state, which encompasses quality of life resilience and capacity for action (WHO, 2021).

Social determinants of health – the social, cultural, political, economic and environmental circumstances across a person's lifespan (non-medical factors) that influence the conditions of daily life (WHO, 2021).

Health inequities – unfair and avoidable differences in health status and distribution of health resources between population groups (WHO, 2021).

sector alone is not able to achieve the changes that need to be made to facilitate and support health. The financial sector, industrial sector, educational sector, transport sector, government sector and so on all have a role to play.

The social determinants of health

The social determinants of health are the circumstances of daily living that influence a person's health and well-being (WHO, 2021). They may act as barriers or enablers (or risk factors and protective factors) to achieving optimal health. These factors are frequently interrelated, which may exacerbate or potentiate the influence they exert. In 1998, the WHO first published a document that identified 10 determinants of health called *The Social Determinants of Health: The Solid Facts*. This document was revolutionary at the time, clearly acknowledging factors beyond biology and physiology relevant to health outcomes. There is no single definitive list of social determinants, as these can be described in various ways by numerous sources. The language around determinants continues to evolve, to reflect current-day influences on health equity, as reflected by the changes in language used in WHO documents published 20 years apart in Table 1.1.

Table 1.1   Comparing WHO social determinants of health

WHO 1998; 2003 (Wilkinson & Marmot, 2003)	WHO 2024
The social gradient	
Stress	Education
Early life	Early childhood development
Social exclusion	Social inclusion and non-discrimination
Social support	
Work	Working life conditions
Unemployment	Unemployment and job insecurity
	Income and social protection
Food	Food insecurity
Transport	
Addiction	
	Housing, basic amenities and the environment
	Structural conflict
	Access to affordable health services of decent quality

The social gradient

Some groups in society have less chance than others of achieving optimal health and well-being due to the circumstances of their lives. The most disadvantaged groups in a society are found to have the poorest health and are more likely to have greater exposure to health-damaging risk factors (Marmot, 2020). Put simply, the greater the disadvantage people face, the harder it becomes to make healthy choices that promote well-being. An individual, group or community may move in either direction along an imaginary continuum of advantage or disadvantage, as life circumstances change, and may move back and forth over time. This imaginary line is referred to as the 'social gradient'. This concept is represented in Figure 1.1.

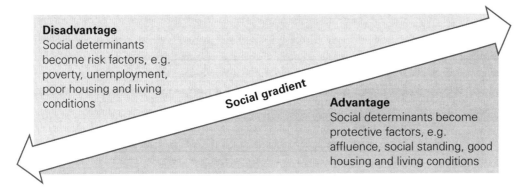

Figure 1.1   The social gradient

Exploring the interrelatedness of the social determinants of health

Although the language used to describe social determinants may be confusing at times, understanding the influence of the associated concept is more important than the terminology used. It is challenging and artificial to contemplate the separate influence of specific social determinants as they are inherently interrelated. Consider economic factors, for example. Income and wealth begin to influence health and well-being from early in life, even before birth (Braveman, 2023). Individual income, as well as employment opportunities (or security) and how they influence a person's well-being, are often more visible than other social factors – this became more apparent during the COVID-19 global pandemic (Armenti et al., 2023).

Income

Income can impact a range of life issues, such as food choices, recreational and social opportunities, access to health care services, educational opportunities and housing options. Housing that is further away from resources, such as schools, shopping centres and health care facilities, is usually cheaper to rent or buy. This means that access to transportation to reach these resources and potential employment opportunities becomes very important. Lack of transportation may limit a person's opportunity for education, and ability to go out with friends or to participate in sporting or other social activities, making them feel isolated or excluded. Depending on personal life circumstances, funding transportation or keeping a car may be prioritised before spending money on food, heating, health care or recreational activities that promote well-being.

Education

Generally, the level of education a person receives influences the type of employment they obtain, which influences how much they may earn. People may be employed, but not necessarily at the level they would like to be – known as being 'underemployed' – and they may also be unemployed. Current employment models find many people working in more than one workplace, and in part-time, contract and/or casual positions. Job insecurity and precarious employment are associated with poorer well-being, physical and mental health (Jaydarifard et al., 2023). Employment opportunities can be influenced by numerous factors, including level of education, geographic location and political conditions (Braveman, 2023).

Prejudice/social exclusion

Other less obvious social factors may similarly influence health outcomes. A person's gender, sexuality or ethnicity may limit educational or employment opportunities, act as a barrier to health care access or contribute to prejudice, leading to social exclusion or isolation (Heise et al., 2019). Social isolation contributes to stress, impacting physical health and mental well-being. Poorly managed stress may lead to unhealthy behaviours, such as illicit substance use. Subsequently, this could affect income, employment, housing and so on (Brandt et al., 2022).

Early life

Early life development and experiences may affect health in many ways. Learned behaviours as diverse as nutritional practices, hygiene, communication style, conflict resolution and stress management can have lifelong consequences. While many protective factors result from positive early life experiences (La Charite et al., 2023), negative factors can lead to lifelong disadvantage. Children whose parents regularly engage in substance use are more likely to initiate similar behaviours at an early age (Kingston et al., 2017). Exposure to intimate partner and family violence is associated with an increased risk of mental health concerns, delinquency and potential for future violence in intimate relationships (Ruddle, Pina & Vasquez, 2017).

Political environment

Extreme political conditions, such as the presence of war or conflict, have obvious impacts on health, such as increased demands on and reduced access to health systems (Hameed, Rahman & Khanam, 2023). However, less obvious political factors, such as government social policies or taxation, are also social determinants of health. Taxation is used by governments to discourage unhealthy behaviours, such as higher taxes on goods like tobacco and alcohol. Revenue raised via taxes is used to fund health care, education and a range of social support programs. Social support provided by governments may include public housing for low-income families, free or subsidised education and universal health care. Socially cohesive societies with social support structures that provide high-quality education and health services demonstrate significant improvements in health that are not apparent in equally affluent but less socially cohesive nations (Taylor et al., 2021).

Physical environment

The built and natural environments can contribute to or negatively impact the health of individuals and communities. The natural environment may influence people's health through extremes in weather conditions such as flood, drought and temperature; events such as earthquakes, tsunamis, cyclones and bushfires influence housing, employment and other opportunities. The impact of climate change on health is increasingly evident and an increasing concern to health professionals (Inglis et al., 2023). Heatwaves are responsible for a significant number of premature deaths (Ballester et al., 2023). Water quality and quantity changes have led to population displacement, loss of agricultural productivity and degraded ecosystems (du Plessis, 2022). Food security is threatened with agriculture, production and food distribution affected globally (Schnitter & Berry, 2019).

The built environment impacts health in terms of access to green spaces, air and noise pollution, road traffic and sanitation. Air pollution, particularly in urban areas, is associated with increases in the incidence of respiratory conditions and exacerbation of respiratory conditions such as asthma (Cohen et al., 2017). Access to basic needs, such as safe food and clean water supplies, adequate housing and transportation systems, clean air and recreational facilities, are environmental factors that affect health and well-being (Patrick, Capetola & Henderson-Wilson, 2021).

REFLECTION

Consider the impact on different members of a community following an event such as an earthquake, flood or bushfire. How might an individual's experience of the event be influenced by factors such as social support, sufficient income to have adequate insurance, ongoing employment, housing and other social determinants?

Some individuals and communities – and even some countries – are socially disadvantaged. Health inequities place these groups at further disadvantage when it comes to their health. Therefore, to achieve the same health outcomes as those who are not disadvantaged, more resources and assistance are required. The effects of social factors, such as gender, class and race, are interconnected and reflect systems of oppression such as sexism and racism. When multiple disadvantages compound, they create further disadvantage. This is known as **intersectionality** (Kelly et al., 2022; Sabik, 2021). For example, all women may experience discrimination based on their gender, but for Indigenous or Māori women, this may be compounded by racism.

Intersectionality – a theoretical framework that considers how people's experiences and access to resources are shaped based on their interacting social identities.

REFLECTION

Consider how you would explain the difference between health equity and health equality to someone who believes that it is not fair if they do not receive the same resources as those given to someone else.

Promoting health

Health promotion is a core principle of PHC. Health promotion focuses on social justice and health equity by providing strategies to enable people to optimise their health via fair and just access to health resources and services (Nutbeam & Muscat, 2021). The guiding framework underpinning health promotion action is referred to as the *Ottawa Charter for Health Promotion* (the Ottawa Charter). This document was developed at the First International Conference on Health Promotion in Ottawa, Canada, in 1986 organised by the WHO. The

Ottawa Charter defined health promotion as 'the process of enabling people to increase control over, and to improve, their health' (WHO, 1981; 1986). Five areas for strategic action, which are still followed today (Wilberg, Saboga-Nunes & Stock, 2021), were designed to improve and maintain the health and well-being of individuals and communities. This is achieved using the primary principles of health promotion activity: to advocate, mediate and enable.

The health promotion activities advocate, mediate and enable, presented in this order, represent a continuum of intervention required to facilitate better health outcomes. Health advocacy is undertaken to change policy and systems to create favourable conditions for better health choices and health outcomes (Chhetri & Zacarias, 2021). When nurses advocate for health, we take a stand on behalf of others who are not able to take this stand for themselves. This may be due to a lack of knowledge or understanding, having little power or authority in the situation or perhaps due to lack of skill and confidence. Advocacy involves some form of effort on behalf of others, whether through speaking, writing, social media or even protesting, and occurs at individual and community levels. It may be required to: protect people's rights; challenge organisational policy, procedure and practice; mobilise resources; or gain political commitment and social acceptance for change (Taylor et al., 2021). Mediation is the process through which competing interests are reconciled to promote and protect health (WHO, 2021). Nurses have a responsibility to ensure that good health remains the priority when competing care requirements might create barriers to better health. However, mediation for health promotion purposes is more likely to relate to actions taken to facilitate cooperation between governments and non-government organisations. In health promotion, enabling refers to taking action in partnership, to empower individuals or communities to become empowered in regard to their health (WHO, 2021). To achieve optimum health outcomes, they must be knowledgeable, skilled and appropriately resourced.

The strategies for action in health promotion

The five key action areas distinguished in the Ottawa Charter (WHO, 1986) provide a comprehensive framework for strategic action in health promotion. These strategies are examined next. When multiple strategies are used simultaneously, the effectiveness of the health promotion intervention is strengthened.

Building healthy public policy

Building healthy public policy directly refers to any set of decisions that can be made by or applied to a specific population. As such, organisations may provide policies, which may take the form of mission statements, procedures, strategic plans and regulations (Taylor et al., 2021). An example of organisational policy might be a kindergarten with a 'no hat, no play' policy in response to sun exposure risk. However, public policy frequently relates to government decision making at various levels (for example, federal, state or local council – in Australia). Governments address health via policy, legislation, fiscal measures and taxation. Public policy devised and enacted by governments directly affects the availability and accessibility of health care services, as well as influencing the sectors that affect health in less obvious ways. Examples of public policy impacting health and well-being include decisions regarding housing regulations, importation of food and road safety.

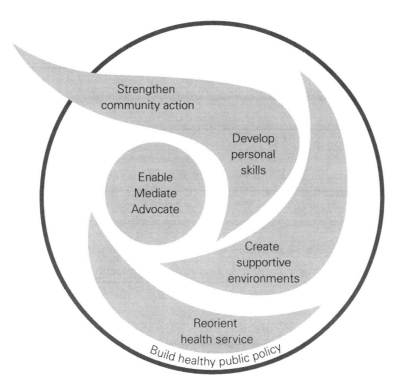

Figure 1.2   The *Ottawa Charter for Health Promotion*
Source: WHO (1986).

Strengthening community action

This key area for action refers to the collective effort by communities aimed at improving health through increasing community control over the social determinants of health that are impacting their community (WHO, 2021). This is achieved by empowering community members to work together to apply their skills and resources in collective efforts to address health priorities and meet health needs. This results in individual and community participation, the development of mutually supportive relationships and the encouragement of cooperation in decision making and action.

REFLECTION

1. Do you participate in any community actions that promote health?
2. How might you, as a registered nurse, strengthen community action in your local area?

Creating supportive environments

Good urban planning for recreation, transportation, health services and educational facilities demonstrates how the built environment can positively support health (Mouratidis, 2021). Conservation of the natural environment also facilitates better health, through clean air and water, minimising the effect of climate change and maintaining biodiversity (Barraclough et al., 2023). However, the environment for health is more than the physical, built and natural environments; it also covers the influence of the social and emotional environments (Magzamen et al., 2017). A supportive environment facilitates individuals, groups and communities to make informed choices and take action to optimise their health. The social environment is enhanced through participation and developing **social capital**. The emotional environment is enhanced through social inclusion and resilience.

Social capital – the degree of social cohesion that exists in communities which is created through everyday interactions between people that establish networks, norms and social trust, facilitating cooperation for mutual benefit (WHO, 2021).

Developing personal skills

Developing personal skills focuses on health education and the development of appropriate life skills to empower an individual's ability to make decisions and have control over their personal health decisions (WHO, 2021). The development of personal skills contributes to improving an individual's **health literacy**.

Health literacy – a sufficient level of personal skill, knowledge and confidence to take action to improve personal and community health, through changing behaviour and living conditions (WHO & United Nations Children's Fund (UNICEF), 2020).

Reorienting health services

Reorienting health services is a necessary response to burgeoning health budgets, the significant increase in chronic conditions and aging populations (Freijser et al., 2023; Maresova et al., 2019). Health care reform in Australia and Aotearoa New Zealand highlights the need to shift health care from a reactive, acute care focus to a greater emphasis on proactive, preventative and health promotion action utilising primary and community care services (Department of Health, 2022; Ministry of Health, 2024).

CASE STUDY 1.1

Jenny is a registered nurse who runs a well women's clinic at a community health centre in a regional city, providing cervical screening and sexual health information. She successfully ran an awareness campaign promoting the need for cervical screening for older women in the community. However, Jenny was disappointed when she realised that, although screening rates had increased locally in the general community, the number of Indigenous women undertaking cervical screening had not altered. She organised a meeting with members of the local Indigenous community service to discuss her concerns.

Following the meeting, Jenny sought funding to run a well women's festival at the local Indigenous service to highlight a range of health services available and to provide educational activities on relevant health issues in a culturally aware manner. Jenny also worked with members of the local community to assist them to become peer support educators, providing information about the importance of cervical screening. Then Jenny negotiated an agreement between her community health centre and the Indigenous community service to run a well women's clinic specifically for Indigenous women at the Indigenous community centre one afternoon per month.

REFLECTION

1. Which of the five Ottawa Charter strategies for action in health promotion does Jenny draw on?
2. Can you think of other ways in which Jenny could promote participation in cervical screening by Indigenous women in her community?

Health prevention

Prevention is a term often associated with health promotion activity, it is sometimes referred to as health prevention, which sounds like it is the opposite of health promotion. However, prevention refers to measures to reduce the occurrence of risk factors, prevent the occurrence of disease, arrest its progress and reduce its consequences once established (WHO, 2021). Depending on where activity is taking place along an illness trajectory, the preventative action may be described as primary, secondary or tertiary prevention.

Primary prevention activities relate to risk factors and risk conditions and stopping a condition before it occurs (Willis et al., 2022). Social marketing and the provision of health information, health education and skill development, community action and creating supportive environments are common health promotion activities associated with primary prevention.

Secondary prevention is associated with early detection and treatment to minimise complications of an existing health issue, recovery from health concerns and prevention of further problems (Willis et al., 2022). Health promotion activities focus on screening and individual risk-factor assessment, personalised health education and skills development. Community action and the creation of supportive environments tend to relate to specific illness concerns, such as the creation of support groups for people who share health problems.

Tertiary prevention is concerned with maximising the quality of life of an individual with an established health issue (Willis et al., 2022). Management and rehabilitation are at the crux of tertiary prevention. Condition-specific health education, skills development and creation of a supportive environment are required.

CASE STUDY 1.2

Kaye is a community health nurse based in a small rural town. The community health service that employs her provides several programs to promote healthy lifestyles in both the small town and for those residing in local smaller townships. Each year the community health service has a stall at the local show to promote the service and the programs they offer. Kaye has been asked to take blood pressure readings for community members attending the show to encourage people to stop at the stall and learn more about the health service.

Andrew is one of the people who stop to have their blood pressure taken. He is a 24-year-old electrician, who plays for the local football and cricket teams. After measuring Andrew's blood pressure, Kaye explains that his reading is within the normal range for someone of his age. Andrew asks Kaye to explain what that means, what result would be considered abnormal and why would abnormal results occur? Kaye provides a quick overview of the physiology related to blood pressure and explains how lifestyle risk factors and underlying conditions might influence blood pressure. Andrew thanks Kaye for her time and the chat and, realising that a queue has formed of people waiting to have their blood pressure taken, hastily says goodbye and leaves.

REFLECTION
Do you consider what Kaye was doing at the show to be health promotion? Why or why not?

Key frameworks underpinning the evolution of PHC

Beyond the Ottawa Charter (WHO, 1986), several other events and documents have contributed to the evolution and integration of PHC globally.

Declaration of Alma-Ata and Astana Declaration

PHC was first defined in the *Declaration of Alma-Ata* (WHO, 1978), developed during the International Conference on Primary Health Care held by the WHO. This Declaration expressed the need for urgent national and international action to protect and promote the health of all people. It identified PHC as an essential component of the health care process. The Declaration states that people have a right participate, individually and collectively, in the planning and implementation of their health care, supporting self-reliance and self-determination. Additionally, health care should be made universally accessible to individuals and families in their community, being delivered as close as possible to where people live and work (WHO, 1978).

Forty years after the Declaration of Alma-Ata, the *Declaration of Astana* (WHO, 2018), reaffirmed the importance of PHC as a fundamental component of achieving universal health coverage and advancing the health and well-being of populations around the world. Delegates made a commitment to orienting health systems towards PHC greater progress towards universal health coverage and the health-related Sustainable Development Goals (SDGs) (WHO & UNICEF, 2020). The Astana Declaration highlights the need for governments, in collaboration with international partners and civil society, to invest in health promotion strategies that prioritise preventative and holistic approaches to health, broadening to consider non-communicable diseases, such as mental health, and climate change impacts.

SDGs and the Shanghai Declaration

Established by the United Nations (UN) in 2015, the SDGs (UN, 2015), are a set of ambitious targets for global economic, social and environmental improvement (Fields et al., 2023) (see Figure 1.3). Of the 17 SDGs, Goal 3 specifically targets 'Good Health and Well-being', aiming to ensure healthy lives and promote well-being for all ages. PHC and health promotion are critical components of achieving this goal. However, the link between the SDGs, PHC and health promotion extends beyond Goal 3. PHC and health promotion play a crucial role in addressing the root causes of health disparities, reducing poverty (Goal 1), promoting gender equality (Goal 5), ensuring quality education (Goal 4) and fostering economic growth (Goal 8).

Despite a clear link between the nursing profession and SDG 3: good health and well-being, Fields and colleagues (2021) report a disconnect between nurses and the relevance of the SDGs to their nursing practice. However, nurses who work using a PHC approach already address many elements of the SDGs including: social justice; health promotion action to address the social determinants of health; encouraging healthy behaviours at individual and community levels; and care of vulnerable populations (Fields et al., 2021). Through PHC, communities receive the necessary health services and support to prevent illness, manage chronic conditions and promote optimal well-being. The integration of health promotion

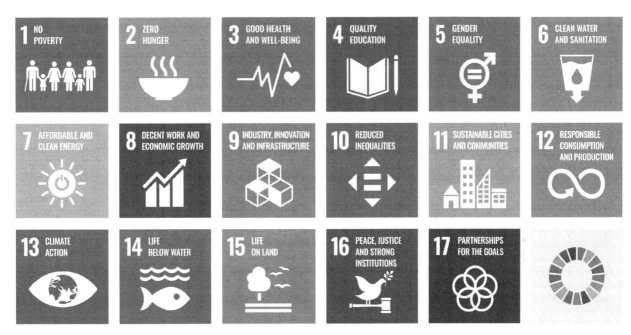

Figure 1.3 The Sustainable Development Goals (SDGs)
Source: UN (2024).

within PHC systems empowers individuals to take an active role in their health, which contributes to the broad aim of Goal 3. Two years following the release of the SDGs, the *Shanghai Declaration* on *Promoting Health in the 2030 Agenda for Sustainable Development* (WHO, 2017) reinforced health promotion efforts in alignment with the SDGs. This re-emphasised health as a universal right and a global political priority. This Declaration focuses on three pillars – healthy cities, enhancing health literacy and good governance – and posits that consideration of the goals of society and new economic approaches will contribute to the success of health promotion for sustainable development.

REFLECTION

Review the SDGs and how they relate to social determinants of health.

1. Which SDGs might influence your practice as a registered nurse?
2. How can nursing, as a profession, contribute to meeting these goals?

Operational Framework for PHC

The WHO and UNICEF (2020) developed an *Operational Framework for Primary Health Care* to guide effective implementation of the *Astana Declaration* commitments. Several core components of PHC are reinforced in the Framework:

- Addressing 'people's health needs through comprehensive promotive, protective, preventive, curative, rehabilitative and palliative care' across the life course.
- Provision of primary care services and public health functions as central elements of integrated health services.
- Empowering individuals and communities to optimise their health, 'as advocates of policies that promote and protect health and well-being, as co-developers of health and social services, and as self-carers and caregivers'.
- 'Systematically addressing the broader determinants of health (including social, economic and environmental factors, as well as individual characteristics and behaviour) through evidence-informed policies and actions across all sectors' (WHO & UNICEF, 2020).

The Framework proposes 14 PHC 'levers' – four core strategic levers and 10 operational levers – designed to work synergistically when they are considered and incorporated into nations' health strategies. To facilitate this, practical, evidence-based actions are proposed for all levers, with accompanying tools and resources to help facilitate the actions. Operational levers are wide-ranging, from models of care to digital technologies for health, to purchasing and payment systems. To use the Framework, countries first assess their needs and capacity then prioritise levers and actions to apply when planning national health policy and strategies.

Global health

Further evolution of PHC philosophy can be seen in the emerging concept of global health. The Global Advisory Panel on the Future of Nursing taskforce explain global health as planetary health, including human, animal, environmental and ecosystem health, with an emphasis on transnational health issues, synthesising population-based prevention and individual holistic care (Wilson et al., 2016). The priorities are health-promoting sustainable sociocultural, political and economic systems to understand emerging health challenges and achieve equity in health for all people and improved health. This is accomplished through individual and population-level care that addresses the social determinants of health, ethical practice and respect for human dignity, rights and cultural diversity. Interdisciplinary collaboration and an interdependent partnership with communities and other health care providers are foundational to global health (Wilson et al., 2016). Transnational health considers issues that go beyond borders, such as climate change and human trafficking, while global public health considers health effects arising from globalisation (Keleher, 2021).

Conclusion

PHC has developed from recognition and improved understanding of the social factors that influence health outcomes. Adopting the social model of health acknowledges the multidimensional interactions that occur within a society and that affect the health of individuals and communities. In this model, health is viewed as being shaped by individual biology, group and family influences, community factors, economic and environmental influences, as well as broader public policy. Social justice underpins the social model of health. Additional support for disadvantaged individuals and communities is necessary to achieve and maintain their optimum level of health and well-being. This is achieved through the equitable distribution of resources and assistance.

PHC emphasises health promotion to reduce health disparity and improve health outcomes. Health promotion is a significant and complex process undertaken to improve and maintain the health and well-being of individuals and communities. Primary care is acknowledged as an important aspect of health care delivery; however, it is not the comprehensive level of care encapsulated in a PHC philosophy. Within the PHC philosophy, principles of accessibility, affordability, sustainability, social justice and equity, self-determination, community participation and intersectoral collaboration drive health care service delivery. The development of sustainable health systems capable of delivering services that are accessible and affordable, and that address the most appropriate health issues in the communities in which people live, can be achieved through the adoption of the PHC approach.

CRITICAL THINKING ACTIVITIES

1. Read the ICN Position Statement, *Health inequities, discrimination and the nurse's role* (2023).
   a. What are the key messages relating to advocacy?
   b. How might the recommendations for individual nurses influence your nursing practice?
2. Consider holistic nursing in terms of practising from a PHC ideology. Access and read the following article:
   Rosa, W.E., Dossey, B.M., Watson, J., Beck, D.M. & Upvall, M.J. (2019). The United Nations Sustainable Development Goals: The ethic and ethos of holistic nursing. *Journal of Holistic Nursing, 37*(4), 381–93. https://doi.org/10.1177/0898010119841723
   a. How do the SDGs relate to the provision of PHC?
   b. How can adopting PHC ideology influence nursing practice across clinical settings?

FURTHER READING

He, J.W., Terry, A.L., Lizotte, D., Bauer, G. & Ryan, B.L. (2024). Understanding intersectional inequality in access to primary care providers using multilevel analysis of individual heterogeneity and discriminatory accuracy. *PloS ONE, 19*(1), e0296657.

Lukewich, J., Martin-Misener, R., Norful, A.A., et al. (2022). Effectiveness of registered nurses on patient outcomes in primary care: A systematic review. *BMC Health Services Research, 22*, 740.

Ranabhat, C.L., Acharya, S.P., Adhikari, C. & Kim, C.B. (2023). Universal health coverage evolution, ongoing trend, and future challenge: A conceptual and historical policy review. *Frontiers in Public Health, 11*, 1041459.

REFERENCES

Armenti, K., Sweeney, M.H., Lingwall, C. & Yang, L. (2023). Work: A social determinant of health worth capturing. *International Journal of Environmental Research and Public Health, 20*(2). https://doi.org/10.3390/ijerph20021199

Ballester, J., Quijal-Zamorano, M., Méndez Turrubiates, R.F., et al. (2023). Heat-related mortality in Europe during the summer of 2022. *Nature Medicine, 29*(7), 1857–66. https://doi.org/10.1038/s41591-023-02419-z

Barraclough, K.A., Carey, M., Winkel, K.D., et al. (2023). Why losing Australia's biodiversity matters for human health: Insights from the latest State of the Environment assessment. *Medical Journal of Australia, 218*(8), 336–40. https://doi.org/10.5694/mja2.51904

Brandt, L., Liu, S., Heim, C. & Heinz, A. (2022). The effects of social isolation stress and discrimination on mental health. *Translational Psychiatry, 12*(1), 398. https://doi.org/10.1038/s41398-022-02178-4

Braveman, P. (2023). *The Social Determinants of Health and Health Disparities*. Oxford University Press.

Chhetri, D. & Zacarias, F. (2021). Advocacy for evidence-based policy-making in public health: Experiences and the way forward. *Journal of Health Management, 23*(1), 85–94. https://doi.org/10.1177/0972063421994948

Cohen, A.J., Brauer, M., Burnett, R., et al. (2017). Estimates and 25-year trends of the global burden of disease attributable to ambient air pollution: An analysis of data from the Global Burden of Diseases Study 2015. *The Lancet, 389*(10082), 1907–18.

Department of Health. (2022). *Future Focused Primary Health Care: Australia's Primary Health Care 10 Year Plan 2022–2032*. Commonwealth of Australia.

du Plessis, A. (2022). Persistent degradation: Global water quality challenges and required actions. *One Earth, 5*(2), 129–31. https://doi.org/10.1016/j.oneear.2022.01.005

Fields, L., Moroney, T., Perkiss, S. & Dean, B.A. (2023). Enlightening and empowering students to take action: Embedding sustainability into nursing curriculum. *Journal of Professional Nursing, 49*, 57–63. https://doi.org/10.1016/j.profnurs.2023.09.001

Fields, L., Perkiss, S., Dean, B.A. & Moroney, T. (2021). Nursing and the sustainable development goals: A scoping review. *Journal of Nursing Scholarship, 53*(5), 568–77. https://doi.org/10.1111/jnu.12675

Freijser, L., Annear, P., Tenneti, N., et al. (2023). The role of hospitals in strengthening primary health care in the Western Pacific. *The Lancet Regional Health Western Pacific, 33*, 100698. https://doi.org/10.1016/j.lanwpc.2023.100698

Hameed, M.A., Rahman, M.M. & Khanam, R. (2023). The health consequences of civil wars: Evidence from Afghanistan. *BMC Public Health, 23*(1), 154. https://doi.org/10.1186/s12889-022-14720-6

Heise, L., Greene, M.E., Opper, N., et al. (2019). Gender inequality and restrictive gender norms: Framing the challenges to health. *The Lancet (British Edition), 393*(10189), 2440–54. https://doi.org/10.1016/S0140-6736(19)30652-X

Inglis, S.C., Ferguson, C., Eddington, R., et al. (2023). Cardiovascular nursing and climate change: A call to action from the CSANZ Cardiovascular Nursing Council. *Heart, Lung and Circulation, 32*(1), 16–25.

International Council of Nurses (ICN). (2023). *Health Inequities, Discrimination and the Nurse's Role*. ICN.

Jaydarifard, S., Smith, S.S., Mann, D., et al. (2023). Precarious employment and associated health and social consequences: A systematic review. *Australian and New Zealand Journal of Public Health, 47*(4), 100074. https://doi.org/10.1016/j.anzjph.2023.100074

Keleher, H. (2021). Global health. In H. Keleher & C. MacDougall (eds.), *Understanding Health* (5th ed.). Oxford University Press.

Kelly, C., Dansereau, L., Sebring, J., et al. (2022). Intersectionality, health equity, and EDI: What's the difference for health researchers? *International Journal for Equity in Health, 21*(1), 182. https://doi.org/10.1186/s12939-022-01795-1

Kingston, S., Rose, M., Cohen-Serrins, J. & Knight, E. (2017). A qualitative study of the context of child and adolescent substance use initiation and patterns of use in the first year for early and later initiators. *PloS ONE, 12*(1), e0170794. https://doi.org/10.1371/journal.pone.0170794

La Charite, J., Khan, M., Dudovitz, R., et al. (2023). Specific domains of positive childhood experiences (PCEs) associated with improved adult health: A nationally representative study. *SSM Population Health, 24*, 101558. https://doi.org/10.1016/j.ssmph.2023.101558

Magzamen, S., Mayer, A.P., Barr, S., et al. (2017). A multidisciplinary research framework on green schools: Infrastructure, social environment, occupant health, and performance. *Journal of School Health, 87*(5), 376–87. https://doi.org/10.1111/josh.12505

Maresova, P., Javanmardi, E., Barakovic, S., et al. (2019). Consequences of chronic diseases and other limitations associated with old age – a scoping review. *BMC Public Health, 19*(1), 1431. https://doi.org/10.1186/s12889-019-7762-5

Marmot, M. (2020). Health equity in England. *British Medical Journal, 368*, 1–4. https://doi.org/10.1136/bmj.m693

Ministry of Health. (2024). *Primary and community care Ngā ratonga hauora mātāmua me ngā ratonga ā-hapori*. New Zealand Government. www.health.govt.nz/strategies-initiatives/programmes-and-initiatives/primary-and-community-health-care

Mouratidis, K. (2021). Urban planning and quality of life: A review of pathways linking the built environment to subjective well-being. *Cities, 115*, 103229. https://doi.org/10.1016/j.cities.2021.103229

Nutbeam, D. & Kickbusch, I. (1998). Health promotion glossary. *Health Promotion International, 13*(4), 349–64. https://doi.org/10.1093/heapro/13.4.349

Nutbeam, D. & Muscat, D.M. (2021). Health promotion glossary 2021. *Health Promotion International, 36*(6), 1578. https://doi.org/10.1093/heapro/daaa157

Patrick, R., Capetola, T. & Henderson-Wilson, C. (2021). Environment, climate change and health. In H. Keleher & C. MacDougall (eds), *Understanding Health* (5th ed.). Oxford University Press.

Rocca, E. & Anjum, R.L. (2020). Complexity, reductionism and the biomedical model. In R.L. Anjum, S. Copeland & E. Rocca (eds), *Rethinking Causality, Complexity and Evidence for the Unique Patient*. Springer. https://doi.org/10.1007/978-3-030-41239-5_5

Ruddle, A., Pina, A. & Vasquez, E. (2017). Domestic violence offending behaviors: A review of the literature examining childhood exposure, implicit theories, trait aggression and anger rumination as predictive factors. *Aggression and Violent Behavior, 34*, 154–65.

Sabik, N.J. (2021). The Intersectionality Toolbox: A resource for teaching and applying an intersectional lens in public health. *Front Public Health, 9*, 772301. https://doi.org/10.3389/fpubh.2021.772301

Schnitter, R. & Berry, P. (2019). The climate change, food security and human health nexus in Canada: A framework to protect population health. *International Journal of Environmental Research and Public Health, 16(14), 253*. https//doi.org/10.3390/ijerph16142531

Taylor, J., O'Hara, L., Talbot, L. & Verrinder, G. (2021). *Promoting Health: The Primary Health Care Approach* (7th ed.). Elsevier Australia.

United Nations (UN). (2015). *Transforming Our World: The 2030 Agenda for Sustainable Development*. UN.

——— (2024). *17 goals to transform our world*. www.un.org/sustainabledevelopment/

United Nations General Assembly (UNGA). (2019). Political declaration of the high-level meeting on universal health coverage. *General Assembly Resolution, 74*(2).

Wilberg, A., Saboga-Nunes, L. & Stock, C. (2021). Are we there yet? Use of the Ottawa Charter action areas in the perspective of European health promotion professionals. *Journal of Public Health, 29*(1), 1–7. https://doi.org/10.1007/s10389-019-01108-x

Wilkinson, R.G., & Marmot, M. G. (2003). *The Solid Facts: Social Determinants of Health*. (2nd ed.). World Health Organization (WHO). https://iris.who.int/handle/10665/326568

Willis, V.C., Thomas Craig, K.J., Jabbarpour, Y., et al. (2022). Digital health interventions to enhance prevention in primary care: Scoping review. *JMIR Medical Informatics, 10*(1), e33518. https://doi.org/10.2196/33518

Wilson, L., Mendes, I.A.C., Klopper, H., et al. (2016). 'Global health' and 'global nursing': Proposed definitions from The Global Advisory Panel on the Future of Nursing. *Journal of Advanced Nursing, 72*(7), 1529–40.

World Health Organization (WHO). (1978). *Declaration of Alma-Ata*. International conference on primary health care, Alma-Ata, USSR, 6-12 September 1978. www.who.int/publications/almaata_declaration_en.pdf

———— (1981). *Global Strategy for Health for All by the Year 2000*. WHO.

———— (1986). *The Ottawa Charter for Health Promotion*. WHO.

———— (1998). *The Social Determinants of Health. The Solid Facts*. WHO.

———— (2017). *Promoting Health in the SDGs*. Report on the 9th Global Conference for Health Promotion, Shanghai, China, 21–24 November 2016: all for health, health for all. WHO.

———— (2018). *Declaration of Astana*. WHO.

———— (2021). *Health Promotion Glossary of Terms 2021*. WHO.

———— (2024). *Social Determinants of Health*. www.who.int/health-topics/social-determinants-of-health#tab=tab_1

World Health Organization (WHO) and United Nations Children's Fund (UNICEF). (2020). *Operational Framework for Primary Health Care: Transforming vision into action*. WHO and UNICEF.

Empowering individuals, groups and communities

Diana Guzys and Melanie Eslick

2

LEARNING OBJECTIVES

At the completion of this chapter, you should be able to:

- explain health literacy, including impacts of media and eHealth (digital health) literacy.
- identify the key principles for effective communication when providing health education.
- describe health-empowering strategies used with individuals, groups and populations.

Introduction

This chapter explores the relationship between primary health care (PHC), health literacy and health education with empowering individuals, groups and communities to improve and maintain optimum health. PHC philosophy encompasses principles of accessibility, affordability, sustainability, social justice and equity, self-determination, community participation and intersectoral collaboration, which drive health care service delivery and health care reform (World Health Organization (WHO) and United Nations Children's Fund (UNICEF), 2018), outlined in Chapter 1. **Empowerment** is a fundamental component of social justice, which seeks to redistribute power so those who are disadvantaged can have more control of the factors that influence their lives. Lack of empowerment is linked to poorer health outcomes due to limited control or agency, associated with poorer social determinants of health (Besnier, 2023). This influences personal resources, agency and participation, as well as limited capacity to access services and opportunities. Health care professionals and systems need to work in ways to promote the empowerment of individuals, groups and communities to achieve better health outcomes.

Health literacy

Health literacy is the ability to access, understand and use health information to make informed decisions (Nutbeam & Lloyd, 2021). It is established as a necessary resource for individual

Empowerment – sharing information, knowledge, skills and resources so people can make decisions, solve problems and have more control over their lives, and are enabled to improve their quality of life and health outcomes (based on the definition by the WHO, 1988).

Health literacy – the knowledge and skills to access, understand and use health information to make informed decisions, including navigating health systems and digital health, to achieve and maintain optimal health.

and collective empowerment (Abel & Benkert, 2022). It enables people to recognise when change is required and to make lifestyle adjustments for improved health. Possessing health literacy facilitates informed choices, as well as awareness of when assistance is needed and how it can be accessed (Coughlin, et al., 2020; van der Gaag et al., 2022). Health literacy is acknowledged as a midstream determinant of health that can be improved to moderate the influence of other social determinants (Nutbeam & Lloyd, 2021).

Individuals with advanced health literacy are more likely to engage in individual and collective actions to address the social determinants that are negatively impacting on health, such as advocacy (Sykes & Wills, 2019). They understand and can navigate the health system they are using, are aware of the right to ask for what they need to stay healthy and have the confidence to act on that right (Sørensen, 2019). When engaging the services of a health care provider, health-literate consumers are more likely to ask for information and understand the information received. They are confident, able to seek and appraise information from a range of sources, seek a second opinion and discuss alternative perspectives with health care providers to determine a suitable course of action, and collaborate on, understand and follow a treatment plan. They can also apply health concepts and information to new situations (Sørensen, 2019).

Health literacy is an issue of equity and social justice as it may negatively influence health outcomes (Besnier, 2023). Lower health literacy levels are often apparent in socially disadvantaged, vulnerable or marginalised groups (Nutbeam & Lloyd, 2021; van der Gaag et al., 2022). Limited health literacy follows the social gradient, reinforcing existing health inequalities, such as living outside of metropolitan areas, to having limited access to health services or to transportation to attend appointments (Abel & Benkert, 2022). This is demonstrated through challenges to self-managing health, navigating health services, understanding available and relevant information, and making informed health-related decisions (Campbell et al., 2019). Those with lower health literacy are less likely to engage in preventative health care and recognise the health needs of others, and tend to poorly self-manage chronic conditions (Nutbeam & Lloyd, 2021; van der Gaag et al., 2022).

Health literacy is a complex concept that is defined and interpreted from multiple perspectives. It is useful to think of health literacy using the typology proposed by Nutbeam (1999), which is based on what health literacy enables a person to do. Functional health literacy refers to basic skills in reading and writing needed for everyday situations. Communicative or interactive health literacy describes cognitive, social and literacy skills necessary to identify, understand and derive meaning from information. The third form – critical health literacy – relates to the ability to critically analyse information and apply this to make changes or take more control over situations and events (Nutbeam, 1999). Abel and Benkert (2022) emphasise the reflective aspect of critical health literacy. They propose that it is the ability to reflect upon health–determining factors and processes, and then apply the results of the reflection for individual or collective action for health that constitute critical health literacy. Critical health literacy has also been used to describe information-seeking and communication skills that advance health knowledge and result in informed decision-making and empowerment, including taking political action (Sykes & Wills, 2019).

Approaches to health literacy have traditionally focused on individual skill deficit (Urstad et al., 2022). This has resulted in strategies to improve the readability of written health materials, enhance the oral communication of health professionals and increase the accessibility and ease of navigation of health care services (Pelikan, 2019). Health care systems need to accommodate the abilities of consumers and ensure easy access to health services and health information. This concept is called 'organisational health literacy' (OHL) (Pelikan, 2019). As with health literacy, there is no single agreed definition of OHL. Efforts to improve OHL target all forms of health service communication with health care consumers. This means that their focus is wider than individual members of the organisation who have direct patient contact, such as nurses, or who develop health information materials and deliver health education.

While there is a strong association between low literacy levels and low health literacy, it is important to remember that the two are not the same thing (Kickbusch, 2001). A person whose first language is not English should not be assumed to have lower health literacy. They may simply need to be provided with information in a different language; this should be viewed as a communication, not a health literacy, issue. An individual's health literacy is situational – it be considered in terms of the demands and resources of the situations in which health-literate decisions or actions need to be made rather than solely on personal skills or competencies (Pelikan, 2019).

Most people struggle to understand information and concepts that they are unfamiliar with. It is not health care consumer's role to know how their body or how a specific health care organisation works. It is the health care professional's role to provide the appropriate information and explain it in a way the patient or client understands. Very few people could explain the function and location of each piece of machinery in cars, except in perhaps vague terms. However, when someone has a car with a recurring mechanical problem, they often become quite knowledgeable about this specific issue. Similarly, people with chronic conditions may become experts about their health issue, yet their health knowledge may be limited in other areas. The best place to start is to ask the person what they understand about their health or condition and work from there.

REFLECTION

Consider how lower health literacy might disempower health care consumers in your clinical environment. What could you do to help address this?

Media and eHealth literacy

We live in a media-saturated and increasingly digitised environment. Digital and non-digital media are subject to commercial and other interests that may conflict with the best health interests of consumers. Increasingly, health-related information and messages are accessed through the media and digital sources, however mass media health content may be implicitly or explicitly health-promoting or health-compromising (Nazarnia, Zarei & Rozbahani, 2022; van Kessel, et al., 2022). The evolution of web-based technologies, including informational websites, blogs, social media platforms, consumer-directed eHealth resources and online interventions, has made people's experience in finding, navigating and interpreting credible health-related information more complex (Kington et al., 2021; van Kessel et al., 2022).

Media and eHealth (also referred to as digital health) literacy require critical thinking. A person's social environment has a significant influence on health, and social media in particular is a complex social environment (Nazarnia et al., 2022; van Kessel et al., 2022). People require skills to identify the social and political context of the information they find. Health information accessed in this manner needs to be considered in terms of how each form of media shapes the message and the relationship it has with the audience. Becoming media health literate requires that we ask ourselves a number of basic questions about what we read and view.

- Who created this message and why?
- Why and how does this message attract my attention?
- What values and points of view are represented in, or omitted from, this message?
- Might other people understand this message differently from me? (Egbert & Neville, 2015).

Individuals may turn to social media for health information or treatment advice and may not possess the skills to evaluate the credibility or veracity of the source (Chen et al., 2018).

Nurses need to consider such questions in relation to the development of their own health literacy and assist health consumers to develop similar skills in assessing the information they may source (Australian Digital Health Agency, 2020).

Health education

Health education – the process of engaging with a person to develop knowledge, understanding or skills to facilitate positive health behaviours.

Belcastro and Ramsaroop-Hansen (2017) argue that health literacy cannot exist without **health education**, as people must have sufficient foundational health knowledge to value and adopt positive health behaviours. The purpose of health education is to encourage the adoption of such behaviours and improve health outcomes. Early efforts to improve health literacy focused on the simplification of language used in health information material and health education. However, how people interpret or understand the meaning of health information is influenced by many factors beyond reading skills. Knowledge is not the only factor influencing health choices and behaviours. A lack of resources, such as access to goods and services, a safe environment, income and other social determinants often influence health behaviours and outcomes (Coughlin et al., 2020). Personal priorities, experiences, histories, culture and beliefs are further factors that must be acknowledged.

The most common way in which health care professionals can facilitate consumers to develop their health literacy is through assisting them to understand and actively manage their own health. Health-literate health professionals and systems encourage consumers to feel welcomed and empowered to ask questions, deliver information in ways that people can use and facilitate informed shared decision-making (Coughlin et al., 2020). People are free to make their own health choices. However, when people are well-informed and understand the mechanisms and processes that affect their health, they are more likely to understand how a proposed treatment plan relates to these (Coughlin et al., 2020). Health knowledge built via effective health education increases the likelihood of people following health care advice that they believe is relevant to their lives and situations.

The way that health information is communicated will vary depending on its purpose. When the intention is to improve awareness of a health issue or concern, we can consider this providing health information. Health information is one strategy used to engage people in health knowledge development through the presentation of content relevant to a health topic. Information on its own rarely results in a change of behaviour or perception; in this way, health information provision differs from health education, which aims to influence behaviour

CASE STUDY 2.1

Vaa is a 28-year-old Samoan migrant to Aotearoa New Zealand. He has followed several of his family there for a 'better life'. While many aspects of life are good, access to health care often presents barriers. Vaa has visited and enrolled at his general practice but finds that many of the facilities and services, and much health information, are Western-centric and not sensitive to cultural considerations. The language is often confusing and at odds with Samoan customs relating to health and health care.

REFLECTION

1. What steps can nurses in the community take to provide clients with culturally competent health information?
2. How could local health care services better support Vaa with 'integrating' into his community and support his cultural health and health care considerations?
3. How might local health care services use Vaa's cultural knowledge to expand their services to the wider community?

change. When information does not connect in a meaningful way to their lives, there may be little motivation to encourage people to engage with it. For example, nearly every secondary school student is provided with information about algebra; some will engage with this information and will apply it to activities in their lives, but many will engage with algebra superficially and, once out of the classroom, will only have vague recollections of the information they have received. It is paramount, therefore, that health care professionals engage with their clients when they are providing them with information about their health, rather than leaving them with vague memories of concepts relevant to maintaining their well-being. Health information that contributes to positive behaviour change underpins health education.

Social marketing

Social marketing techniques have been used as a tool for health promotion in public health at a population level for several decades. Although many of the strategies used in social marketing are drawn from traditional marketing concepts, the underlying goal is to confront health-related behaviours and convey concepts that create positive behaviour change for socially desirable goals (Akbar, et al., 2022; Shawky, et al., 2019). Large social marketing campaigns may target public safety issues such as driving under the influence of alcohol or other drugs, and texting while driving and speeding. The adoption of SunSmart behaviours, healthy eating and quit smoking campaigns are other well-established long-term social marketing efforts evaluated as effective. Social marketing has evolved as an approach to promote people's well-being and social welfare through social change, tackling social issues such as domestic violence, gambling, climate change, energy and water efficiency, sustainability and citizen engagement.

There is strong evidence that public health social marketing campaigns conducted through mainstream media, such as print, radio and television, have a direct and positive effect on behaviour (Shawky et al., 2019). Subsequently, there is growing interest in the use of social media as a tool for awareness raising, information sharing and behaviour change as an adjunct to these traditional forms of social marketing (Shawky et al., 2019).

Delivering health education

Health education relies on engaging with an audience, which is facilitated through a range of skills and techniques. Whether delivered to an individual or group, health education requires planning. Opportunistic moments for health education occur for every health professional. These moments are most effective when the health professional is well-versed in the content and has the benefit of prior experience in planning its delivery. Prior planning of the delivery of health information facilitates construction of a coherent scaffolding of the content, which reduces the cognitive load experienced by the health information recipient (Albrecht & Karabenick, 2018).

The guiding principles in providing health education are to keep the messages simple, use everyday English and avoid jargon. This is even more important when working with culturally and linguistically diverse people. When information is translated into another language, the same principles need to be applied. Consideration of cultural perspectives on health and illness, health practices and the media being used is essential (Coughlin et al., 2020). Content delivered through health education activities needs careful consideration and planning if it is to achieve its intended purpose. Effective education requires that the content is communicated in an appropriate manner (Coughlin et al., 2020). Some foundational aspects of communicating effectively when engaging in health education are highlighted here.

Providing health information verbally

Health care professionals provide health information verbally in many settings, informally or in formal conversations with individuals or small groups. As the number of participants increases, so does the level of formality usually required in delivery. In all situations, speaking clearly, facing the audience, avoiding jargon and using everyday language works best. Slowing the rate of speech slightly when talking to a large group of people, such as in a class or during a public lecture, ensures that what is said is clear. A modulated tone adds interest for the audience (Henderson, 2019), so speaking in a monotone should be avoided, and intonation should be used to emphasise significant points. It is best to use short sentences, as long sentences are often more complex and may obscure the point trying to be made.

The ability to clarify whether participants understand the information presented is a key advantage of providing information verbally. Monitoring non-verbal cues for distraction, confusion or misunderstanding is essential. Opportunities to ask questions should be provided and participants should be asked if their questions have been adequately answered (Henderson, 2019). Learning is improved through people being engaged with the content and with the process of learning. Participants appreciate simple explanations but do not appreciate being treated as simpletons, so care should be taken to consider the pitch of the information. Plain language used with family and friends who do not have a health care background provides a useful guide to the level at which information should be provided. The need for further simplification can be assessed by checking understanding with participants. A further word of caution to consider about oversimplification is to be highly selective with the words used, particularly if their meanings could be misinterpreted. It is not only children who become distressed when told that they will be 'put to sleep' during their medical procedure or operation, given that their only previous experience with something being 'put to sleep' was their pet dog being euthanised!

Tailoring the presentation to the individual needs of participants is more challenging with very large groups. However, tailoring a presentation to the needs of participants could be as simple as suggesting an appropriate modification of a technique or activity for an elderly person, or someone with a disability. Personalising information makes it relevant to the individual, and that person is more likely to engage with the information presented (Henderson, 2019). If a participant is having difficulty grasping an important concept, it may be useful to find a circumstance in that person's life or situation to demonstrate the concept (Henderson, 2019). Following up with individuals after the presentation ensures that information has been clarified sufficiently for them.

Written information

Providing written health information allows people to refer back to it in their own time. However, if this is the only way the information is presented, the main disadvantage is the inability to clarify the person's understanding. Care needs to be taken when producing written health information so that it is comprehensive yet simple. As written information is less personal, it may be difficult for some people to see how it can apply to their own lives (Henderson, 2019). Given that written information is less likely to be personally engaging, it should be used to supplement other forms of health education. The same key principles of keeping it simple, avoiding jargon and using plain language apply to written resources.

The volume of content will determine the format required for written information. Less detailed content may be presented as a poster or pamphlet, while more detailed content might best be presented as a booklet or website. If you are writing health information, it may be useful to consider the profile of the target audience when contemplating its format (Scrimshaw, 2019).

The readability of the information is imperative, regardless of the format selected. Three of the most commonly used readability tools are the Flesch-Kincaid Index (FKI), the Gunning-Fog Index (GFI), and the Simple Measure of Gobbledygook (SMOG). These involve looking at the number of syllables, words or sentences in a text to calculate a score using a specific weighted formula that corresponds to a particular school level (Szabó, Bíró & Kósa, 2021). Unfortunately, reading comprehension levels are difficult to label accurately, as they vary within and between countries. Material written for the general population is often described as being presented at the expected educational level of a 13- to 14-year-old (Szabó et al., 2021). A rough guide is to model written material at the same level as popular reading materials, such as magazines on popular culture, local newspapers and articles in television guides. Alternative resources are also available to address barriers to health literacy among consumers with intellectual and developmental disorders and communication difficulties (Shady, Phillips & Newman, 2022). Using resources specially designed for consumers by peak organisations, such as the Heart Foundation or Diabetes Australia, may ensure that the written material is appropriate.

Presenting written information

Nurses providing written health information to patients and clients must consider that the reader's engagement will be influenced by how easy it is to read and how interesting it is, regardless of the media. Some fonts are easier to read than others and the overuse of different fonts can also be off-putting and sometimes visually nauseating (O'Sullivan, et al., 2020). Small-sized texts are difficult for most people to read and may make the information appear dense. The use of white space – which contains no text or images – also influences how dense the material will appear. The more white space, the less intimidating the information will be to read (Walsh, Hill & Waterhouse, 2019).

Colour and images can be used to attract attention or emphasise certain aspects of the information being presented. However, the overuse of colour can detract from the appeal of the document and some colours – particularly certain shades of green, red and yellow – are more difficult to read. Images increase visual appeal but more importantly can clarify or emphasise key information (Walsh et al., 2019). The information they depict must be clear; simplicity is the best option. Copyright laws and the requirement to seek permission to use photos and other images must be considered. Although some images are royalty-free or accessible through Creative Commons options, it is essential that the copyright owner of the image is acknowledged.

Working with individuals

Health education provided to individuals usually addresses issues associated with managing a specific health concern (Henderson, 2019). As the purpose of health education is to empower individuals to make positive behaviour changes for optimal health, two tools to assist with this are 'teach back' and motivational interviewing (MI). Teach back is a person-centred approach to assess and promote an individual's understanding of health education (Yen & Leasure, 2019). It is a quick and effective method that allows the health care professional to assess a person's understanding of the health information provided, correct any misunderstanding and re-teach if necessary. Most importantly, this approach enables personalisation of education through the identification of individual learning needs. MI is a strategy used to encourage behavioural change to improve health status, particularly to encourage clients to engage with recommended treatments and reduce lifestyle risk factors (Bischof, Bischof & Rumpf, 2021). MI is a technique commonly used with people with long-term chronic conditions of significant lifestyle risk factors. Nurses work in a non-judgemental manner assisting people to activate their own personal resources and overcome obstacles in working towards achieving the goals set by the client (Rethorn, Bezner & Pettitt, 2022; Singh, Kennedy & Stupans, 2022).

Teach back

Shersher and colleagues (2021) report that 40–80 per cent of verbally delivered clinical information is forgotten instantly, and that almost half of what can be recalled is incorrect. Teach back is a simple communication technique to confirm that what the health care professional has explained has been understood by their client (Nutbeam & Lloyd, 2021). The technique involves asking a person to explain in their own words the educational information they have just received. If the person's response omits important information or contains mistakes, these can be corrected, or additional information can be provided at that time. A key feature of the technique is to avoid closed questions such as 'Do you understand?'. Instead, the health care professional frames their question as if they are checking up on the completeness of their own delivery of health information (Shersher et al., 2021). It is useful to forewarn the person that you will ask them to explain the information back to you after you have delivered it to them to ensure that you have included everything they need to know.

MI

MI is an evidence-based, person-centred approach to behaviour change that acknowledges the clients' expertise about their own health and circumstances (Bischof, et al. 2021). It originated as a form of therapy in the field of substance abuse but has since been used widely across a range of settings. The guiding principles of MI are expressing empathy, developing discrepancy, rolling with resistance and supporting **self-efficacy** (Rethorn et al., 2022). MI is a collaborative method for addressing issues, involving activities that help individuals reflect on their circumstances, pinpoint areas they wish to alter, and explore potential pathways for achieving those changes. MI aims to empower consumers to make changes by eliciting what is meaningful and a priority for them, and their capacity to change (Motivational Interviewing Network of Trainers (MINT), 2019).

Miller and Rollnick (2013, p. 29), the developers of MI, describe it as 'a collaborative, goal-oriented style of communication with particular attention to the language of change. It is designed to strengthen personal motivation for and commitment to a specific goal by eliciting and exploring the person's own reasons for change within an atmosphere of acceptance and compassion.' MI requires that nurses engage with the person as an equal partner and do not give unsolicited advice, be confronting or instruct/direct their behaviour. An 'ask-tell-ask' approach is used to seek the person's permission to discuss a health behaviour, for example 'Is it okay if we discuss…'. This approach is respectful of the person's autonomy and is supportive by working in a collaborative manner (Cole, 2023). The nurse should not proceed with providing information if the client declines or appears reluctant as this is likely to be counterproductive. When the client expresses a willingness for information exchange, the sharing or 'telling' of information relevant to health improvement should occur as the next step in the 'ask-tell-ask' process. This is followed by the nurse 'asking' the client what they think and feel about what they have then been told (Cole et al., 2023). It is imperative for the nurse to resist telling the clients what they need to change to improve their health. Rather, the nurse should assist them to see the positives and negatives of the issue or health concern (Dobber et al., 2019). Individuals are more likely to change their behaviour when they perceive that they themselves are making the decisions and setting the goals (Dobber et al., 2019; MINT, 2019).

The MI approach seeks to enhance client empowerment, self-esteem and self-efficacy, encouraging and supporting change rather than forcing it. Using empathy, the clients' individual needs for change are explored through providing information and asking them what the effects and possible outcomes of change would be (Dobber et al., 2019; MINT, 2019). Empathy is demonstrated by using a reflective listening style facilitating a non-judgemental, collaborative and therapeutic relationship (Rethorn et al., 2022). Listening rather than telling communicates respect and acceptance, reinforcing to the client that they are being listened to and understood. Reflective listening is displayed through repeating or rephrasing what the person is communicating. Open questions are used to draw out and explore the client's experiences, perspectives and ideas. The questions guide the client to reflect on how change may be meaningful or possible. Affirmation of the person's strengths, effort and past successes is given to help build the person's self-esteem and self-efficacy (MINT, 2019). Summarising is also a component of reflective listening, ensuring a shared understanding and reinforcing key points made by the client (Dobber et al., 2019; MINT, 2019).

The purpose of MI is to assist individuals to recognise and understand the connection between their current lifestyle behaviours, their health status and/or levels of health risk (Lim et al., 2019). Nursing can clarify what the client is saying by asking in a non-confrontational way how their views or comments fit in with wider goals or objectives that they have previously expressed. Any discrepancy needs to be acknowledged, as it provides an opportunity to

Self-efficacy – an individual's beliefs in their capacity to impact events affecting their lives (Bandura, 2000). Unless individuals are confident in their ability to achieve a desired outcome, there is limited incentive to engage in it.

develop consciousness for a need to change. From this understanding, individuals are motivated to choose to adopt healthier behaviours and reduce their modifiable risks. Clients are encouraged to express their reasons for and against behavioural change and identify personal health goals that can be achieved through self-management.

There are four fundamental processes within MI, each of which has a specific purpose in the behaviour change process as outlined in Table 2.1.

Table 2.1 Fundamental processes of motivational interviewing

Process	Goal
Engaging	Establishing a relationship with the client
Focusing	Developing a directed conversation about behaviour change
Evoking	Identifying the individual's motivations for change
Planning	Developing a commitment to change and establishment of an action plan

Source: Adapted from Miller & Rollnick (2013).

Intrinsic motivation – a person's inner desire to change a behaviour; behaviour that is driven by internal rewards.

Extrinsic motivation – a person's behaviour that is driven by external factors such as approval/ reward or disapproval/ punishment from others.

The process of engaging, focusing, evoking and planning are sequential and may occur in a single therapeutic interaction or be revisited over a longer period of care involving short-term and long-term goals (Rethorn et al., 2022). By exploring and addressing individuals' ambivalent attitudes and perceived barriers to behaviour change, MI seeks to enhance their **intrinsic motivation** (Dobber et al., 2019). Intrinsic motivation exists when the individual is driven by internal rewards, such as enjoyment in the task itself or personal satisfaction. In contrast, **extrinsic motivation** is external approval/disapproval from peers or health professionals. Change driven by intrinsic motivation has been demonstrated to be more sustainable and enduring than that driven by extrinsic motivation. More information relating to behaviour change, specifically the stages of change model, is discussed in relation to managing chronic illness in Chapter 14.

Change talk is a very important part of MI and behavioural change. It is an important predictor of successful change and is apparent by the increasing use of phrases that move speech from 'I could' or 'I might' to 'I will' or 'I do'. The client's own desires and goals can be used as the catalyst in MI to assist in adopting healthy behaviours. When there is a specific behaviour identified for change, MI is more effective than when the goal of change is less specific.

CASE STUDY 2.2

Ken is a 68-year-old self-funded retiree, who has lived alone since his wife died from breast cancer a few years ago and his adult children left home. After his wife died, Ken started smoking cigarettes again. Ken has joined a walking group that provides him with the opportunity to exercise and socialise. However, he often becomes breathless during and after these walks and he is considering whether it is worth the effort to keep attending. Recently, Ken has had episodes of asthma, a condition he has not experienced since he was a child. His doctor has prescribed him a preventer and a reliever to assist him in

managing his condition. The preventer medication is not covered by his national pharmacological scheme so is expensive. To save money, Ken relies on his reliever medication when
he becomes breathless as it is a lot cheaper, and only uses his preventer medication when
he starts to feel unwell. Ken has been referred to Quitline to help with smoking cessation
and an asthma education nurse to assist him in better identifying his asthma triggers and
managing his condition.

REFLECTION

1. What are the issues for Ken?
2. What health education content would be valuable in this scenario?
3. What would be the best way to deliver this education?
4. How could teach back help Ken understand the relationship between his increasingly
   frequent breathlessness and his behaviours?

Working with groups

Health education may be provided in a group setting as it is an efficient way to reach multiple
people and enables participants to share information and resources as well as strengthen
community networks. Some education groups may continue to have a life of their own when
the delivery of the educational content has concluded and may develop into support groups.
Support groups have a different purpose to that of an educational group and may also be
formed specifically for that purpose (McCarthy et al., 2022). These groups provide support
to group members who are experiencing some form of stress or who share a common illness;
in some circumstances they may be formally facilitated by a specifically qualified health care
worker. A task group is another type of group that develops to achieve a specific purpose
and may evolve out of an educative or support group, or simply in response to a shared concern. A task group has a fixed and specific purpose resulting in the group processes being
highly structured with a strong focus on decision-making and action (McCarthy et al., 2022).
Groups can often also act as a resource for their members when health knowledge and health
literacy are distributed across the group (Muscat et al., 2022), which can further assist individuals develop their personal health literacy.

   Groups can be described as open or closed. Support groups are often open, meaning participants can come and go as they choose. Closed groups generally do not allow new people
to join once they have commenced. Education groups and some support groups are closed
groups so that the group dynamic that forms is not disrupted. Open groups tend to be less
cohesive in nature as their memberships may fluctuate. The ideal number of people involved
in a group is determined by its purpose. Smaller numbers are particularly appropriate for
groups that meet over an extended period as this tends to facilitate building trust, greater
intimacy and discussion between members (van Diggele, Burgess & Mellis, 2020). When the
development of trust is an important requirement to achieve the purpose of the group, having
between 6 and 12 members is appropriate.

   Setting group rules is an essential part of any group process. This can occur in a variety
of ways such as discussion, brainstorming and contracting. The purpose of this process is to
obtain agreement from participants about what behaviour is acceptable to keep the session
on track (van Diggele et al., 2020). Rules of behaviour ensure that communication is open and

friendly, everyone is included, no individual dominates or side-tracks the session and time is managed appropriately. It is also important that the facilitator acknowledges that they, too, are bound by the group rules.

The group process

Understanding a group process enables the facilitator to assess the health and engagement of the group. This is most relevant for groups that are run over time but can also be observed in shorter time frames. Groups have a predictable life cycle. Despite some open groups such as Alcoholics Anonymous appearing to live on in perpetuity, the group process follows a well-established sequence. Tuckman (1965) identifies distinct stages in the group process. The early stage is often referred to as 'forming'. The group leader or facilitator needs to provide direction for the group, demonstrate good communication skills and create interaction between participants. The focus is on organisation and clarity of purpose. The following stages are referred to as the 'storming' and 'norming' phases. Participants develop an understanding and appreciation of each other and bonds are established. While remaining influential, the group leader or facilitator is seen less as an authority figure during this middle phase. Originally, Tuckman (1965) concluded the stages of group process with 'performing', referring to the group's ability to focus its purpose once a relatively stable structure has developed. In later work, he replaced this with 'adjourning' or 'mourning', a stage which describes when the group has concluded its primary purpose and prepares for the end of the group and separation. A skilled facilitator manages this stage by keeping the focus on the benefits of having participated in the group.

Facilitating group education

Effective small group teaching and learning strategies increase participant engagement, deeper understanding of content and retention of knowledge (Poort, Jansen & Hofman, 2022; van Diggele et al., 2020). When developing a group education session or program, the nurse needs to consider who will be participating, their potential background knowledge and their learning needs. It is also necessary to consider the resources that are available to the nurse and to the learners, including a suitable venue, potential transportation requirements and appropriate timing of sessions. Consider environmental factors such as seating, lighting, heating, ease of access to amenities and potentially the provision of refreshments. Show respect for the participants by starting and finishing on time.

When planning the session, focus on achievable learning outcomes. A reasonable expectation is 3–6 learning outcomes in a session (van Diggele et al., 2020). Be clear in explaining these to participants and what can be realistically achieved in the time available. Make sure what you teach is relevant to the participants and pitched at their anticipated level of background knowledge. Ask questions to check participant understanding and to keep participants actively involved. The average adult attention span is 10 to 20 minutes (van Diggele et al., 2020). Deliver information in a way that is engaging and succinct. Provide a clear explanation of any activities the participants are required to engage in and ensure that these activities are not likely to embarrass them or make them feel uncomfortable. Conclude the session with a summary of what has been covered. It can be useful to ask participants to identify the most important knowledge or skill/s that they have learnt during the session (van Diggele et al., 2020).

REFLECTION

Consider the groups in which you have participated. These might be sporting teams, your class at school or a group that shares a common interest.

1. Would you describe them as open or closed groups?
2. If possible, compare the level of trust or intimacy between large groups and small groups in which you have taken part. Is there a difference? Why or why not?
3. Do you think it is easier or more difficult to ask a question to a group of 10 or 100 people?

Working with populations

Social marketing is a concept that was introduced earlier in this chapter. Mass media campaigns are the most common approach to providing health information and potentially health education to whole populations or when targeting specific populations. Such campaigns rely on exposing large audiences in the population repeatedly to specific health messages using both traditional media, such as television, radio and newspapers, and evolving forms of social media. Other forms of working at the population level involve community development and facilitating public participation.

Community development

Community development is more than a process; it can be considered a philosophy of practice and a means of empowerment. Collective or community empowerment is the process of developing the ability to make decisions and take action as a group on life issues to achieve shared objectives (WHO, 2024). Empowerment is limited by social structure; however, empowered people understand this structure and are aware that through collective action they are able to bring change to their community to address shared needs or common problems (Nutbeam & McGill, 2019; Žganec & Opačić, 2021). Consultation to inform goals or strategies; community advisory groups or committees; and leadership training may be part of a community development strategy, however they are not in themselves community development (Australian Institute of Family Studies, 2023).

The concept of community development is multidisciplinary, therefore, community development work is perceived in several different ways. The term is used in relation to physical resources, economic resources, social resources and human resources (Hasan, 2022). Fundamentally, community development refers to a wide range of processes used to improve a community. Power and disadvantage are complex concepts that are integral to community development practice. Community development is strongly linked to the concept of empowerment. Empowerment emphasises participation as a means for the redistribution of resources and power to redress inequity and social injustice (Hasan, 2022; Žganec & Opačić, 2021). Ife (2016) argues that shifting community development from rhetoric to reality is challenging particularly as it threatens assumptions that professionals, politicians and people in positions of power know what is best. Central to the philosophical ideal of community development is the idea that change should be initiated by the community itself. This is referred to as 'grassroots' or 'bottom-up activism' and acknowledges that the community knows itself and what is needed locally (Ife, 2016).

Community development principles are considered useful in supporting individuals and communities to become familiar with local health issues and services (Australian Institute of Family Studies, 2023). By creating this interest, they develop an understanding of the determinants of health and health inequalities and the skills necessary for critical health literacy (Nutbeam & McGill, 2019). From a health promotion perspective, the links between community development and the need to take action to address the social determinants of health are easily identifiable. Physical resources relate to the built and natural environment, emphasising local infrastructure. Economic resources refer to employment opportunities and income. Social resources describe interpersonal relationships and social capital, which are associated with inclusion and early life experiences. Human resources can be viewed as an opportunity for education, personal capacity, participation and leadership. The importance of understanding the social determinants of health and engagement in collective action is underlined when considering critical health literacy (Nutbeam & McGill, 2019). The essential aspect of critical health literacy is its relationship with decision-making.

A fundamental goal of health promotion activity is to create a healthy community in which its members have the knowledge and skills to take action to be healthy (Haldane et al., 2019; Nutbeam & McGill, 2019). The involvement of people in making decisions on issues that impact their community is beneficial to health outcomes and a core value underpinning health promotion practice. Community development should aim to build social capital and strengthen the social bonds and interactions within the community (Hasan, 2022). Communities with good social capital have been found to be healthier and are more likely to engage in actions that improve their community. Social capital contributes to personal well-being and happiness and provides the foundation for empowerment and the development of community capacity (Gilchrist, 2019).

Involving local citizens in processes to identify problems – particularly those related to complex social issues – and contributing to determining solutions achieves enduring social benefits (Haldane et al., 2019; Hasan, 2022). Valuing local knowledge, culture, resources, skills and processes is necessary for effective community development work, even when local community members do not recognise these in themselves (Ife, 2016). In this approach to community development, local input and involvement in the process result in high levels of learning and interpersonal outcomes for the community. Community members develop self-reliance, increasing their capacity to direct change and achieve sustainable outcomes. Community capacity is associated with participation and leadership, critical reflection, social and interorganisational networks, appropriate resources, skills and a sense of community that includes an understanding of community history, community power and community values (Gilchrist, 2019).

Public participation

Public participation can be viewed as a process and a goal. As a process, participation is seen as a means to achieve externally developed predetermined objectives. As a goal, people are directly involved in shaping, deciding and taking part in the development process, resulting in a 'bottom-up' approach. Participation as a process can help to develop people's capacities or abilities and provide them with opportunities to influence and share power (Haldane et al., 2019). The International Association for Public Participation (IAP2) distinguishes five main types of processes: informing, consulting, involving, collaborating and empowering citizens (IAP2 Australasia, 2019–2024).

Informing refers to provision of balanced and objective information to assist the public in understanding the problem, alternatives and possible solutions, whereas consultation refers to obtaining public feedback on analysis, alternative options or decisions. However, working directly with the public throughout the process to ensure that their concerns and desires are understood and considered is identified as public involvement. Collaboration occurs through partnership in every aspect of decision-making with the public, including developing alternatives and identification of the preferred solution. Finally, empowerment is when the public is responsible for making the final decision (IAP2 Australasia, 2019–2024).

Conclusion

PHC principles, such as equity, access and sustainability, are closely linked to improving the health of individuals and communities. Effective health education contributes to the development of health literacy, enabling improved access to and navigation of health care services. Health literacy empowers individual and community participation in decisions that impact health and improve health outcomes. Health education requires planning to ensure that the audience engages with the content being presented. The starting point, when planning a health education activity, is to understand the needs and characteristics of the intended audience, and to tailor the activity to meet these. A variety of skills and techniques for facilitating effective health education have been discussed in this chapter. The key principles to remember when providing health education are to keep it simple, avoid jargon and use everyday English. The value of appropriate and effective health education as a means of empowering people to maintain and improve their health and the health of their communities should not be underestimated. When working at a population level, public participation and community development – which focuses on building social capital – along with critical health literacy are recognised as essential components required to empower communities.

CRITICAL THINKING ACTIVITIES

1. What marketing strategies do you think could be used to attract the following groups of participants to attend health education activities:
   - adolescents
   - the elderly
   - Aboriginal and Torres Strait Islander or Māori men
   - Islamic women
   - homeless people
   - people with an intellectual disability?
2. What specific considerations might need to be addressed for each of these groups when developing and delivering health education programs?
3. As effective education requires sufficient motivation to engage with the information being provided, is it possible to identify shared motivation within groups, or is motivation required at an individual level? If specific groups have common or shared motivators, identify one potential shared motivator for each group.

FURTHER READING

Bell, K. & Reed, M. (2022). The tree of participation: A new model for inclusive decision-making. *Community Development Journal*, *57*(4), 595–614. https://doi.org/10.1093/cdj/bsab018

Hayward, B., Sinclair, S., Martin-Babin, M., Villa, L. & Madell, D. (2020). Creating health literate consumer resources: Insights from a professional development program. *Health Literacy Research and Practice*, *4*(3), e185–e189. https://doi.org/10.3928/24748307-20200806-01

Kavanagh, S., Shiell, A., Hawe, P. & Garvey, K. (2022). Resources, relationships, and systems thinking should inform the way community health promotion is funded. *Critical Public Health*, *32*(3), 273–82. https://doi.org/10.1080/09581596.2020.1813255

Osborne, R.H., Cheng, C.C., Nolte, S., et al. (2022). Health literacy measurement: Embracing diversity in a strengths-based approach to promote health and equity, and avoid epistemic injustice. *BMJ Global Health*, *7*(9), e009623. http://dx.doi.org/10.1136/bmjgh-2022-009623

REFERENCES

Abel, T. & Benkert, R. (2022). Critical health literacy: Reflection and action for health. *Health Promotion International*, *37*(4), daac114. https://doi.org/10.1093/heapro/daac114

Akbar, M.B., Garnelo-Gomez, I., Ndupu, L., Barnes, E. & Foster, C. (2022). An analysis of social marketing practice: Factors associated with success. *Health Marketing Quarterly*, *39*(4), 356–76. https://doi.org/10.1080/07359683.2021.1997525

Albrecht, J.R. & Karabenick, S.A. (2018). Relevance for learning and motivation in education. *The Journal of Experimental Education*, *86*(1), 1–10. https://doi.org/10.1080/00220973.2017.1380593

Australian Digital Health Agency. (2020). *National Nursing and Midwifery Digital Health Capability Framework*. Australian Digital Health Agency. www.digitalhealth.gov.au/healthcare-providers/initiatives-and-programs/workforce-capability/nursing-and-midwifery

Australian Institute of Family Studies. (2023). *What is community development?* Resource Sheet. Australian Government. https://aifs.gov.au/resources/resource-sheets/what-community-development#:~:text=Community%20development%20is%20a%20holistic,Kenny%20%26%20Connors%2C%202017

Bandura, A. (2000). Self-efficacy: The foundation of agency1. In W. J. Perrig & A. Grob (eds), *Control of Human Behavior, Mental Processes, and Consciousness* (pp. 16-30). Psychology Press.

Belcastro, P.A. & Ramsaroop-Hansen, H. (2017). Addressing the antinomy between health education and health literacy in advancing personal health and public health outcomes. *Journal of School Health*, *87*(12), 968–74.

Besnier, E. (2023). Women's political empowerment and child health in the sustainable development era: A global empirical analysis (1990–2016). *Global Public Health*, *18*(1), 1849348. https://doi.org/10.1080/17441692.2020.1849348

Bischof, G., Bischof, A. & Rumpf, H.J. (2021). Motivational interviewing: an evidence-based approach for use in medical practice. *Deutsches Arzteblatt International*, *118*(7), 109–15. https://doi.org/10.3238/arztebl.m2021.0014

Campbell, P., Lewis, M., Chen, Y., et al. (2019). Can patients with low health literacy be identified from routine primary care health records? A cross-sectional and prospective analysis. *BMC Family Practice*, *20*(1), 101. https://doi.org/10.1186/s12875-019-0994-8

Chen, X., Hay, J.L., Waters, E.A., et al. (2018). Health literacy and use and trust in health information. *Journal of Health Communication*, *23*(8), 724–34. https://doi.org/10.1080/10810730.2018.1511658

Cole, S.A., Sannidhi, D., Jadotte, Y.T. & Rozanski, A. (2023). Using motivational interviewing and brief action planning for adopting and maintaining positive health behaviors. *Progress in Cardiovascular Diseases*, *77*, 86–94. https://doi.org/10.1016/j.pcad.2023.02.003

Coughlin, S.S., Vernon, M., Hatzigeorgiou, C. & George, V. (2020). Health literacy, social determinants of health, and disease prevention and control. *Journal of Environment and Health Sciences*, *6*(1), 3061.

Dobber, J., Latour, C., Snaterse, M., et al. (2019). Developing nurses' skills in motivational interviewing to promote a healthy lifestyle in patients with coronary artery disease. *European Journal of Cardiovascular Nursing*, *18*(1), 28–37.

Egbert, J. & Neville, C. (2015). Engaging K–12 language learners in media literacy. *TESOL Journal*, *6*(1), 177–87.

Gilchrist, A. (2019). *The well-connected community 3E: A networking approach to community development.* Policy Press.

Haldane, V., Chuah, F.L., Srivastava, A., et al. (2019). Community participation in health services development, implementation, and evaluation: A systematic review of empowerment, health, community, and process outcomes. *PloS ONE*, *14*(5), e0216112.

Hasan, M. (2022). *Community Development Practice: From Canadian and Global Perspectives.* Pressbooks. https://ecampusontario.pressbooks.pub/communitydevelopmentpractice/

Henderson, A. (2019). *Communication for Health Care Practice.* Oxford University Press.

International Association for Public Participation Australasia (IAP2). (2019–2024). *IAP2 Public Participation Spectrum.* https://iap2.org.au/resources/spectrum/

Ife, J. (2016). *Community Development in an Uncertain World* (2nd ed.). Cambridge University Press.

Kickbusch, I.S. (2001). Health literacy: Addressing the health and education divide. *Health Promotion International*, *16*(3), 289–97. https://doi.org/10.1093/heapro/16.3.289

Kington, R.S., Arnesen, S., Chou, W.S., et al. (2021). Identifying credible sources of health information in social media: principles and attributes. *NAM Perspectives*, *2021*, 10.31478/202107a. https://doi.org/10.31478/202107a

Lim, D., Schoo, A., Lawn, S., & Litt, J. (2019). Embedding and sustaining motivational interviewing in clinical environments: A concurrent iterative mixed methods study. *BMC Medical Education*, *19*, 1–12.

McCarthy, C.J., Bauman, S., Choudhuri, D.D., et al. (2022). Association for specialists in group work guiding principles for group work. *The Journal for Specialists in Group Work*, *47*(1), 10–21. https://doi.org/10.1080/01933922.2021.1950882

Miller, W.R. & Rollnick, S. (2013). *Motivational Interviewing: Helping People to Change* (3rd ed.). Guilford Press.

Motivational Interviewing Network of Trainers (MINT). (2019). *Understanding motivational interviewing.* https://motivationalinterviewing.org/understanding-motivational-interviewing

Muscat, D.M., Gessler, D., Ayre, J., et al. (2022). Seeking a deeper understanding of 'distributed health literacy': A systematic review. *Health Expectations*, *25*(3), 856–68. https://doi.org/10.1111/hex.13450

Nazarnia, M., Zarei, F. & Rozbahani, N. (2022). Development and psychometric properties of a tool to assess Media Health Literacy (MeHLit). *BMC Public Health*, *22*(1), 1839. https://doi.org/10.1186/s12889-022-14221-6

Nutbeam, D. (1999). Literacies across the lifespan: Health literacy. *Literacy and Numeracy Studies*, *9*(2), 47.

Nutbeam, D. & Lloyd, J.E. (2021). Understanding and responding to health literacy as a social determinant of health. *Annual Review of Public Health*, *42*(1), 159–73. https://doi.org/10.1146/annurev-publhealth-090419-102529

Nutbeam, D. & McGill, B. (2019). Improving health literacy in clinical and community populations. In O. Okan, U. Bauer, D. Levin-Zamir, P. Pinheiro & K. Sørensen (eds), *International Handbook of Health Literacy* (pp. 219–32). Policy Press.

O'Sullivan, L., Sukumar, P., Crowley, R., McAuliffe, E. & Doran, P. (2020). Readability and understandability of clinical research patient information leaflets and consent forms in Ireland and the UK: A retrospective quantitative analysis. *BMJ Open*, *10*(9), e037994.

Pelikan, J.M. (2019). Health-literate healthcare organisations. In O. Okan, U. Bauer, D. Levin-Zamir, P. Pinheiro & K. Sørensen (eds), *International Handbook of Health Literacy* (pp. 539–54). Policy Press.

Poort, I., Jansen, E. & Hofman, A. (2022). Does the group matter? Effects of trust, cultural diversity, and group formation on engagement in group work in higher education. *Higher Education Research & Development*, *41*(2), 511–26. https://doi.org/10.1080/07294360.2020.1839024

Rethorn, Z.D., Bezner, J.R. & Pettitt, C.D. (2022). From expert to coach: Health coaching to support behavior change within physical therapist practice. *Physiotherapy Theory and Practice*, *38*(13), 2352–67. https://doi.org/10.1080/09593985.2021.1987601

Scrimshaw, S.C. (2019). Science, health, and cultural literacy in a rapidly changing communications landscape. *Proceedings of the National Academy of Sciences*, *116*(16), 7650–5. https://doi.org/10.1073/pnas.1807218116

Shady, K., Phillips, S. & Newman, S. (2022). Barriers and facilitators to healthcare access in adults with intellectual and developmental disorders and communication difficulties: An integrative review. *Review Journal of Autism and Developmental Disorders*, 1–13. Advance online publication. https://doi.org/10.1007/s40489-022-00324-8

Shawky, S., Kubacki, K., Dietrich, T. & Weaven, S. (2019). Using social media to create engagement: A social marketing review. *Journal of Social Marketing*, *9*(2), 204–24. https://doi.org/10.1108/JSOCM-05-2018-0046

Shersher, V., Haines, T.P., Sturgiss, L., Weller, C. & Williams, C. (2021). Definitions and use of the teach-back method in healthcare consultations with patients: A systematic review and thematic synthesis. *Patient Education and Counseling*, *104*(1), 118–29. https://doi.org/10.1016/j.pec.2020.07.026

Singh, H.K., Kennedy, G.A. & Stupans, I. (2022). Competencies and training of health professionals engaged in health coaching: A systematic review. *Chronic Illness*, *18*(1), 58–85. https://doi.org/10.1177/1742395319899466

Sykes, S. & Wills, J. (2019). Critical health literacy for the marginalised: Empirical findings. In O. Okan, U. Bauer, D. Levin-Zamir, P. Pinheiro & K. Sørensen (eds), *International Handbook of Health Literacy: Research, Practice and Policy Across the Life-Span* (pp. 167–81). Policy Press.

Szabó, P., Bíró, É. & Kósa, K. (2021). Readability and comprehension of printed patient education materials. *Frontiers in Public Health*, *9*, 725840. https://doi.org/10.3389/fpubh.2021.725840

Tuckman, B.W. (1965). Developmental sequence in small groups. *Psychological Bulletin*, *65*(6), 384–99.

Urstad, K.H., Andersen, M.H., Larsen, M.H., et al. (2022). Definitions and measurement of health literacy in health and medicine research: A systematic review. *BMJ Open*, *12*(2), e056294.

van der Gaag, M., Heijmans, M., Spoiala, C. & Rademakers, J. (2022). The importance of health literacy for self-management: A scoping review of reviews. *Chronic Illness*, *18*(2), 234–54. https://doi.org/10.1177/17423953211035472

van Diggele, C., Burgess, A. & Mellis, C. (2020). Planning, preparing and structuring a small group teaching session. *BMC Medical Education 20*(Suppl 2), 462. https://doi.org/10.1186/s12909-020-02281-4

van Kessel, R., Wong, B.L.H., Clemens, T. & Brand, H. (2022). Digital health literacy as a super determinant of health: More than simply the sum of its parts. *Internet Interventions*, *27*. https://doi.org/10.1016/j.invent.2022.100500

Walsh, L., Hill, S., Waterhouse, T. (2019). *Guide to Producing and Sourcing Quality Health Information.* Centre for Health Communication and Participation, La Trobe University. https://doi.org/10.26181/5cda55cdaca30

World Health Organization (WHO). (1998). *Health promotion glossary.* www.who.int/publications/i/item/WHO-HPR-HEP-98.1

——— (2024). *Health promotion.* www.who.int/teams/health-promotion/enhanced-wellbeing/seventh-global-conference/community-empowerment

World Health Organization (WHO) and United Nations Children's Fund (UNICEF). (2018). *A Vision for Primary Health Care in the 21st Century: Towards Universal Health Coverage and the Sustainable Development Goals.* WHO and UNICEF.

Yen, P.H. & Leasure, A.R. (2019). Use and effectiveness of the teach-back method in patient education and health outcomes. *Federal Practitioner, 36*(6), 284–9.

Žganec, N. & Opačić, A. (2021). Principles of community development and challenges facing deprived communities. In A. Opačić (ed.), *Practicing Social Work in Deprived Communities. European Social Work Education and Practice* (pp. 69–88). Springer. https://doi.org/10.1007/978-3-030-65987-5_3

3

Developing a career in primary health care

Kaara Ray B. Calma, Anna Williams and Elizabeth Halcomb
With acknowledgement to Susan McInnes

LEARNING OBJECTIVES

At the completion of this chapter, you should be able to:

- discuss how primary health care (PHC) is represented in contemporary nursing curricula.
- understand pre-registration nursing students' clinical placement exposure to PHC during undergraduate education.
- discuss pre-registration nursing students' perceptions and attitudes towards the nursing role and working in PHC.
- describe the opportunities and challenges of new graduate employment in PHC.
- identify the challenges faced by acute care nurses transitioning to PHC employment and factors that facilitate the transition.

Introduction

Despite current and predicted ongoing PHC nursing workforce shortages (Heywood & Laurence, 2018), the undergraduate nursing curricula in Australasia and internationally remain largely directed towards acute care (Calma, Stephens & Halcomb, 2019). Additionally, the efforts of schools of nursing in supporting the career development of new graduate nurses and their transition to practice also remain largely focused on employment in acute care tertiary settings. Registered nurses (RNs) are integral members of the multidisciplinary PHC team and fulfil various roles. These roles include managing acute presentations, coordinating care for people with complex chronic conditions, providing preventive care, promoting the health of individuals and communities, and supporting end-of-life care (Bauer & Bodenheimer, 2017; Halcomb et al., 2017). Nurses are ideally positioned to undertake these roles due to their close therapeutic relationships and ongoing engagement with clients and their families that promote continuity of care (Karam et al., 2021).

While some nurses will enter their careers with a passion for PHC, others will develop an interest in the field because of exposure to the sector or when seeking a career change. This chapter provides an overview of the extent to which current undergraduate nursing curricula prepare RNs to work in PHC. In presenting this information, it is acknowledged that nursing curricula are developed according to accreditation cycles and thus the material may not reflect changes in the health care system that might be occurring at present. The chapter also explores the nursing students' perceptions and attitudes towards working in a PHC setting and the challenges RNs face when transitioning between acute and PHC practice environments. Understanding these factors and the extent to which pre-registration nurses are prepared during their education for a PHC career is important to promote recruitment and retention of a PHC nursing workforce – notably an area of predicted future shortages.

Pre-registration nursing education

Nursing education in Australia was historically hospital-based, delivered via an apprenticeship system where student nurses gained clinical skills training and theoretical education in employing hospitals (Currie et al., 2019). In 1994, pre-registration nursing training in Australia was transferred to the tertiary education sector (Ralph et al., 2015). University nursing programs must be approved by the **Australian Nursing and Midwifery Accreditation Council (ANMAC)** to be accredited to provide courses that lead to registration as a nurse with the Nursing and Midwifery Board of Australia (NMBA) (2019). The ANMAC assesses programs against accreditation standards to ensure the content and program delivery meet minimum standards.

Aotearoa New Zealand became the first country to register nurses, via the New Zealand Nurses Act of 1901 (Lusk et al., 2001). Presently, nursing registration and program accreditation in Aotearoa New Zealand are under the governance umbrella of the **Nursing Council of New Zealand (NCNZ)**, working with national tertiary organisations such as the New Zealand Qualifications Agency (NCNZ, 2020a).

While some aspects of nursing curricula are mandated to meet the accreditation standards (ANMAC, 2019; NCNZ, 2020a), including the minimum clinical placement hours, targeted specialty areas (for example, national health priority areas and the extent to which PHC is considered a focus) or priority groups (for example, Aboriginal and Torres Strait Islander peoples, Māori and Pacifica), are less well articulated (ANMAC, 2019; NCNZ, 2020b). Universities independently determine if and to what extent these aspects are incorporated into their curricula. To date, PHC has not been a mandated component of undergraduate curricula and, as a result, variations are found between universities regarding the degree of PHC content included, and generally undergraduate nursing curricula are reported to have limited PHC content (Murray-Parahi et al., 2020). Furthermore, and in general, there is a lack of consistency regarding the specific PHC content that needs to be included in undergraduate nursing education to support the development of a PHC workforce. This observation was highlighted in a national review of nursing education in Australia (Schwartz, 2019).

Some universities limit PHC content due to a belief that pre-registration nursing education should prepare students to work in an acute care setting (Wojnar & Whelan, 2017). Additionally, the limited availability of suitable PHC clinical placements (compared to the number of pre-registration nursing students requiring placements) and the lack of academics with PHC expertise to inform the design and delivery of course/subject content impact on PHC content being a priority in undergraduate education (Calma et al., 2019; Schwartz, 2019). Nursing students also have expectations that their pre-registration courses will prepare them to work in acute care settings and this is also a barrier for universities developing an

Australian Nursing and Midwifery Accreditation Council (ANMAC) – an independent accrediting authority for nursing and midwifery education that operates under Australia's National Registration and Accreditation Scheme (ANMAC, 2019).

Nursing Council of New Zealand (NCNZ) – the accrediting authority for bachelor of nursing programs in Aotearoa New Zealand, working in collaboration with the New Zealand Qualifications Authority and the committee on University Academic Programmes (NCNZ, 2024).

increased curriculum focus on PHC (Calma et al., 2021b; Wojnar & Whelan, 2017). However, in recent years, a growing number of nursing schools internationally have recognised the important role of RNs who engage in practice outside a hospital setting and have correspondingly shifted the focus of curricula to better prepare nurses for diverse practice. However, to date, there has been limited investigation into how this should best be achieved and its impact on graduate nurses (Calma et al., 2019).

The inconsistent integration of PHC knowledge, skills and clinical exposure into undergraduate nursing curricula has resulted in new graduate RNs reporting feeling somewhat underprepared for employment in a PHC setting (Calma et al., 2019). Feelings of being unprepared may impact students' confidence and career choices (Calma et al., 2022a). Given the current and future PHC nursing workforce shortages, pre-registration nurses must be supported to develop the skills, knowledge and capabilities to work in a diverse range of settings following graduation. This opens up the vast array of career opportunities that exist for nurses outside the walls of the hospital. As part of their undergraduate education, pre-registration students need to be encouraged to explore the range of clinical practice and career opportunities available, to understand the significant diversity of the nursing role and to determine which areas of practice may be best suited to their individual skills and interests as well as personal needs.

REFLECTION

Consider how PHC is being covered in your undergraduate education.

1. To what extent has PHC been addressed in your undergraduate education?
2. What skills have you learnt that could be applied in a PHC setting?
3. What career opportunities have you come across in the PHC sector? Where could you find out more about employment opportunities in PHC?

Pre-registration clinical placement experiences

As nursing is a practice-based discipline, new graduate nurses must be work-ready and possess a level of knowledge, skills and capabilities to ensure safe practice as beginning nurses (Schwartz, 2019). Clinical-based learning in real-life settings provides opportunities to expose pre-registration nurses to the realities of the nursing profession and to challenge preconceived ideas about the clinical areas in which they wish to work (McInnes et al., 2015). Pre-registration **clinical placements** expose nursing students to a diverse range of experiences in a supportive environment and, in doing so, provide valuable opportunities to consolidate theoretical knowledge, develop confidence and competence in newly acquired skills and promote interdisciplinary socialisation (Carr, Taylor & Pitt, 2018; McInnes et al., 2015).

Clinical placements – the successful completion of a minimum of 800 clinical placement hours in diverse health care settings is a mandatory requirement for registration as an RN in Australia (ANMAC, 2019). The NCNZ (2020b) stipulates a minimum of 1100 clinical placement hours as mandatory for registration as a nurse in Aotearoa New Zealand.

PHC offers a diverse range of settings for clinical placement experience including justice health, refugee centres, community health centres, Indigenous community-controlled health centres, aged care facilities and general practices. The opportunities to secure a PHC clinical placement differ between universities and are dependent on the number of placements locally available, the university's model of clinical facilitation and the ability of the PHC facility to support student placements. The timing of a PHC placement within a degree program can also vary, from a placement in the first year that focuses on the development of communication and basic care skills (for example, therapeutic relationships and vital signs), to a placement in the third year that engages the student in complex chronic disease case management. Before undertaking clinical placements in PHC, students must understand the context of the setting and the preparation required to perform the role of a nurse within their scope of practice (McInnes et al., 2015). This might require students to investigate the role of the nurse within a specific PHC setting, the profile of the community that is served and the core functions of different members of the multidisciplinary team. Students might also want to consider any preconceptions, expectations and attitudes that they might have before attending a placement and consider what impact these might have on the way that they present during the placement.

Commonly students indicate some reluctance to undertake a clinical placement in PHC, as they believe that there will be insufficient opportunity to practise or complete necessary clinical skills and that their time will be wasted doing basic skills and therefore not be challenging (Calma et al., 2021c; McInnes et al., 2015). These perceptions are often confronted during PHC placements, with students reporting more positive learning experiences than they had expected (McInnes et al., 2015; Peters, McInnes & Halcomb, 2015). Indeed, students often report that they develop a variety of clinical and communication skills and engage in broad and rewarding practice during their PHC placements (McInnes et al., 2015). Students are often surprised by the diversity of clinical presentations in PHC, the advanced nursing practice and the high levels of autonomy in these settings (Calma et al., 2021a; Calma et al., 2021b; McInnes et al., 2015; Peters et al., 2015). At all times, however, activities undertaken during a PHC placement should be consistent with the skills and knowledge of the student at the specific point in their undergraduate education (scope of practice).

In many cases, pre-registration nursing students describe feeling well supported by mentors when completing a PHC placement, when the mentors express a genuine interest in their learning and facilitate time for them to consolidate their clinical skills (Peters et al., 2015). However, in some cases, given the professional isolation of many nurses working in PHC roles, there may be a need to ensure that mentors understand the specific scope of the nursing students' practice and the activities expected of them during the placement experience (Zulu, du Plessis & Koen, 2021).

Community and PHC placements provide valuable opportunities for pre-registration nurses to develop an understanding of the nurse's role, the philosophies that underpin PHC, approaches to person-centred care and working with families and communities (Byfield, East & Conway, 2019). PHC placements offer nursing students a myriad of opportunities to develop clinical reasoning skills through exposure to the assessment, treatment and management of diverse health conditions across the lifespan, within traditional and innovative models of care (Byfield et al., 2019; McInnes et al., 2015). Additionally, real-life experience working within PHC environments exposes students to the complexities associated with funding small business enterprises and the impact of these on interprofessional relationships and health service delivery.

Perceptions and attitudes

The perceptions of others, clinical placement experiences and personal factors can influence pre-registration nursing students' knowledge of and attitudes towards working in PHC (van Iersel et al., 2018a). Collectively, these factors influence the pre-registration nursing students' perceived value of PHC within the health care system, as part of their undergraduate education and as a potential career opportunity (Mackey et al., 2018; van Iersel et al., 2018a). Although pre-registration nursing students may appreciate the important contribution PHC makes to the maintenance and promotion of health and well-being in the community (Mackey et al., 2018; van Iersel et al., 2018a), many fail to fully appreciate the value of working in a community or PHC setting (Calma et al., 2022b). Furthermore, students commonly consider curriculum content related to PHC as the least important component of their undergraduate education (Calma et al., 2019). Developing such views at a pre-registration level can ultimately affect students' enthusiasm and interest in PHC more broadly, which can potentially have a detrimental impact on the recruitment and retention of nurses to work in community and PHC settings (Calma et al., 2022a), immediately post registration and during their careers.

Some studies report pre-registration nursing students having a positive attitude towards working in PHC (Mackey et al., 2018), whereas others have found that many nursing students did not consider PHC as 'real nursing' or an attractive future employment option (Calma et al., 2019). Some pre-registration nursing students perceive employment in a PHC setting following graduation as a 'low-status' job (van Iersel et al., 2018a) that will limit future career advancement and the ability to develop nursing skills (van Iersel et al., 2018a; Wojnar & Whelan, 2017). Calma and colleagues (2022b) found that final-year pre-registration nursing students prioritised wages and opportunities for advancement when choosing an employment setting but considered these to be limited in a primary care setting.

Tertiary institutions are well positioned to inform the career choices of nursing students and to raise the profile of PHC through the provision of quality undergraduate education and clinical exposure to the diverse range of PHC settings and practice opportunities (van Iersel et al., 2018b). Pre-registration nursing students should also be encouraged to seek more information regarding PHC and the possibility of a clinical practice placement in a PHC setting. Identifying nurse academics with expertise and/or an interest in PHC can assist students to identify local opportunities for education, experience and networking. Alternatively, professional and PHC organisations such as the Australian Primary Health Care Nurse Association (APNA), Primary Health Networks (PHNs) and the New Zealand Nurses Organisation (NZNO), offer detailed information regarding PHC nursing careers, support networks and ongoing professional development opportunities.

CASE STUDY 3.1

Emma is a student nurse commencing her final, five-week clinical placement at Greenleaf Community Health Centre. Emma had initially planned on completing her final placement in a hospital medical ward. However, completion of the PHC unit at university has influenced her decision to take up her longest and final clinical placement in PHC. On her first day, Emma feels a mixture of excitement and nervousness as she becomes aware of the complexities of the community health nurse's role.

REFLECTION

1. If you were Emma, what aspects of the community health nurse's role would you want to know about prior to commencing your placement?

2. What are some potential challenges Emma might expect as a student nurse working in community health?
3. What skills and experience do you think Emma might gain during her placement? Would any of these be transferable to work in a medical ward?

Working in PHC

In 2023, 26.2 per cent of Australian nurses worked in a PHC setting (Department of Health and Aged Care, 2023). In 2020, 23 per cent of RNs in Aotearoa New Zealand worked in PHC, of which 16 per cent were Aotearoa New Zealand-qualified RNs and 7 per cent had received their qualifications overseas (NCNZ, 2020c). In comparison to acute care nurses, who are commonly employed by state/territory/regional health services or private hospitals, PHC nurses are employed by a range of different organisations. These may include non-government organisations and charities (e.g. Royal District Nursing Service in Australia and Hospice New Zealand), government organisations (local health districts, departments of education) and small and large private businesses (solo, small and corporate general/family practices). Working in smaller private organisations means that PHC nurses are faced with several challenges compared to their counterparts working in publicly funded hospital settings or larger health and non-health government-funded organisations. The provision of services may be more constrained by funding issues and wages and employment conditions are more frequently negotiated on an individual basis rather than covered by an industrial award (Halcomb et al., 2018). This creates a need for nurses seeking employment in this sector to be informed about industrial issues and develop skills in negotiating wages and conditions with prospective employers (Halcomb et al., 2018). In addition, the general practice setting has several reported challenges for new graduate nurses including their employer (e.g. GPs) not fully understanding the nursing scope of practice, lack of access to support from other nurses and the need for the general practice environment to support the transition of the graduate into their role and provide opportunities for ongoing professional development (McInnes et al., 2019) (see also Chapter 24). An evaluation of a PHC transition program found that there were varying levels of responsibilities for new graduates across general practices, and that some of the new graduates believed that there were limited opportunities to develop professionally as they progressed through the primary care program (Aggar et al., 2017). Despite these challenges, Aggar and colleagues (2018) reported that more than half of the graduate nurses intended to extend their careers in PHC. As the graduate nurse experience accumulated and the level of supervision naturally declined as the transition program advanced, independence and confidence were fostered among the new graduates. The quality of preceptor support that new graduates received was identified as a key facilitator in the program (Aggar et al., 2018).

While the number of nurses working in community and PHC settings has increased in recent decades, there is a current and predicted future shortage of nurses working in PHC (Department of Health and Aged Care, 2022; Halcomb & Bird, 2020) It is vital that new graduate nurses see PHC as a viable career opportunity and experienced nurses consider future employment in PHC. Policymakers and PHC organisations have a great responsibility in providing clarity around nurse remuneration and opportunities for advancement in PHC settings, establishing equity by ensuring that these are commensurate with other areas of nursing (Calma et al., 2022b).

REFLECTION

1. What is your attitude towards working in PHC?
2. Would you be suited to work in a PHC environment? Why? Why not?
3. What challenges do you think you might face when starting a career in PHC?
4. What might be some of the challenges or disadvantages to working in PHC?

Transitioning to new graduate practice

The stage at which a pre-registration nursing student transitions into an RN is an exciting and potentially intimidating period. Formal transition to practice programs must have the capacity to guide and support the new graduate within situated learning experiences and real-life challenges (Weller-Newton et al., 2022). Structured preceptorship models of transition support have been found to positively influence the retention and recruitment of nurses (Aparício & Nicholson, 2020). The majority of Australian new graduates enter the nursing workforce via 'transition to professional practice' (TPP) programs commonly managed by state/territory health departments and implemented in acute hospital settings (Schwartz, 2019). However, there is a focus on supporting and promoting new graduate nurses to work in PHC settings, in particular general practice and aged care. In Aotearoa New Zealand, the national Nurse Entry to Practice Programme governs new graduate programs through district health boards (Doughty et al., 2018), and later merged with Health New Zealand (2022). While many of these programs offer graduate rotations through several clinical areas, others support the transition into a single clinical environment.

Although limited evaluations have been undertaken regarding the transition to practice programs, in general, they report positive outcomes including the confidence to work autonomously within the scope of practice (McInnes et al., 2019). Before completing their transition program, many new graduate nurses report a limited understanding of general/family practice nursing and a perception that the transition program provided a supportive environment in which to transition into their professional role. The program also facilitated building their confidence in their ability to work more autonomously and to a full scope of practice (McInnes et al., 2019).

Due to the diversity of settings and employment opportunities in PHC, not all employers can offer formal transition-to-practice programs, and some may only provide limited or informal support. New graduate nurses interested in pursuing a career in PHC should actively investigate the extent of support available to assist the transition process and inform their employment decisions. This should include understanding the willingness of the employer to provide support during the period of transition; access to education and ongoing professional development opportunities; availability of mentors, wages and other employment conditions; and prospects for career advancement. Connecting with professional and local PHC organisations, such as the APNA, the NZNO and local PHNs, can assist in networking and identifying opportunities for support and mentoring. The future looks bright for those new graduate nurses who wish to work in PHC as opportunities continue to grow. However, individual nurses need to seek these career opportunities and invest in connecting with others to ensure that they are well-supported during their transition into PHC practice.

In Australia, the supply of transition-to-practice programs does not meet demand, with many new graduate nurses being unsuccessful in securing a placement each year (Russell & Juliff, 2021). For those graduating nurses who are unsuccessful in obtaining a place in an acute care transition program, PHC may be an alluring career option (McInnes et al., 2019).

New graduates are increasingly successful in gaining employment in PHC settings and developing a career outside the hospital setting. Experienced PHC nurses value the contribution that new graduate nurses bring to the workplace including up-to-date knowledge of best practice principles and the ability to source evidence-based information (McInnes et al., 2019).

Nurses transitioning from acute care

Nurses may also enter the PHC workforce after gaining experience in hospital settings. Experienced nurses move to PHC employment for various reasons including a better work-life balance, improved working hours, greater work satisfaction and to experience a more autonomous role (Ashley et al., 2017). Transitioning into a new workplace requires adaptation to a new role, team members and a different environment and context, which may cause a degree of career disruption (Ashley et al., 2018c). For some, PHC is 'a whole different ball game' that requires a significant reshaping of practice and application of clinical knowledge and skills (Ashley et al., 2018a).

A study of experienced Australian nurses transitioning into PHC employment found that many of these RNs had positive experiences in their new employment, valuing the work-life balance, diversity of the PHC role and interactions with clients and their families (Ashley et al., 2018a; 2018b). However, participants also struggled with prioritising workload, adapting to new technology, familiarising themselves with the workplace and gaining organisational knowledge. Approximately half of the RNs also described feeling isolated or overwhelmed in their new job (Ashley et al., 2018c). The RNs in the same study identified that improved orientation, workplace-specific skills practice and enhanced preceptor support could all have assisted in the transition process. In more recent studies, the expanded responsibilities around triaging, greater autonomy with decision-making and having to adapt from the more 'controlled' hospital environment to the unpredictable community-based settings have been reported as significant challenges to nurses moving into PHC roles (Koh et al., 2022; Muhsin et al., 2020). These studies highlight that, regardless of professional background, moving into a new clinical setting requires adjustment, development and adequate support. Indeed, several papers report that informal, clinical and professional mentoring is a key enabling factor in the transition to PHC practice (Cox et al., 2023; Koh et al., 2022).

Given that there are no current national requirements for nurses transitioning in specific clinical settings to undertake post-graduate studies or formal graduate programs (Schwartz, 2019), there is a need for higher education institutions, professional associations, registration bodies and government health departments to identify the role of PHC-focused transition to practice programs that centralises on competency-based education, opportunities for certification and microcredentialing (Cox et al., 2023). Ensuring that a PHC position is well supported by management and other team members has educational and training opportunities and a potential for career advancement is essential before accepting a position.

CASE STUDY 3.2

Alvin has recently joined a general practice, and it is his first job as an RN. He is pleased to get this job and knows that the practice has a very experienced RN, Danica, who can support him in his new role. Danica is an RN with over 20 years experience as a general practice nurse (GPN). James presented to the treatment room with a 7cm burn on his right forearm. He explains to Alvin that he accidentally scalded himself while cooking two days ago and needs help to manage the wound because it is 'very painful'. Alvin, although familiar with basic first aid principles, feels uncertain about the appropriate management of burn wounds.

Danica is currently completing a health assessment with another patient, leaving Alvin to handle the situation independently. Recalling their previous discussions about wound care principles and guidelines, Alvin feels pressured to provide James with effective treatment. Drawing upon his knowledge of burn management, Alvin assesses the severity of the injury and cleanses the wound with a sterile saline solution. However, Alvin is unsure how to proceed following cleansing the wound.

REFLECTION

1. How should Alvin approach the management of the wound?
2. Who could he reach out to for support?

Conclusion

A nursing career in PHC provides significant opportunities for autonomy and diversity in practice. Nursing in PHC involves working within a multidisciplinary team and in partnership with individuals and communities to maintain and promote health and well-being. PHC is a valid and valuable career path for new graduates and experienced RNs, especially with the support of transition-to-practice programs. PHC offers RNs a diverse, exciting and rewarding career path that provides care across the lifespan to individuals, families and communities.

CRITICAL THINKING ACTIVITIES

1. Commonly, formal transition to professional practice programs takes place in acute care facilities. How does this impact the career choices of new graduate nurses?
2. What are some of the considerations that nurses should take into account when seeking employment in a PHC setting?
3. What challenges do you anticipate as a new graduate nurse entering employment in PHC?
4. How do you think nursing education programs can better prepare students to navigate these challenges and succeed in PHC settings?

FURTHER READING

Calma, K., Stephens, M. & Halcomb, E.J. (2019). The impact of curriculum on nursing students' attitudes, perceptions and preparedness to work in primary health care: An integrative review. *Nurse Education in Practice*, *39*, 1–10. https://doi.org/10.1016/j.nepr.2019.07.006

Halcomb, E., Smyth, E. & McInnes, S. (2018). Job satisfaction and career intentions of registered nurses in primary health care: An integrative review. *BMC Family Practice*, *19*(136). https://doi.org/10.1186/s12875-018-0819-1

Hunt, G., Verstappen, A., Stewart, L., Kool, B. & Slark, J. (2020). Career interests of undergraduate nursing students: A ten-year longitudinal study. *Nurse Education in Practice*, *43*, 102702. https://doi.org/10.1016/j.nepr.2020.102702

Stainsby, H.L. & Vintis, J. (2023). General practice nursing: Student-led health check roadshows raising career profile. *Primary Health Care*, *33*(1). https://doi:10.7748/phc.2023.e1792

REFERENCES

Aggar, C., Bloomfield, J., Thomas, T.H. & Gordon, C.J. (2017). Australia's first transition to professional practice in primary care program for graduate registered nurses: A pilot study. *BMC Nursing*, *16*(14), 1–11. https://doi.org/10.1186/s12912-017-0207-5

Aggar, C., Thomas, T.H.T., Gordon, C.J., Bloomfield, J. & Wadsworth, L. (2018). Evaluation of a community transition to professional practice program for graduate registered nurses in Australia. *Nurse Education in Practice*, *32*(1), 101–7. https://doi.org/10.1016/j.nepr.2018.03.005

Aparício, C. & Nicholson, J. (2020). Do preceptorship and clinical supervision programmes support the retention of nurses? *British Journal of Nursing*, *29*(20), 1192–7. https://doi.org/10.12968/bjon.2020.29.20.1192

Ashley, C., Brown, A., Halcomb, E. & Peters, K. (2018a). Registered nurses transitioning from acute care to primary healthcare employment: A qualitative insight into nurses' experiences. *Journal of Clinical Nursing*, *27*(3/4), 661–8. https://doi.org/10.1111/jocn.13984

Ashley, C., Peters, K., Brown, A., & Halcomb, E. (2018b). Work satisfaction and future career intentions of experienced nurses transitioning to primary health care employment. *Journal of Nursing Management*, *26*(6), 663–70. https://doi.org/10.1111/jonm.12597

Ashley, C., Halcomb, E., Brown, A. & Peters, K. (2018c). Experiences of registered nurses transitioning from employment in acute care to primary health care-quantitative findings from a mixed-methods study. *Journal of Clinical Nursing, 27*(1/2), 355–62. https://doi.org/10.1111/jocn.13930

Ashley, C., Halcomb, E., Peters, K. & Brown, A. (2017). Exploring why nurses transition from acute care to primary health care employment. *Applied Nursing Research, 38*, 83–7. https://doi.org/10.1016/j.apnr.2017.09.002

Australian Nursing and Midwifery Accreditation Council (ANMAC). (2019). *Registered Nurse Accreditation Standards 2019*. ANMAC. https://anmac.org.au/sites/default/files/2024-06/registerednurseaccreditationstandards2019_0.pdf

Bauer, L. & Bodenheimer, T. (2017). Expanded roles of registered nurses in primary care delivery of the future. *Nursing Outlook*, *65*(5), 624–32. https://doi.org/10.1016/j.outlook.2017.03.011

Byfield, Z., East, L. & Conway, J. (2019). An integrative literature review of pre-registration nursing students' attitudes and perceptions towards primary healthcare. *Collegian*, *26*(5), 583–93. https://doi.org/10.1016/j.colegn.2019.01.004

Calma, K., Halcomb, E., Williams, A. & McInnes, S. (2021a). Final-year undergraduate nursing students' perceptions of general practice nursing: A qualitative study. *Journal of Clinical Nursing, 30*(7–8), 1144–53. https://doi.org/10.1111/jocn.15662

Calma, K., McInnes, S., Halcomb, E., Williams, A. & Batterham, M. (2022a). Confidence, interest and intentions of final-year nursing students regarding employment in general practice. *Collegian, 29*, 220–7. https://doi.org/10.1016/j.colegn.2021.08.005

Calma, K., Stephens, M. & Halcomb, E.J. (2019). The impact of curriculum on nursing students' attitudes, perceptions and preparedness to work in primary health care: An integrative review. *Nurse Education in Practice, 39*, 1–10. https://doi.org/10.1016/j.nepr.2019.07.006

Calma, K., Williams, A., McInnes, S. & Halcomb, E. (2021b). New graduate employment in general practice: Perceptions of final-year nursing students. *Nurse Education in Practice, 54*, 103115. https://doi.org/10.1016/j.nepr.2021.103115

Calma, K.R.B., Halcomb, E.J., Fernandez, R., Williams, A. & McInnes, S. (2022b). Understanding nursing students' perceptions of the general practice environment and their priorities for employment settings. *Nursing Open, 9*(5), 2325–34. https://doi.org/10.1002/nop2.1242

Calma, K.R.B., Halcomb, E.J., Williams, A. & McInnes, S. (2021c). Final-year undergraduate nursing students' perceptions of general practice nursing: A qualitative study. *Journal of Clinical Nursing, 30*(7–8), 1144–53. https://doi.org/10.1111/jocn.15662

Carr, J., Taylor, R. & Pitt, M. (2018). Supporting student nurses who have their first clinical placement in the community nursing team. *British Journal of Community Nursing, 23*(10), 496–500. https://doi.org/10.12968/bjcn.2018.23.10.496

Cox, R., Robinson, T., Rossiter, R., Collison, L. & Hills, D. (2023). Nurses transitioning to primary health care in Australia: A practice improvement initiative. *SAGE Open Nursing*, 1–9. https://doi.org/10.1177/23779608231165695

Currie, J., Grootemaat, P., Samsa, P., Halcomb, E. & Thompson, C. (2019). *Topic 3: Clinical Skill Development.* Australian Government: Department of Health and Aged Care. www.health.gov.au/resources/publications/topic-3-clinical-skill-development?language=en

Department of Health and Aged Care. (2022). *Future Focused Primary Health Care: Australia's Primary Health Care 10 Year Plan 2022–2032.* Commonwealth of Australia. www.health.gov.au/resources/publications/australias-primary-health-care-10-year-plan-2022-2032

———— (2023). *Data tool.* Commonwealth of Australia. https://hwd.health.gov.au/datatool/.

Doughty, L., McKillop, A., Dixon, R. & Sinnema, C. (2018). Educating new graduate nurses in their first year of practice: The perspective and experiences of the new graduate nurses and the director of nursing. *Nurse Education in Practice, 30*(1), 101–5. https://doi.org/10.1016/j.nepr.2018.03.006

Halcomb, E., Ashley, C., James, S. & Smyth, E. (2018). Employment conditions of Australian primary health care nurses. *Collegian, 25*(1), 65–71. https://doi.org/10.1016/j.colegn.2017.03.008

Halcomb, E.J. & Bird, S. (2020). Job satisfaction and career intention of Australian general practice nurses: A cross-sectional survey. *Journal of Nursing Scholarship, 52*(3), 270–80. https://doi.org/10.1111/jnu.12548

Halcomb, E.J., Stephens, M., Bryce, J., Foley, E. & Ashley, C. (2017). The development of professional practice standards for nurses working in Australian general practice. *Journal of Advanced Nursing, 73*(8), 1958–69. https://doi.org/10.1111/jan.13274

Health New Zealand (2022). *How our health system is changing/E panoni ana tō tātou hātepe hauora.* New Zealand Government. www.futureofhealth.govt.nz/health-nz/

Heywood, T. & Laurence, C. (2018). An overview of the general practice nurse workforce in Australia, 2012–15. *Australian Journal of Primary Health, 24*(3), 227–32. https://doi.org/10.1071/PY17048

Karam, M., Chouinard, M.-C., Poitras, M.-E., et al. (2021). Nursing care coordination for patients with complex needs in primary healthcare: A scoping review. *International Journal of Integrated Care, 21*(1), 16. https://doi.org/10.5334/ijic.5518

Koh, H.M.D., Lee, C.S.C., Anna, C. & Lau, Y. (2022). Perceptions and experiences of nurses transitioning to primary care: A qualitative study. *International Nursing Review*, *69*(2), 201–10. https://doi.org/10.1111/inr.12691

Lusk, B., Russell, R.L., Rodgers, J. & Wilson-Barnett, J. (2001). Preregistration nursing education in Australia, New Zealand, the United Kingdom, and the United States of America. *Journal of Nursing Education*, *40*(5), 197–202. https://doi.org/10.3928/0148-4834-20010501-04

Mackey, S., Kwok, C., Anderson, J., et al. (2018). Australian student nurse's knowledge of and attitudes toward primary health care: A cross-sectional study. *Nurse Education Today*, *60*(1), 127–32. https://doi.org/10.1016/j.nedt.2017.10.003

McInnes, S., Halcomb, E.J., Huckel, K. & Ashley, C. (2019). The experiences of new graduate registered nurses in a general practice based graduate program: A qualitative study. *Australian Journal of Primary Health*, *25*(4), 366–73. https://doi.org/10.1071/PY19089

McInnes, S., Peters, K., Hardy, J. & Halcomb, E. (2015). Clinical placements in Australian general practice: (Part 1) the experiences of pre-registration nursing students. *Nurse Education in Practice*, *15*(6), 437–42. https://doi.org/10.1016/j.nepr.2015.04.003

Muhsin, M.G.B., Goh, Y.S., Hassan, N., Chi, Y. & Wu, X.V. (2020). Nurses' experiences on the road during transition into community care: An exploratory descriptive qualitative study in Singapore. *Health and Social Care in the Community*, *28*(6), 2253–64. https://doi.org/10.1111/hsc.13038

Murray-Parahi, P., Digiacomo, M., Jackson, D., Phillips, J. & Davidson, P.M. (2020). Primary health care content in Australian undergraduate nursing curricula. *Collegian*, *27*(3), 271–80. https://doi.org/10.1016/j.colegn.2019.08.008

Nursing and Midwifery Board of Australia (NMBA). (2019). *About NMBA*. www.nursingmidwiferyboard.gov.au/About.aspx

Nursing Council of New Zealand (NCNZ). (2020a). *Education*. www.nursingcouncil.org.nz/Education

——— (2020b). *Handbook for Pre-registration Nursing Programmes*. https://nursingcouncil.org.nz/Public/NCNZ/Education-section/Schools_Handbook.aspx

——— (2020c). *The Nursing Cohort Report*. www.nzdoctor.co.nz/sites/default/files/2021-07/Nursing%20Council%20%20Cohort%20Report%202020.pdf

——— (2024). *Home page*. www.nursingcouncil.org.nz/

Peters, K., McInnes, S. & Halcomb, E. (2015). Nursing students' experiences of clinical placement in community settings: A qualitative study. *Collegian*, *22*, 175–81. https://doi.org/10.1016/j.colegn.2015.03.001

Ralph, N., Birks, M. & Chapman, Y. (2015). The accreditation of nursing education in Australia. *Collegian*, *22*(1), 3–7. https://doi.org/10.1016/j.colegn.2013.10.002

Russell, K. & Juliff, D. (2021). Graduate nurse transition programs pivotal point of participants' practice readiness questioned during the COVID-19 pandemic crisis: A scoping review. *Journal of Continuing Education in Nursing*, *52*(8), 392–6. https://doi.org/10.3928/00220124-20210714-09

Schwartz, S. (2019). *Educating the Nurse of the Future: Report of the Independent review of nursing education*. Department of Health and Aged Care, Australian Government. www.health.gov.au/resources/publications/educating-the-nurse-of-the-future?language=en

van Iersel, M., Latour, C.H.M., de Vos, R., Kirschner, P.A. & Scholte op Reimer, W.J.M. (2018a). Perceptions of community care and placement preferences in first-year nursing students: A multicentre, cross-sectional study. *Nurse Education Today*, *60*, 92–7. https://doi.org/10.1016/j.nedt.2017.09.016

van Iersel, M., Latour, C.H.M., van Rijn, M., et al. (2018b). Factors underlying perceptions of community care and other healthcare areas in first-year baccalaureate nursing students: A focus group study. *Nurse Education Today*, *66*, 57–62. https://doi.org/10.1016/j.nedt.2018.04.004

Weller-Newton, J.M., Murray, M., Phillips, C., Laging, B. & McGillion, A. (2022). Transition to practice programs in nursing: A rapid review. *Journal of Continuing Education in Nursing*, *53*(10), 442–50. https://doi.org/10.3928/00220124-20220907-05

Wojnar, D.M. & Whelan, E.M. (2017). Preparing nursing students for enhanced roles in primary care: The current state of prelicensure and RN-to-BSN education. *Nursing Outlook*, *65*(2), 222–32. https://doi.org/10.1016/j.outlook.2016.10.006

Zulu, B.M., du Plessis, E. & Koen, M.P. (2021). Experiences of nursing students regarding clinical placement and support in primary healthcare clinics: Strengthening resilience. *Journal of Interdisciplinary Sciences*, *26*(2), 1–11. https://doi.org/10.4102/hsag.v26i0.1615

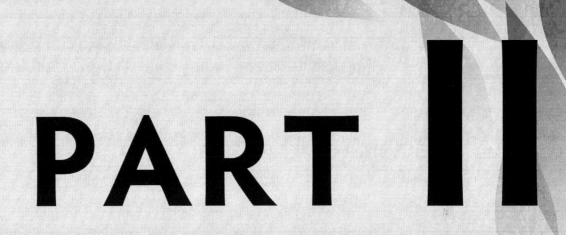

PART II

Diverse communities

4

Disability: issues for primary care nurses

Nathan J. Wilson, Natasha Jojo and Henrietta Trip
With acknowledgement to Rhonda Brown and Nick Arnott

LEARNING OBJECTIVES

At the completion of this chapter, you should be able to:

- define the different types of disabilities and approaches to providing care and support.
- understand a range of contemporary issues facing people with a disability.
- identify the range of disparate health problems in people with a disability.
- apply the principles of person-centred care to your daily practice with people with a disability.

Introduction

Approximately one in every six people have some form of disability and about one-third of these people have a severe or profound limitation to their daily activities and function (Australian Institute of Health and Welfare (AIHW), 2022). As a subgroup, they are some of the most marginalised and disadvantaged, often experiencing disparate chronic and complex health problems when compared to the general population. In addition, they sometimes encounter disabling challenges accessing the health system and have experienced poor quality care from health professionals whose capacity to understand their needs, and how to best respond to them, is limited. This chapter seeks to inform health care professionals about the intersection of health and disability so that they can better work with people with a disability no matter the health context. Firstly, the chapter defines disability and offers content to broaden insights into the lives of people with a disability. Next, the chapter unpacks a range of key considerations that all health professionals should be aware of. The critical intersection of health and disability is then explored in detail. Finally, the roles of nurses, regardless of context, in the lives of people with a disability are described and discussed.

Defining and understanding disability

Disability is a multifaceted concept with different definitions based on context and perspective. Disability is a condition affecting the mind or body that causes functional limitations on a person to perform certain activities, challenges to interact with other people or access certain services and opportunities.

REFLECTION

Consider your own personal understanding of what disability is and what it means for an individual with a disability.

1. Would having a disability differ depending on whether the person lived in a developed country or a developing country? If so, in what ways would it differ and why?
2. Think about any people you know who have a disability and reflect on how it affects their participation in society, if at all? If it does not affect some aspect of their participation, consider why this might be.

Defining disability

There are several well-established definitions of disability, however for the purposes of health care workers, a functional model of disability and health is often most useful to know about and understand. The *International Classification of Functioning, Disability and Health* (ICF) (World Health Organization (WHO), 2001) is a functional model that defines disability as impairments in body structures or functions, limitations in activities and restrictions in participation in various domains of life. The *United Nations Convention on the Rights of Persons with Disabilities* (United Nations (UN), 2006) is an international convention that all health workers should be aware of, and this defines persons with disabilities as 'those who have long-term physical, mental, intellectual, or sensory impairments which, in interaction with various barriers, may hinder their full and effective participation in society on an equal basis with others'. In the Australian context, a useful definition of disability is provided by the *Disability Discrimination Act 1992* (Australian Government, 1992), which defines a person with a disability as someone who has a physical, intellectual, sensory, neurological or psychiatric impairment that has lasted for a continuous period of at least six months or is likely to stay for a continuous period of at least six months or is permanent. In the context of Aotearoa New Zealand, the Public Health and Disability Act 2000 (New Zealand Legislation, 2000) defines disability as: 'A significant limitation in a person's ability to carry out day-to-day activities, lasting or expected to last for six months or more, and which is likely to continue indefinitely. This includes physical, sensory, psychiatric, intellectual, and neurological impairments.'

Types of disabilities

Although there are some arguments against categorising disability types, appreciating the different types of disabilities is important for the purposes of health and other service provision, as well as for funding for disability-related supports. Disability can be visible or non-visible, with a higher prevalence of non-visible disability in Australia. Some examples of invisible disabilities can include learning disabilities or hearing impairments.

Physical disability

Physical disability refers to impairments that affect a person's mobility, coordination or functioning. It involves long-term or permanent loss of part of the body's physical function. It includes conditions such as paralysis, amputation, muscular dystrophy and chronic illnesses that limit physical abilities. Assistive devices and accommodations, such as wheelchairs or prosthetic limbs, are often used to mitigate the impact of physical disabilities (AIHW, 2022).

Intellectual disability

Intellectual disability encompasses limitations in intellectual functioning and adaptive behaviour. Individuals with intellectual disability may struggle with learning, problem solving, communication and social skills. This can include conditions such as, but is not limited to, intellectual developmental disorder, Down syndrome, autism spectrum disorder and specific learning disabilities (American Association on Intellectual and Developmental Disabilities (AAIDD), 2020).

Sensory disability

Sensory disability includes impairments that affect a person's senses, such as vision or hearing. Visual impairments include blindness, low vision or conditions like macular degeneration or cataracts. Hearing impairments encompass varying degrees of hearing loss, including deafness. Assistive technologies like hearing aids or Braille systems can support individuals with sensory disabilities (Abdullah et al., 2021).

Psychiatric disabilities

Psychiatric disabilities refer to impairments related to mental health conditions, such as depression, anxiety disorders, bipolar disorder, schizophrenia and other psychosocial disabilities (AIHW, 2022).

Neurological disabilities

Neurological disabilities encompass impairments of the nervous system, including conditions like multiple sclerosis, epilepsy, cerebral palsy and acquired brain injury (National Disability Services, 2023).

Language and historical terms

Society's understanding and attitudes towards disability have evolved, leading to the recognition of the importance of inclusion, accessibility and equal rights for individuals with disabilities. It is essential, therefore, to be mindful of historical terms and language that are now considered offensive and outdated. Words such as 'cripple', 'handicapped' or 'mentally retarded' were once commonly used but are now considered derogatory and stigmatising, and have been replaced by more appropriate and less offensive terminologies such as intellectual developmental disorder (Cluley, 2018). To foster inclusivity and respect, it is recommended to use person-first language, which highlights the person rather than their disability. For instance, instead of 'a disabled person', it is usually considered more appropriate to say, 'a person with a disability'. That being said, there are some people who prefer identify-first language (e.g. autistic youth, deaf people) and so it is imperative that nurses seek to understand these differences and refer to individuals in the manner that they request.

Lifelong and acquired disability: understanding the differences

Lifelong disabilities are present from birth or early in life and persist throughout an individual's lifetime. These disabilities are typically of a congenital or developmental nature, resulting from genetic conditions, prenatal factors or early childhood injuries or illnesses. Lifelong disabilities can manifest in various ways and impact individuals differently. Examples of lifelong disabilities include Down syndrome, cerebral palsy, intellectual disability and spina bifida. Lifelong disabilities can impact an individual's physical, cognitive, communication and social abilities. They may require ongoing support, therapies, rehabilitation, habilitation and accommodation to promote optimal functioning and inclusion. Education, employment and independent living can be areas where lifelong disabilities may present unique challenges that require targeted support (National Disability Services, 2023).

Acquired disabilities develop or are acquired later in life, usually due to an injury, illness or other factors. They can occur suddenly or gradually and significantly impact an individual's functioning and quality of life (Lourida et al., 2022). Examples of acquired disabilities include spinal cord injury, traumatic brain injury, debilitating chronic illnesses, stroke and conditions like multiple sclerosis or amyotrophic lateral sclerosis (ALS) that worsen over time, leading to increasing disability and functional limitations. Acquired disabilities often require adjustments and adaptations to the individual's lifestyle, environment and daily routines. Rehabilitation, medical interventions, assistive technologies and psychological support are crucial in helping individuals with acquired disabilities regain or adapt to their abilities and enhance their overall well-being (Borg et al., 2023; Lourida, 2022).

Rehabilitation and habilitation

Rehabilitation and habilitation are essential, but uniquely different, components of health care that aim to support individuals with disabilities in maximising their functioning, independence and quality of life (Arslanov et al., 2020). Nurses play a crucial role in these processes, employing various approaches and utilising biopsychosocial models to address the multifaceted needs of individuals with disabilities (Olli, Vehkakoski, T. & Salanterä, 2014). Rehabilitation focuses on restoring or enhancing an individual's physical, cognitive and psychosocial functioning after an injury, illness or acquired disability. Nurses in rehabilitation settings employ a holistic approach, integrating medical, psychological and social interventions to promote recovery and functional improvement. On the other hand, habilitation focuses on developing specific new skills, abilities and adaptive strategies in individuals with lifelong disabilities or developmental conditions. It aims to enhance functioning, promote independence and optimise participation in daily activities and social interactions (Arslanov et al., 2020). For example, early childhood therapy to support walking and talking at a developmentally appropriate time is an example of habilitation. Conversely, learning to talk and walk again after a stroke is an example of rehabilitation.

The biopsychosocial model recognises that biological, psychological and social factors influence disability. Focusing on rehabilitation, rehabilitation nurses utilise this model by addressing individual rehabilitation needs through person-centred therapies, medications and adaptive devices, while also considering psychological factors such as mental health, coping strategies and adjustment to disability. Additionally, social aspects are addressed through support systems, community integration and vocational rehabilitation to facilitate successful reintegration into society. This approach involves collaborative care, addressing the individual's goals, providing therapeutic interventions and family support and connecting individuals with appropriate community resources (Olli et al., 2014). Importantly, rehabilitation and habilitation require a multidisciplinary team approach, with nurses collaborating closely with physicians, therapists, psychologists, social workers and other health care professionals. They critically assess functional abilities, implement interventions, educate patients and their families, monitor progress and coordinate care across different settings (Gutenbrunner et al., 2021).

Diverse nursing roles in primary care contexts

In the Australian and Aotearoa New Zealand contexts, nurses play a significant role in providing primary care and support for people with disabilities. By employing a holistic approach and collaborating with interdisciplinary teams, nurses contribute significantly to the well-being and functional outcomes of individuals with disabilities. Nurses in Australia work across various health care settings, including hospitals, community health centres, disability-specific services and home care. It is important to note that the specific roles and responsibilities of nurses may vary depending on their level of training, specialisation and the health care setting in which they work. Their role encompasses various responsibilities and interventions to address the unique needs of individuals with disabilities, some of which are now described.

Comprehensive assessment and monitoring

Comprehensive assessment and monitoring include gathering information about the individual's health history, functional abilities, support systems and specific challenges related to their disability. This assessment helps in developing personalised care plans and identifying appropriate interventions. They also provide ongoing health surveillance, identify potential health issues or complications, track progress and provide preventive care (Wilson et al., 2020).

Intersectoral collaboration and case management

Nurses often serve as care coordinators, working collaboratively with other health care professionals, support services and community organisations to ensure coordinated and holistic care. They facilitate referrals, schedule appointments and advocate for the individual's needs across various health care settings and community resources (Khanlou et al., 2023; Swanson et al., 2020.; Wilson et al., 2020).

Rehabilitation and supportive interventions

Nurses contribute to the rehabilitation and supportive interventions for individuals with disabilities. They collaborate with rehabilitation professionals, such as physiotherapists, occupational therapists and speech-language therapists, to facilitate the individual's rehabilitation goals. Nurses provide support and guidance for activities of daily living, mobility and assistive device management (Khanlou et al., 2023).

Health promotion and education

Health promotion and education can include offering guidance on preventive care, healthy lifestyle choices and disease management strategies. Nurses empower individuals with disabilities and their families to participate in their health care and make informed decisions actively (Wilson et al., 2020).

Capacity building support

Capacity building involves strengthening individuals, organisations and communities, by building knowledge, skills, resources and infrastructure to improve their effectiveness and sustainability. Nurses play a significant role in training and supervising a delegated disability support worker to respond efficiently to the complex care needs of people with disabilities (Wilson et al., 2020).

Advocacy and support

Nurses have a clear and strong **advocacy** role. They support individuals and their families in navigating health care systems, accessing appropriate services and addressing barriers to care. Nurses act as a voice for individuals with disabilities, promoting their autonomy and ensuring that their preferences and choices are respected (Wilson et al., 2020).

Advocacy –when a nurse speaks on behalf of, or in support of, someone who is unable to speak on their own behalf.

Emotional support

Nurses provide emotional support and counselling to individuals with disabilities and their families, acknowledging the psychosocial impact of disability. They assist in addressing emotional challenges, facilitating coping mechanisms and promoting mental health and well-being, as well as liaising with the GP to ensure appropriate referrals are made.

Key considerations about disability

There are many personalised and community-wide considerations when working with people with a disability, all of which are not possible to cover concisely in a short book chapter. Therefore, this section focuses on four key considerations that are arguably more common, with nurses and other health professionals more likely to encounter these issues during their day-to-day practice.

Cultural differences and disability

It is important that health and social care services are culturally informed. In the Australian and Aotearoa New Zealand context, this includes, but is not limited to, indigenous perspectives and the range of diverse issues relevant to providing culturally competent care to immigrants from different parts of the world. Importantly, different cultures will understand and respond to disability in different ways. Crucially, nurses need to be abreast of these nuances and always seek to offer culturally appropriate care and support, yet many services in Australia are not as culturally competent as they should be (King et al., 2016). Recent Australian research points to the vital role that refugee health services offer refugee families who have a family member with a disability, in particular by navigating families to access a range of disability-specific services and supports (Dew et al., 2023).

CASE STUDY 4.1

Abdul is a six-year-old boy who was a refugee with his family from Iraq. The family does not speak English well, and Abdul knows only a few English words such as 'no', 'drink' and 'car'. Abdul's father takes him to the GP practice, where you work as a practice nurse, without an appointment. Abdul has some bruising and swelling to his wrist that Abdul's father states was from a behavioural outburst where Abdul was hitting the walls and furniture. As the practice nurse, you need to assess Abdul before he sees the GP.

REFLECTION
1. What is the range of cultural-specific issues that you will need to consider?
2. What information do you need to gather and who are you going to get this from?
3. Irrespective of the extent of the injury, what types of services would you consider referring Abdul and his family to?

Gender and disability

Disability, whether lifelong or acquired, disproportionately affects more males than females. For instance, approximately 60 per cent of all people with intellectual disability are male, there is twice the prevalence of boys with developmental disabilities, and even more so with autism (Wilson, Smidt & Tehan, 2018a). Males are more likely to experience spinal cord (Harrison,

O'Brien & Pointer, 2021) and brain injuries (AIHW, 2007). Although drawing attention to these gendered differences is important, this does not mean that women and girls with disabilities don't have unique gendered issues that must be considered. For instance, women and girls with disabilities experience greater violence than women without disabilities (Dowse et al., 2013) and in addition, they encounter access and other barriers to mainstream health and social services (Dyson, Frawley & Robinson, 2017). It should also be noted that women and men with disabilities are less likely to be aware of and to access gender-specific health prevention services, such as breast and cervical screening for females, and prostate and testicular screening for males. Of note is that research points to a higher prevalence of testicular cancer and hypogonadism in males with intellectual disability, and they often present with noticeable symptoms much later in relation to communication and health literacy difficulties (Wilson et al., 2018b). In their parallel randomised trial, Wilson and colleagues demonstrated that direct teaching about or the provision of an accessible leaflet about conducting routine testicular self-examination was effective in increasing knowledge about this practice in a group of young males with mild degrees of intellectual disability. This shows that by giving the right amount of information, at the right time and with the right approach, people with intellectual disability can learn about their health with primary health nurses uniquely positioned to lead such health promotion activities.

CASE STUDY 4.2

Sarah, a 19-year-old woman with mild intellectual disability, lives in a flat with drop-in support from support workers and has recently started a sexual relationship with a colleague in her vocational education class. Sarah has many fears about pregnancy and sexually transmitted infections (STIs), some of which she learnt at a sex education class and others she heard about from friends while she was at school. Sarah's support worker learns about the new relationship and Sarah tells the support worker that she has had sexual intercourse several times. Sarah's support worker is very concerned for Sarah as she has an intellectual disability and often needs help with decision-making. Sarah's support worker has booked an appointment for Sarah at the GP practice, and you are the practice nurse who conducts initial assessments and conducts some health education activities.

REFLECTION

1. What are the most important ethical issues that you will need to consider when assessing Sarah?
2. How will you determine if Sarah is making informed decisions about this new relationship?
3. What types of health education would you support Sarah to engage with and how would you follow this up over time?

Aging and disability

Not only is the overall population aging, but so is the population of people with disabilities, meaning that there will be more aging-related and disability-specific issues emerging in the years ahead. Often-forced retirement of aging people with a disability from employment (Brotherton et al., 2020) is one issue that has started to receive some attention and has had a particular impact on paid and family caregivers Usually from health-related issues, forced retirement means that the primary care nurse has a role to play in supporting the individual's changing health needs, particularly when the caregiver's capacity to provide support is strained. More research will be needed in the years ahead as more people with a disability experience age-related health problems and face changes to their support networks.

The increased incidence of dementia, particularly for people with Down syndrome who are genetically predisposed to early onset Alzheimer's disease (McGlinchey et al., 2019), is an added challenge facing many older people with intellectual disability and it has received a greater amount of research and practice attention People with Down syndrome who are over 40 years of age will have the neuropathology of Alzheimer's disease, most likely as the 21st chromosome, which is over-expressed in people with Down syndrome, also hosts the amyloid precursor protein. Once diagnosed, individualised support is required to help primary care nurses work more effectively with the individual, the family and any caregivers.

Dodd and colleagues (2018) led the development of a person-centred dementia model that is based around regular reviews and paying attention to the needs of caregivers. These components include:

- post-diagnostic counselling, support and education to the person and their caregivers
- routine surveillance of psychological and medical status
- regular care plan reviews that take account of changes and the pace of change
- early identification of psychological and behavioural changes
- once the person is nearing end-of-life, care practices and supports are reviewed and modified as needed
- advice and support are offered to caregivers at every stage
- all decisions are based on the person's quality of life.

Crucially, these issues are heavily intersected in the context of primary health with primary health nurses being key players in the pursuit of good outcomes that are based on individual quality of life.

CASE STUDY 4.3

John is a 38-year-old man with Down syndrome who lives with his aging parents in a suburb of a large city. John works part-time at a sheltered workshop where he performs a range of manual labour tasks. Staff at the sheltered workshop have reported that John is falling asleep at work in the mid-afternoon and have noted that his productivity seems to be less than it has been. John's parents have also noticed that John has fallen a few times at home, in particular, in doorways where carpeted areas change to tiled areas of the house. You are a community nurse and have received a referral to your service for a review of changes to John's overall health and well-being as there is a concern that he may have some early symptoms of dementia.

REFLECTION

1. What types of assessments do you think you will conduct when visiting John and his parents?
2. What sorts of underlying health problems might you be looking for that could explain the changes that John is experiencing?
3. How would you involve John's family in your assessment?

Disability and health

The research literature is unequivocal that people with a disability experience greater morbidity and earlier mortality when compared to people without a disability. There are also subgroups who have far worse outcomes and experiences, such as people with intellectual disabilities and Aboriginal and Torres Strait Islander peoples with a disability. Health disparities include being more at risk of under or overweight (Slevin & Northway, 2014), poorer oral health status and outcomes (Wilson et al., 2019) and higher rates of diabetes (Flygare Wallén et al., 2018). Crucially, recent Australian research identified that people with intellectual disability are also more likely to die from potentially avoidable causes (Trollor et al., 2017).

A functional model of disability and health: the ICF

The ICF (WHO, 2001) offers the most useful and non-ideological model to understand the intersection of disability and health. Consisting of a diagrammatic framework that illustrates the relationships between each domain, the ICF not only notes the impairments and health conditions of the individual, but also the context and environment within which the person lives and the association with activity and participation. The ICF fits perfectly with nurses' biopsychosocial world view and offers them a logical and meaningful way to conceptualise not only the person's disability, as noted by their level of function, but also the intersection of this with every facet of their life, such as family life, work, socialising with friends and participating in society.

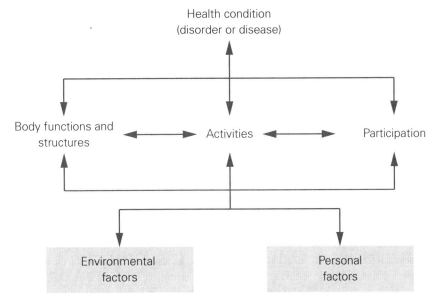

Figure 4.1   The ICF
Source: Reproduced from WHO (2001).

The main causes of intellectual disability

Approximately 2 per cent of the population has intellectual disability (Department of Health, 2021). Intellectual disability often has an unclear cause. However, advances in genetic and other screening processes mean that more is being uncovered every year. Common causes that would be well-known to most nurses include Down syndrome, Fragile X syndrome, Williams syndrome and Rett syndrome. These are all examples of chromosomal disorders, with Rett syndrome being more common in girls and Fragile X syndrome more common in boys (Hellings, Butler & Grant, 2010). Cerebral palsy is another common cause, however, it is not attributed to chromosomal disorders but rather often caused by brain injury before or during the time of birth (Wilson-Jones & Morgan, 2010). Less common causes include metabolic disorders such as phenylketonuria and infections during pregnancy such as toxoplasmosis and cytomegalovirus. Less common nowadays is intellectual disability caused by lead and mercury exposure. Accidents such as drowning and poisoning can also cause intellectual disability.

Common health problems in people with intellectual disability

Overall, people with intellectual disability not only have more health problems than the general population, but they also encounter disparities in the level of health care they receive and they have greater rates of premature death (Davis et al., 2014). In addition, it is probable that the range of health problems is under-reported as many health and research studies either exclude people with intellectual disability or rely on data from other people. Nurses working in primary care have a unique role to play as they are able to conduct health assessments and screening that could uncover some health problems that the person may be unaware that they have. Some of the reasons for such health disparities are specific to the underlying syndrome or condition of the person and have a genetic cause. For example, people with Down syndrome have greater rates of cardiac problems, endocrine disorders, and are prone to obesity and have low muscle tone (Hellings et al., 2010). Dysphagia and epilepsy are common conditions in people with Angelman or velocardiofacial syndrome and ataxia is very common in people with Rett syndrome. For people with cerebral palsy, in addition to having physical disabilities that can affect all or only some parts of the body's movement, common health problems include scoliosis, underweight, epilepsy, dysphagia and vision or hearing problems (Wilson-Jones & Morgan, 2010). Primary care nurses need to not only be aware of these unique and diagnosis-specific risks, but also the disadvantaged context of their lives where they have fewer choices and little control over their health care (Wullink, et al., 2009).

Nursing and people with a disability: a diverse nursing role

The National Disability Insurance Scheme (NDIS) (Australia) and Enabling Good Lives (EGL) (Aotearoa New Zealand)

The intention of each disability care and support system is to enable the disabled person and their networks access to funding more directly, and to have greater choice, control and flexibility about using these funds. The Australian NDIS funds a range of disability-related supports, for example, equipment, environmental and vehicle modifications, respite care, transportation to promote participation, access to therapies, assistance with household tasks and personal care, and employment support. A key factor is the determination of supports that are 'reasonable and necessary', which will impact upon the scope, level of care and support available, as well as the roles and responsibilities of individuals and families therein regarding 'maintaining co-ordination of care, or for making up the shortfall in care' (Foster et al., 2016, p. 38). This can be additionally challenging for people who have a psychosocial disability as it may be episodic in nature and impedes a person with symptoms of mental illness from connecting and consistently engaging with the mechanisms designed to support the impact of the 'disability and recovery disconnect' (Mellifont et al., 2022). Likewise, for people with a cognitive impairment, such as intellectual disability, navigating the NDIS and managing one's own care coordination can be a challenge. Notwithstanding, NDIS has been shown to provide greater choice and control for many people with a disability (Goode et al., 2018).

Similarly, EGL in Aotearoa New Zealand is starting to have a positive impact for people with lived experience of disability. Of note, it was not designed simply as a funding pathway for disability support as it can also capture a range of supports through education, health and disability funding to enable the disabled person to have 'control over how they use their personal budget to help them achieve their goals and aspirations as part of having a good everyday life' (Enabling Good Lives, 2014, p. 2). Philosophically, however, there are eight principles that all health and disability service providers have a responsibility to embed and promote in the way that they support the everyday lives of people with a disability:

1. Self-determination
2. Beginning early
3. Person-centred
4. Achieving ordinary life outcomes
5. Mainstream first
6. Mana enhancing (i.e. recognising inherent knowledge)
7. Easy to use
8. Relationship building.

The existing system of needs assessment and service coordination continues to be in place to work alongside people and their networks of support who may have higher and more complex needs and/or may be less able to manage the practicalities of sourcing services, staff and budgets (www.enablinggoodlives.co.nz/about-egl/egl-approach/principles).

Person-centred care

A key question to ask people with disabilities and/or their caregivers, is 'What matters to you?' or explore what is of value and important to them rather than what might be impaired for the person (Kebede, 2016). This opens up an entirely different approach to health care delivery that is not driven by the health professional; instead, it is about partnering with people about their own health and well-being, thereby informing self-management (Whitehead, 2016). Despite some key differences, the NDIS and EGL approaches both reflect fundamental considerations in working with people regardless of their condition, contingencies or context. Person-centred care is integral, imperative and intrinsic to the role of any health and disability support professional. Many health professionals would argue that this is the basis of their practice, yet the essence of partnership and joint decision-making can easily go astray, meaning that person-centred care should be embedded across all levels of an organisation for it to be truly genuine and effective (Moody et al., 2018). Santana and colleagues' (2018) conceptual framework for person-centred care reflects this and is a timely reminder that the values of person-centred care extend not only to the disabled person, but also to those in their network of support. Collaborative, or relational-centred care, is also an important consideration and tensions exist about what this looks like in practice. It should include not only the person with the lived experience and their significant others, but also a reciprocal interrelationship between health professionals and agencies involved to support, inform and enable accessible care coordination and delivery (Hebblethwaite, 2013).

Negotiated autonomy is essential in order to optimise inclusion for people with a disability in making choices and having control in and about their own lives (Whitehead et al., 2016). Therefore, as health professionals, the paradigm shift posited by the *United Nations Convention on the Rights of Persons with Disabilities* (UN, 2006) to move from a 'best interests' and 'substituted judgement' approach to one of 'will and preference' underpins supported decision making (Article 12). This is a mechanism by which self-determination, autonomy, choice and control intersect and can be implemented and actualised (Mirfin-Veitch, 2016).

Practical communication tools, tips and reasonable adjustments

People with a disability experience both greater health needs and barriers to health care than the general population. These include transportation challenges, waiting lists, financial implications for consultation and/or medication (Sakellariou & Rotarou, 2017). However, there has been a renewed focus in recognising the role of all registered and unregistered health professionals alongside disabled people across primary and community health care contexts. For instance, the *Equality Act 2010* in the United Kingdom expects that public services make anticipatory 'reasonable adjustments' which may include 'changing a policy practice of procedure... physical feature... [or] providing additional aids or services' to assist with access and communication (Heslop et al., 2019). Heslop and colleagues (2019) further advise that:

> Nurses have a significant role in identifying disabled people and their specific needs for reasonable adjustments, through holistic, person-centred assessments involving discussion with the person and/or their carers, through any records in the patient's notes or referral letters, via any existing computerised flagging system, or through new patient registration forms. As part of a humanistic approach to nursing care, disabled people must have their need for reasonable adjustments clearly recorded in their nursing and medical records, along with a summary of the required adjustments to their care, which is available to all relevant health and social care providers.

Other examples of reasonable adjustments include the provision of more appropriate time frames for appointments (e.g. less waiting and longer appointments), disability awareness education for all professionals, and environments that are disability sensitive and promote supported decision-making (Doherty et al., 2020). Alongside personalised reasonable adjustments, there are communication tools that people with disabilities can use to promote inclusion and equitable access to health care and enable them to participate in their communities. These include:

- health passports
- easy-to-read materials that are appropriate for the local context
- resources such as Beyond Words: https://booksbeyondwords.co.uk/
- tips for better communication, such as these listed in Fisher et al., 2022: https://ojin.nursingworld.org/table-of-contents/volume-27-2022/number-3-september-2022/international-nursing-actions-to-reduce-health-inequities/
- communication passports that incorporate sounds, gestures, signs and assistive technologies that are specific to the person (Burke et al., 2023).

Contemporary nursing roles supporting people with a disability

Recent research has started to map the outcomes of nursing-led models of care and support in primary health contexts, which show that nursing interventions can and do avoid acute exacerbations of chronic illnesses that can otherwise lead to admission to an acute hospital setting (Wilson et al., 2021). While this research is based on nursing roles within disability services, many nurses work outside these contexts. NDIS, which commenced about 10 years ago, has created many opportunities for nurses working in primary care to expand into disability-specialised roles, many of which are created by nurses setting up their own private practice. Triggers for these opportunities have partly come from funding categories within the scheme, but others from unmet needs. For instance, the funding around continence support has enabled many specialised continence nurses to expand into disability-specific roles. Other condition-specific roles have also emerged, such as epilepsy and diabetes nurse specialists who can write plans of care and provide training to the disability workforce. Nurses with expertise in behaviour support and counselling are also operating within the NDIS landscape providing behaviour support plans and therapeutic services. One funding area that is yet to be fully engaged with is for nurse practitioners, as there are very few who are working in the disability sector. This has the potential to be a huge growth area and nurses wishing to expand into fully autonomous roles specialising in disability care and support have several pathways to choose from.

Conclusion

This chapter has taken a deliberately pragmatic and applied approach to describing and discussing the key issues facing people with a disability with respect to their health and well-being. Crucially, a number of health disparities have been articulated that all nurses need to be aware of, including disparities at the individual and system levels. Nurses working in primary care contexts have a vital role to play in improving the health outcomes of and access to health services for people with a disability. Consider that a challenge has been set for all nurses, to increase their capacity to work with people with a disability and champion strategies in their workplace to effect positive change. That many people with a disability are dying unavoidably and that these issues have been explored in depth at the recent Royal Commission should alert all nurses to the challenges ahead and their role in countering these problems.

CRITICAL THINKING ACTIVITIES

1. Consider your context of nursing practice. What types of reasonable adjustments might you be able to make at a systems and/or policy level that will increase the accessibility of your service to people with a disability? What is needed to get these adjustments in place and sustainable?
2. You are working as a community nurse and have been given the task of being a disability nurse champion for your team. Where would you start to increase your capacity, and that of your colleagues, to work more effectively with people with a disability? What areas need addressing the most? What would you tackle first?
3. After reading this chapter, have your views on the health needs of people with a disability changed? Why or why not?

FURTHER READING

Department of Social Services. (2021). *Australia's Disability Strategy 2021–2031*. Australian Government. www.disabilitygateway.gov.au/document/3106

Royal Commission into Violence, Abuse, Neglect and Exploitation of People with Disability. (2022). *Public Hearing Report. Public Hearing 10: Education and training of health professionals in relation to people with cognitive disability.* https://disability.royalcommission.gov.au/public-hearings/public-hearing-10

Wilson, N.J., Howie, V. & Tomsic, G. (2020). Nursing and people with intellectual disability. In N.J. Wilson, P. Lewis, L. Hunt & L. Whitehead (eds), *Nursing in Australia Contemporary Professional and Practice Insights*. Routledge.

World Health Organization (WHO). (2011). *The World Report on Disability 2011*. www.who.int/teams/noncommunicable-diseases/sensory-functions-disability-and-rehabilitation/world-report-on-disability

REFERENCES

Abdullah, N., Low, K.E.Y. & Feng, Q. (2021). Sensory disability. In D. Gu & M.E. Dupre (eds), *Encyclopedia of Gerontology and Population Aging*. Springer. https://doi.org/10.1007/978-3-030-22009-9_480

American Association on Intellectual and Developmental Disabilities (AAIDD). (2020). *Intellectual Disability: Definition, Classification, and Systems of Supports* (11th ed.). AAIDD.

Arslanov, K.M., Varlamova, A.N., Khabirov, A.I. & Khamitova, G.M. (2020). On the procedure for the rehabilitation and habilitation of persons with disabilities. *Archivos Venezolanos De Farmacologia y Terapéutica, 39*(7), 813–16. https://doi.org/10.5281/zenodo.4421990

Australian Government. (1992). *Disability Discrimination Act 1992*. Australian Government. www.legislation.gov.au/Details/C2018C00125

Australian Institute of Health and Welfare (AIHW). (2007). *Disability in Australia: Acquired Brain Injury.* (Bulletin no. 55. Cat no. AUS 96.) Australian Government. www.aihw.gov.au/reports/disability-services/disability-australia-acquired-brain-injury/summary

—— (2022). *People with Disability in Australia*. Australian Government. www.aihw.gov.au/reports/disability/people-with-disability-in-australia/contents/people-with-disability/prevalence-of-disability

Borg, S.J., Borg, D.N., Foster, M.M., et al. (2023). Use and cost of Medicare Benefits Schedule and Pharmaceutical Benefits Scheme services following inpatient rehabilitation for acquired disability in Australia. *Australian Health Review, 47*(2), 165–74. https://doi.org/10.1071/AH22118

Brotherton, M. Stancliffe, R.J., Wilson, N.J. & O'Loughlin, K. (2020). Australians with intellectual disability share their experiences of retirement from mainstream employment. *Journal of Applied Research in Intellectual Disabilities, 33*(5), 905–16. https://doi.org/10.1111/jar.12712

Burke, É.A., Fleming, S., Doyle, C., et al. (2023). Using verbal and non-verbal communication to support people with learning disabilities. *Learning Disability Practice, 26*(3).

Cluley, V. (2018). From "Learning disability to intellectual disability" – Perceptions of the increasing use of "intellectual disability" in learning disability policy, research and practice. *British Journal of Learning Disabilities, 46*(1), 24–32. https://doi.org/10.1111/bld.12209

Davis, R., Proulx, R. & van Schrojenstein Lantman-de Valk, H. (2014). Health issues for people with intellectual disabilities: the evidence base. In L. Taggart & W. Cousins (eds), *Health Promotion for People with Intellectual and Developmental Disabilities.* McGraw Hill Education.

Department of Health. (2021). *National Roadmap for Improving the Health of People with Intellectual Disability.* Commonwealth of Australia. www.health.gov.au/sites/default/files/documents/2021/08/national-roadmap-for-improving-the-health-of-people-with-intellectual-disability.pdf

Dew, A., Lenette, C., Wells, R., et al. (2023). 'In the beginning it was difficult, but things got easier': Service use experiences of family members of people with disability from Iraqi and Syrian refugee backgrounds. *Journal of Policy and Practice in Intellectual Disabilities, 20*(1), 33–44. https://doi.org/10.1111/jppi.12424

Dodd, K., Watchman, K., Janicki, et al. (2018). Consensus statement of the International Summit on Intellectual Disability and Dementia related to post-diagnostic support. *Aging and Mental Health, 22*(11), 1406–15. https://doi.org/10.1080/13607863.2017.1373065

Doherty, A.J., Atherton, H., Boland, P., et al. (2020). Barriers and facilitators to primary health care for people with intellectual disabilities and/or autism: An integrative review. *BJGP Open, 4*(3), 1–10. https://doi.org/10.3399/bjgpopen20X101030

Dowse, L., Soldatic, K., Didi, A., Frohmader, C. & van Toorn, G. (2013). *Stop the violence: Addressing violence against women and girls with disabilities in Australia* Background Paper. Women With Disabilities Australia. http://wwda.org.au/wp-content/uploads/2013/12/STV_Background_Paper_FINAL.pdf

Dyson S., Frawley P. & Robinson S. (2017). *"Whatever t Talkes": Access for Women with Disabilities to Family/Domestic Violence Services: Final report. Horizons Research Report.* Australia's National Research Organisation for Women's Safety. https://d2rn9gno7zhxqg.cloudfront.net/wp-content/uploads/2019/02/19024645/Disability_Horizons_FINAL-1.pdf

Enabling Good Lives (EGL). (2014). *Enabling Good Lives Newsletter* (Issue 4, February/March). www.enablinggoodlives.co.nz/assets/ResourceSnippets/4-EGL-Newsletter-Feb-Mar14.pdf

Fisher, K., Desroches, M.L., Marsden, D., et al. (2022). International nursing actions to reduce health inequities faced by people with intellectual and developmental disability. *The Online Journal of Issues in Nursing, 27*(3). https://ojin.nursingworld.org/table-of-contents/volume-27-2022/number-3-september-2022/international-nursing-actions-to-reduce-health-inequities/

Flygare Wallén, E., Ljunggren, G., Carlsson, A.C., et al. (2018). High prevalence of diabetes mellitus, hypertension and obesity among persons with a recorded diagnosis of intellectual disability or autism spectrum disorder. *Journal of Intellectual Disabilities Research, 62*(4), 269–80.

Foster, M., Henman, P., Tilse, C., et al. (2016). 'Reasonable and necessary' care: The challenge of operationalising the NDIS policy principle in allocating disability care in Australia. *Australian Journal of Social Issues, 51*(1), 27–46.

Goode, A., Walton, H., Smith, L., Wei, Z. & Flavel, J. (2018). *Evaluation of the NDIS: Final report.* https://apo.org.au/sites/default/files/resource-files/2018-04/apo-nid143516_1.pdf

Gutenbrunner, C., Stievano, A., Stewart, D., Catton, H. & Nugraha, B. (2021). Role of nursing in rehabilitation. *Journal of Rehabilitation Medicine, Clinical Communications, 4*, 1000061. https://doi.org/10.2340/20030711-1000061

Harrison, J., O'Brien, D. & Pointer, S. (2021). *Spinal Cord Injury, Australia, 2017–18.* (Injury research and statistics series no. 136. Cat. no. INJCAT 219.) AIHW. www.aihw.gov.au/getmedia/5b4a8579-a010-40f0-9ad6-31522a4fcc12/aihw-injcat-219.pdf.aspx?inline=true

Hebblethwaite, S. (2013). "I think it could work but...": Tensions between the theory and practice of person-centred and relationship-centred care. *Therapeutic Recreation Journal, XLVII*(1), 13–34.

Hellings, J.A., Butler, M.G. & Grant, J.A. (2010). Congenital causes. In J. O'Hara, J. McCarthy & N. Bouras (eds), *Intellectual Disability and Ill Health: A Review of the Evidence.* Cambridge University Press.

Heslop, P., Turner, S., Read, S., et al. (2019). Implementing reasonable adjustments for disabled people in healthcare services. *Nursing Standard, 34*(8), 29–34. https://researchspace.bathspa.ac.uk/11520/7/11520.pdf

Kebede, S. (2016). Ask patients "What matters to you?" rather than "What's the matter?" *British Medical Journal, 354*, i4045. https://www.bmj.com/content/354/bmj.i4045

Khanlou, N., Khan, A., Kurtz Landy, C., et al. (2023). Nursing care for persons with developmental disabilities: Review of literature on barriers and facilitators faced by nurses to provide care. *Nursing Open, 10*(2): 404–23. https://doi.org/10.1002/nop2.1338

King, J.A., Edwards, N., Correa-Velez, I., Hair, S. & Fordyce, M. (2016). Disadvantage and disability: Experiences of people from refugee backgrounds with disability living in Australia. *Disability and the Global South, 3*(1), 844–5.

Lourida, I., Bennett, H.Q., Beyer, F., Kingston, A. & Jagger, C. (2022). The impact of long-term conditions on disability-free life expectancy: A systematic review. *PLOS Global Public Health, 2*(8), e0000745. https://doi.org/10.1371/journal.pgph.0000745

McGlinchey, E., Reilly, E., McCallion, P., et al. (2019). Dementia and intellectual disability: Prevalence, assessment and post-diagnostic support. In J.L. Matson (ed.), *Handbook of Intellectual Disabilities: Integrating Theory, Research and Practice* (pp. 965–86). Springer.

Mellifont, D., Hancock, N., Scanlan, J.W. & Hamilton, D. (2023). Barriers to applying to the NDIS for Australians with psychosocial disability: A scoping review. *Australian Journal of Social Issues, 58*, 262–78. https://doi.org/10.1002/ajs4.245

Mirfin-Veitch, B. (2016). *Exploring Article 12 of the United Nations Convention on the Rights of Persons with Disabilities: An Integrative Literature Review.* Donald Beasley Institute. www.odi.govt.nz/assets/Whats-happening-files/exploring-article-12-literature-review-october-2016.pdf

Moody, L., Nicholls, B., Shamji, H., et al. (2018). The person-centred care guideline: From principle to practice. *Journal of Patient Experience, 5*(4), 282–8. https://doi.org/10.1177/2374373518765792

National Disability Services. (2023). *Disability types and description.* www.nds.org.au/index.php/disability-types-and-description

New Zealand Legislation. (2000). *Public Health and Disability Act 2000.* New Zealand Government. www.legislation.govt.nz/act/public/2000/0091/latest/DLM80051.html

Olli, J., Vehkakoski, T. & Salanterä, S. (2014). The habilitation nursing of children with developmental disabilities: Beyond traditional nursing practices and principles? *International Journal of Qualitative Studies on Health and Well-being, 9*, 23106. https://doi.org/10.3402/qhw.v9.23106

Sakellariou, D. & Rotarou, E.S. (2017). Access to healthcare for men and women with disabilities in the UK: Secondary analysis of cross-sectional data. *BMJ Open, 7*(8), e016614.

Santana, M., Manalili, K., Jolley, R.J., et al. (2018). How to practice person-centred care: A conceptual framework. *Health Expectations, 21*, 429–40. https://doi.org/10.1111/hex.12640

Slevin, E. & Northway, R. (2014). Obesity. In L. Taggart, & W. Cousins (eds), *Health Promotion for People with Intellectual and Developmental Disabilities.* McGraw Hill Education.

Swanson, M., Wong, S.T., Martin-Misener, R. & Browne, A.J. (2020). The role of registered nurses in primary care and public health collaboration: A scoping review. *Nursing Open, 7*(4), 1197–207. https://doi.org/10.1002/nop2.496

Trollor, J.N., Srasuebkul, P., Xu, H. & Howlett, S. (2017). Cause of death and potentially avoidable deaths in Australian adults with intellectual disability using retrospective linked data. *BMJ Open, 7*(e013489). https://doi.org/10.1136/bmjopen-2016-013489

United Nations (UN). (2006). *United Nations Convention on the Rights of Persons with Disabilities.* www.un.org/disabilities/documents/convention/convention_accessible_pdf.pdf

Whitehead, L. (2016). The effects of personalized care planning for adults living with chronic conditions. *International Journal of Nursing Practice, 22*(2), 138–40. https://doi.org/10.1111/ijn.12429

Whitehead, L.C., Trip, H.T., Hale, L.A. & Conder, J. (2016). Negotiating autonomy in diabetes self-management: The experiences of adults with intellectual disability and their support workers. *Journal of intellectual Disability Research, 60*(4), 389–97.

Wilson, J., Adeline, P., Bungaroo, D., et al. (2018b). Promoting testicular self-examination and awareness amongst young men with intellectual disabilities: A parallel intervention randomized study. *Journal on Developmental Disabilities, 23*(3), 57–70.

Wilson, N.J. Collison, J., Feighan, S.J., et al. (2020). A national survey of nurses who care for people with intellectual and developmental disability. *Australian Journal of Advanced Nursing, 37*(3), 4–12. https://doi.org/10.37464/2020.373.120

Wilson, N.J., Lin, Z., Villarosa, A. & George, A. (2019). Oral health status and reported oral health problems in people with intellectual disability: A literature review. *Journal of Intellectual and Developmental Disability, 44*(3), 292–304. https://doi.org/10.3109/13668250.2017.1409596

Wilson, N.J., Reeve, R., Lin, Z. & Lewis, P. (2021). The financial costs of registered nurse led relationship centred care: A single-case Australian feasibility study. *Disabilities, 1*, 331–46. https://doi.org/10.3390/disabilities1040023

Wilson, N.J., Smidt, A. & Tehan, M. (2018a). Health and social policies for Australian men and boys with intellectual and developmental disability: A health and wellbeing double jeopardy? *International Journal of Social and Community Men's Health, 1*(Special Issue 1), e6–e13.

Wilson-Jones, M. & Morgan, E. (2010). Cerebral palsy. In C.L. Betz & W.M. Nehring (eds), *Nursing Care for Individuals with Intellectual and Developmental Disabilities: An Integrated Approach.* Paul H Brookes Publishing Company.

World Health Organization (WHO). (2001). *International Classification of Functioning, Disability and Health.* https://apps.who.int/iris/bitstream/handle/10665/42407/9241545429.pdf?sequence=1

Wullink, M., Widdershoven, G., van Schrojenstein Lantman-de Valk, H., et al. (2009). Autonomy in relation to health among people with intellectual disability: A literature review. *Journal of Intellectual Disability Research, 53*(9), 816–26.

5

First Nations' health and well-being: culturally responsive practice in primary health care

Susan Mlcek, Jessica Biles and Rhonda Wilson
With acknowledgement to Kerry Taylor, Wayne Rigby,
Basseer Jeeawody and Maree Meredith

ACKNOWLEDGEMENTS OF COUNTRY

Susan: I am Māori from Aotearoa – a member of the Ngāiterangi Iwi – I acknowledge being part of the settler community here in Australia, where I am a 'guest' living and working on the First Nations lands of the Gundungurra and Dharug peoples in the Blue Mountains. I pay respect to all First Nations Elders for they are the custodians and care-takers of the knowledges of these unceded lands.

Jessica: I would like to acknowledge the Wiradjuri people, who are the traditional own-ers and custodians of the lands, skies and waters where I live and work. I would like to acknowledge the links that I have through marriage to the Murrawarri people and pay respect to Elders both past and present. I acknowledge these lands are unceded lands.

Rhonda: As a Wiradjuri descendent, I pay yindyamarra (respect) to Elders past, present and leaders emerging. Living on Darkinjung land, I extend respect to the Traditional Custodians of the land and language where I live and work. I pay respect to First Nation peoples and allies who are reading this book. As a matter of cultural obligation and urgency, I aim to con-tinuously produce culturally safe scientific evidence towards strengthening and improving the health and social and emotional well-being outcomes of First Nation peoples.

LEARNING OBJECTIVES

At the completion of this chapter, you should be able to:

- identify key historical influences on contemporary health and health outcomes for First Nations.
- explain the relevance and appropriateness of primary health care (PHC) and culturally responsive practice for First Nations' contexts.
- articulate the principles of cultural safety and culturally responsive practice.
- identify the main focus of the community nursing role when engaging in deliv-ery of PHC with First Nations communities in a health-promoting way.

Introduction

A note on terminology before proceeding: as readers navigate the appropriate use of terms, they will come across different ways that groups of people are referenced – Indigenous, Aboriginal, First Nations. In the Australian context, the term 'First Nations' is used to refer to Aboriginal and Torres Strait Islander peoples and, '... with due respect, these terms are used interchangeably and acknowledge the diversity of languages and cultures that characterise Australian indigeneity' (Rigby & Jeeawody, 2014, p. 283). In Aotearoa New Zealand, Māori are First Nations who can trace their ancestry and genealogy (*whakapapa*) right back to those who arrived from the Tahitian and Hawaiki regions in the early canoe fleet migrations of the mid-fourteenth century (Ministry for Culture and Heritage, 2005). From an international perspective, if the actual cultural or tribal names are not known, then individuals and communities can be referred to as being 'Indigenous'. However, there is a cautionary consideration to make; 'Indigenous' is seen by many to be a colonising Whiteness term that labels people in an inferior manner as the 'other'. This labelling contributes to the diminishment of cultural identity, and may create a deep sense of shame and blame for Indigenous peoples (Wingard, Johnson & Drahm-Butler, 2015) underpinned by an ongoing legacy of grief and loss. For this reason, the best option is always to ask the community – *what term or name is the most appropriate to use*?

This chapter introduces First Nations approaches to health care that have relevance for the Australian and Aotearoa New Zealand contexts. It examines the historical influences that impacted the health and well-being of First Nations in these countries and considers the need for adopting First Nations approaches to health care practice such as **cultural safety**, **cultural responsiveness** and other cultural frameworks. Several of the principles for practice are transferrable to international First Nations communities as well as culturally and linguistically diverse populations. Future thinking determines that knowledges and understandings in health needs to start with being responsive to the needs of First Nations. To this end, this chapter also examines the role of the community nurse in First Nations PHC.

A common question asked by students and even staff involved in nursing education is: 'Why do we need a separate topic/chapter/course on First Nations or Indigenous health?' While this should be self-evident considering a greater contemporary awareness of the impact of social determinants of health on Indigenous lives, it is not always clear. First Nations countries, such as Australia and Aotearoa New Zealand, although diverse in languages, cultures and histories, often share a common experience of being colonised that had a detrimental and ongoing impact on health and well-being. However, despite these common experiences, there is also a resilience and capacity among Indigenous peoples and First Nations groups that provides the community/PHC nurse, as well as health and well-being professionals, with an opportunity to effect real change towards better health outcomes. When considerations about the choice of inclusive practice are driven by culturally competent and systemically informed knowledge about the different *access* and *accessibility* situations for Indigenous peoples, then there is a better chance that all populations of minorities, intersectionalities and diversities will benefit. Keeping a focus on the user and service alignment (synthesis) is critical. Haggerty and colleagues (2014) suggest that the idea of 'access' relates to the capacity (knowing) and capability (choice) of Indigenous individuals and communities to obtain relevant health care services, while 'accessibility'

Cultural safety – a philosophy and practice that seeks to engage effectively with Indigenous peoples.

Cultural responsiveness – being knowledgeable and aware of the changing nature of behaviours and skills required to work with diverse communities, groups and individuals.

is best understood as the ability and responsiveness of the service provider or system to respond effectively to those needs and expectations. Furthermore, for any PHC organisation, contributing to cultural safety is the main part in a culturally responsive and wise practice framework (Muller, 2014).

Historical influences on contemporary health

According to Taylor and Guerin (2019), health professionals are required to take a client's history before they attempt to engage in any therapeutic relationship. In the First Nations health context, this history-taking necessitates knowing more than the immediate individual medical or health story.

Aotearoa New Zealand and Australia share histories of colonisation that are implicated in the contemporary health of each country's First Nations. Although these histories differ, the experience of colonisation itself has been clearly linked to health outcomes today. That is, social determinants of health can be identified and analysed against the reality of Indigenous situations whereby *accessibility* plays an important part. When considering PHC services, you need to ask yourself the following questions about their accessibility:

- Are services available? What is the location of these services? Where are these services placed in proximity to communities?
- Are services approachable? Even when located near communities, are they welcoming of Indigenous individuals? How can you tell?
- Are services acceptable? Are they inclusive of culturally autonomous decision–making (self-determination = own decision–making)?
- Are services appropriate? Do they fit the environmental and political situations of the time? For example, would responses to a pandemic situation embrace the complexities that make up an Indigenous community?
- Are services affordable? When so many Indigenous communities around the world experience ongoing poverty and the effects of global food price rises, how will the additional cost of accessing health care provision be provided against the cost of basic needs?

The social determinants of health can be seen in the shorter life expectancy (LE) of First Nations Australians with a gap of 8.6 years for First Nations males and 7.8 years for First Nations females (Australian Institute of Health and Welfare (AIHW), 2023). First Nations generally have higher infant mortality and other health indicators such as cardiovascular disease, diabetes and renal disease (AIHW, 2023).

In Aotearoa New Zealand and Australia, LE is often determined through looking at adult mortality. Phillips and colleagues (2017, p. 1) advise that, 'In Australia and NZ (New Zealand), First Nations LE and adult mortality are improving in absolute terms, but not relative to the entire or non-Indigenous populations, causing gaps in life expectancy to persist.' Furthermore, while LE is a common population health indicator, there are challenges around interpreting data.

Overall, evidence suggests that access to an integrated and comprehensive PHC system with a strong primary and preventative focus, which promotes equity and addresses social determinants of health, can deliver better outcomes for First Nations populations (Butler et al., 2022).

Comprehensive PHC services in Australia are best typified by the Aboriginal community-controlled health services (ACCHS). These health services are designed to deliver holistic, comprehensive, and culturally appropriate health care for First Nations Australians. (Percival et al., 2016, p. 2)

In Aotearoa New Zealand, most PHC services adopt a model of *whānau*(family)-centred care that embraces the three principles of the *Te Tiriti ō Waitangi* (Treaty of Waitangi). In practical terms, this could mean at the very least:

- partnership – working together with *iwi, hapū, whānau* and Māori communities to develop strategies for improving the health status of Māori
- participation – involving Māori at all levels of the organisation in planning, development and delivery of health and disability services that are put in place to improve the health status of Māori
- protection – ensuring Māori well-being is protected and improved as well as safe-guarding Māori cultural concepts, values and practices (summarised from the Taranaki District Health Board, 2014, p. 3).

Australia does not have a treaty, being one of the few colonised places claimed under the doctrine of terra nullius ('nobody's land'). This meant that the colonising powers at the time saw First Nations Australians as having no recognisable sovereignty over their land.

As with Māori well-being, First Nations Australians have a profound relationship to land which differs from European notions. Land is not 'owned' in a European sense, but people have a responsibility for looking after Country and Country will also look after us (Bulloch, Goarty & Bellchambers, 2019, p. 38). People have a deep spiritual relationship with land, cosmos and Country; they belong to the land and derive health, connection, identity and well-being from this belonging (Bulloch, et al., 2019).

In First Nations communities, the social determinants of health are often used to frame health outcomes and continue to inform a deficit discourse of First Nations health. First Nations land management transforms an alternative narrative to the deficit discourse and advocates for cultural determinants of health (The Lowitja Institute, 2014). The reality of this type of wellness transformation is linked to other Indigenous connections to place and land, for example, the way that these factors contribute to the spiritual-cultural identity of native Hawaiians (Kana'iaupuni & Malone, 2006).

Cultural responsiveness: at the 'heart' of PHC for First Nations

When analysing the characteristics of Indigenous PHC delivery models, *culture* was the most prominent characteristic underpinning all of the other seven 'accessible health services, community participation, continuous quality improvement, culturally appropriate and skilled workforce, flexible approach to care, holistic health care and self-determination and empowerment' (Harfield et al., 2018, para 22). Along with professional skills and knowledge, working across these types of cultural interfaces requires a genuine engagement with cultural principles that are the foundation of wise practice: *to respect, to do slowly, to be gentle, to be polite, and to honour.* These are the five main tenets of *Yindyamarra Winhanganha* – a First Nations Wiradyuri approach to an Indigenous way of thinking, being and doing as espoused by Dr Stan Grant Snr OAM (Charles Sturt University (CSU), 2016).

PHC is seen as an appropriate model for addressing health disparities between populations because of its emphasis on preventative and health-promoting practices and implies a broader responsibility for health to include housing, education and employment. All of these areas are referred to as the social determinants of health. Additionally, the cultural determinants associated with positive health and well-being outcomes might include the absence of racism, and the cultural connections to people, place and the environment are also important considerations (Wilson & Waqanaviti, 2021). PHC is considered relevant to First Nations health because of its inherent and purposeful practice framework that engages with aspects of social justice – **E**quity, **A**ccess, **P**articipation, **R**ights – further defined as fairness in resource distribution and equality of access to essential services such as health, housing and education, and community participation, incorporating inter-sectoral collaboration that recognises that health is socially determined, and a balance in focus to include high-technology tertiary care with health promotion and prevention. That is, a holistic model of care is required to ensure that physical and social, as well as emotional well-being outcomes, can be achieved at individual and community levels (Wilson & Waqanaviti, 2021).

Best practice indicates that the principles of PHC should enable co-design and/or co-production methodology, whereby complex and wicked problems are solved by collaboration with key stakeholders. Within First Nations Australian approaches to PHC this would involve shared decision, community control and First Nations leadership, as well as the implementation of First Nations methods such as Yarning (Butler et al., 2022).

CASE STUDY 5.1

Sue is a nurse in a remote Aboriginal community who works closely with Aboriginal health care workers at a local clinic. Together, they have devised a program to educate people about skin infections after one of the health care workers asked why so many people had scabies and other skin infections at the clinic. This program involves Sue and the health care workers sharing information, collaborating and working in partnership to address the problem with Community members. As a result, clinic attendance has fallen. In response, health managers have suggested that the clinic will no longer need the same level of staffing, rather than seeing the valuable work that has been done and ensuring ongoing resources to support the program.

REFLECTION
1. What elements and characteristics of PHC are evident in this brief scenario?
2. What implicit message can be found in management's response?
3. What would your response be as a manager to the outcomes demonstrated for this one issue of skin health?

Practising cultural safety and cultural responsiveness: *is there a difference?*

As noted above, 'culture' is the defining consideration for any effective PHC professional practice framework. That is, while clinical applications must be applied where relevant, so too must these skilled interventions be exercised with deep understanding of the realities for First Nations alongside whom we work. Cultural responsiveness is 'simply' about meeting the needs and expectations of individuals and communities, and one way that this can be achieved is to engage in creating spaces of cultural safety.

First Nations' ways of thinking, being and doing

How is cultural safety enabled? Ways of communicating, of *thinking, being* and *doing* (Martin, 2003), are critical considerations when working alongside First Nations communities. For example, in nearly all First Nations contexts, credibility and acceptance come from a keen sense of self-awareness; from being quiet, reserved and respectful, engaging in truth listening as well as truth telling, and by fitting in with the rules and protocols of the people and situation. For example, in Māori communities, a credible and competent communicator is one who is able to connect with others as a member of a wider *whānau*, knows and uses correct behaviours and procedures for the context, establishes trust through an auto-ethnographic (*pūrākau*) telling of their own personal story, shares other relevant stories and is attentive to the comfort of all communicators in a particular communication event. Furthermore, self-monitoring of appearance, language and behaviour can indicate not just communication competence but cultural responsiveness as well.

There are many ways for nurses and health professionals to enhance and build their understanding of culturally appropriate practice, including taking a local cultural tour, reading the work of First Nations scholars or visiting the local museums and art galleries to get an appreciation for the history and cultural context of the place (Biles, 2017). Visiting the local communities for sporting events and community open days is also a good option. Students can be proactive and educate themselves by immersing themselves in the local culture by undertaking cultural awareness training with First Nations organisations as the preferred service provider. Taking time to learn the basics of the local language is also advantageous and is often met with appreciation by the local people.

In Australian First Nations settings, there are numerous examples of respectful engagement conceptualised both in language and practice. *Dadirri*, for instance, is a Northern Australian concept of 'deep listening' (Ungunmerr-Baumann, 2015). Pitjantjatjara people use a singular word for thinking, listening and understanding over a period of time – *kulilkatinyi* (personal communication with M. Heffernan, Renal Consumer Group, Alice Springs, 2016). This sits alongside other concepts of observing closely, reflecting and then doing. Nurses who want to affect change would be well served by embracing such thoughtful approaches to health education and health promotion. First Nations histories, through storytelling, Indigenous literacies and artworks, can be successfully employed as education and health promotion tools that recognise existing knowledges and offer a platform for the laying down of new knowledges.

At the very outset of working alongside First Nations communities, intuitive links have to be made between levels of practice such as: *knowing what, knowing how, knowing why* and *knowing whether to* (Mlcek, 2011) that draw on transformational and sustainable methodologies. Practice needs to be developed from a blend of Western and First Nations world views, engagement and relationship building. As PHC workers, our epistemologies (how we know what we know) may straddle both world views (First Nations and non-Indigenous) (Smith, 2000, p. 230).

CASE STUDY 5.2

Margie is 40 years old and part of the Māori diaspora population living in Australia, a 'guest' on First Nations lands, and feels the keenness of being away from home, but thankful that there are those left 'behind' who 'keep the home-fires burning'. When she does go home to visit, there are spiritual and bodily connections that provide essential fuel for her ongoing well-being, *mana*, identity, connectedness, and that of significant others in her community. Her mother has also long left Aotearoa for her spiritual place in Hawaiki but continues to guide Margie to first go and visit the cemetery (*urupa*) to reconnect and talk to all the ancestors and those who have passed before her. She then allows plenty of time to visit her *kaumatua* (Elders) with food that they enjoy –*to feed their sense of well-being*. Margie knows that when she leaves, these are the *pūrākau* (stories) that will be shared among *whanau* for many months to come, and in a way, she is contributing to *ahi ka* (keeping the home-fires burning).

REFLECTION

1. What are the 'knowing what' messages that resonate with the cultural considerations for effective PHC?
2. Reflect on the origin of other 'knowing whether to' stories of cultural obligations, and how important they are for meeting the needs and expectations of individuals and community.

There are countless stories to demonstrate the 'largeness' of situations that are bound together by so many diverse cultural threads that relate to spirituality, knowledge, life and death – the world in which we live – and especially for Māori, *Te Āo Māori* – 'the Māori World'. As one *whakatauki* (proverb) emphasises:

> *Titiro whakamuri hei arahi mō āpōpō.* We walk backwards into the future, our eyes fixed on the past. We look to the past so we can move forward understanding where we have come from in order to understand who we are today. (Gordon-Burns & Campbell, 2014, p. 24)

For First Nations Australians, the following Aboriginal Wiradjuri phrase, *Yindyamarra Winhanganha*, captures the essence of deep spiritual connections to place and space; of *having the wisdom to live respectfully in a world worth living* (CSU, 2016). *Yindyamarra Winhanganha* is built on values of reciprocity and trustful relationships; it asks practitioners to respectfully contribute to the world in which we live and to develop knowledge and wisdom for the benefit of all (CSU, 2016). The term indicates a culturally responsive practice that values human dignity and self-worth (Dominelli, 2010).

A suggested approach for effective PHC nursing in a First Nations context is offered through engagement from a Kaupapa Māori Theoretical (KMT) stance that conceptualises Māori Indigenous (Smith, 2012) and privileges serious storytelling, reciprocity, humility and inclusion as precursors for similar wise practice in First Nations communities (Muller, 2010; 2014). The story of one person is never just that in a First Nations context but includes stories of connection to all aspects of living: linkage to ancestors and Elders both past and present; ecological practices among people sharing culture; and spiritual alignment to the land, its life-forces, geography and environmental structures.

A fundamental factor contributing to First Nations health is the presence and sense of well-being among individuals (Ministry of Health, 2023). The community setting plays an integral part in establishing this well-being because of the strong relationships already formed between family members, and PHC workers must understand that care of individuals does not happen in isolation to the rest of the clan, mob, *iwi* (tribe), *hāpori* (community) or *whānau* (family unit). There could be several groups to be aware of, and the extent and level of PHC success may have to be measured against the care also shown to all and not just the individual.

It could be argued that one of the early limitations of PHC approaches was in the introduction of selective PHC that focused on singular issues and sometimes singular groups to the exclusion of whole families and communities.

CASE STUDY 5.3

Jane, a nurse in an urban PHC setting, has obtained funding to run a quit smoking campaign because she has noted how many young women, in particular, are smoking. She has devised a health promotion program and has invited some guest speakers and young women from the community to a lunch gathering. Only a couple of women have turned up. Jane is disappointed and feels that the people are not interested in their health.

REFLECTION
1. What might Jane have done differently to encourage people in the community to participate in this program?
2. What are the key points in Jane's approach that have moved away from PHC principles?
3. What key skills or attributes might help Jane turn the program around to become a genuine PHC activity?

Clinical yarning

Incorporating clinical yarning as a model of therapeutic care in the PHC (and beyond) is increasingly discussed in the literature (Bessarab & Ng'andu, 2010; Burke et al., 2022). Cultural safety and respect are fundamental, as without them, positive health outcomes are unlikely (McGough et al., 2022). A number of steps can be extrapolated to guide a clinical approach to yarning (see Table 5.1).

Table 5.1   Clinical yarning cycle

Stages of clinical yarning cycle	Activities associated with stage	Examples	Ways of knowing being, doing and belonging
Preparation	Attend to any hospitality or material requirements.	Is there sufficient seating? Is water available? Are toilets nearby? Are all the relevant people available to gather? Is transport available?	Hosts (clinical settings) should ensure that visitors (patients) are comfortable in their surroundings and promote cultural safety with the people they encounter. Are there any cultural activities that clash with appointment times: e.g. sorry business/ sad news; corroboree; music festivals; football knockouts?
Cultural protocol	Acknowledgement of Country Do you know who the traditional custodians of the land where you are conducting your work today? What steps have you taken to inform yourself about the Country, Culture and Language where you work?	Are you prepared to adopt a First Nation standpoint? How will you position yourself with agency to privilege the perspective of First Nations in this encounter? Cultural humility Be prepared to respond to: 'What's your name? Who's your Mob? Where are you from?'	Recognise the cultural expertise in the room/setting. Recognise allyship in the room. Establish connections. Establish cultural safety and humility.
Social yarning	Establish social trust.	Share something of your own personal story with each other. Authenticity is valued.	Reflexivity: listen deeply to yourself while simultaneously paying present attention to others around you. Maintain safe cultural responsiveness
Topical yarning	Listen deeply to each other – with each having time to speak and time to be fully heard.	Identify the health or social and emotional well-being topic that is the focus of the yarn. Discuss it fully together.	Have two-way understanding and respect as everyone is equal in the yarning relationship. No hierarchy exists.

Table 5.1   (cont.)

Stages of clinical yarning cycle	Activities associated with stage	Examples	Ways of knowing being, doing and belonging
New shared understanding emerges	Priorities, actions and plans are agreed to address health matters.	Create a new health-focused story (knowledge). It takes time to develop and tell a new story, and to be confident with it as a new knowledge. The story can only be shared with others after sufficient consolidation and safety are established. Plan sufficient, unhurried and respectful time to develop a healthful story.	Stories are narratives of knowledge. They are often shared and passed on to others. Self-determination is a priority – the story must make real-world sense to the one who must live it. It must be holistic. The new story will need application across the whole of life and connections.
Respectful conclusions	Affirm trust in the yarning relationship.	Agree on a course of therapeutic action.	Express gratitude.
Remember (repeat the yarning cycle if needed – or a variation to the healthful plan is required)	Leave to pursue the agreed therapeutic action. Invite the possibility to yarn again if and when needed.	*'If you would like to return to the clinical yarn, we can listen to feedback and yarn again to improve the story'.* Provide access strategies for any practical resources required to carry out the plan.	Remain in harmony with each other.

Source: Rhonda Wilson.

CASE STUDY 5.4

Rhonda is a First Nations woman and a registered nurse, working as a professor of nursing at a regional university. During the COVID-19, pandemic she heard the alarming news that a first case of the infection had emerged in an isolated rural Aboriginal community in Australia where she had worked and had cultural connections. As a matter of cultural obligation, and equipped with clinical expertise, she reached out to the community (an Aboriginal Medical Service (AMS)) to see if her skills could be of assistance during the impending emergency. It was early days, and Australia was in lockdown with movement restrictions limited to a 5 km radius within local government areas, with physical distancing and mask-wearing mandatory. The Chief Executive Officer (CEO) of the AMS said, 'Yes Sis, please come, and soon as you can'. The CEO arranged for the Royal Flying Doctors service to collect Rhonda, and a further two nurses that Rhonda had invited to join the emergency vaccination clinic. Rhonda

CASE STUDY 5.4 Continued

and another Aboriginal nurse, Donna shared a heightened sense of obligation and worry for Aboriginal communities, particularly as they were going to Donna's ancestral Country. No one knew what might happen, with death rates climbing across the world. The outlook could be grim, and risk was unknown, yet their capacity to serve community with their nursing and health skills compelled them forward. Arrangements were made quickly, with the fly-in team required to apply for travel permits, complete online COVID-19 vaccination immunisation certification, and return negative COVID-19 PCR results prior to departure.

Vaccinations were in short supply in Australia at this time, and cold chain transportation requirements made delivery logistics for vaccination challenging. On delivery, vaccination refrigeration needed to be maintained. The multi-dose vials of vaccination were another challenge to manage carefully in light of the limited national stock of vaccines. They arrived in full personal protective equipment (PPE) and set to work vaccinating hundreds of community members under the leadership of the AMS. The CEO of the AMS was fielding calls from the public health and other government sectors, while simultaneously working with community at a time of high anxiety for the community.

Listening to community, the CEO was able to collaborate with community Elders and leaders, leveraging cultural connection and trust to focus on safety planning and infection prevention and control matters. The Mob 'grape vine' has a way of working that effectively communicates urgent messaging. Aboriginal ways of communicating are frequently oral, and ways of being are holistic, prioritising caring for one another, especially the most vulnerable, and with utmost respect. So, it was no surprise that the community rallied quickly with their established ways of knowing, being, doing and belonging that were a great asset when fast and decisive action was needed in the face of a potentially catastrophic threat such as COVID-19. The holistic and organic way in which the community behaved was at odds with the corporate ways of working for government agencies, who were interested in delivering intervention to the community but did not have the relationship with the community or social agency to achieve timely outcomes. For example, the AMS had no trouble with the community accessing testing and vaccination clinics. Established as a trusted health provider, and at a time of high suspicion about the safety of vaccinations, they were able to navigate successfully towards positive outcomes at relative speed. Government agencies, with little local knowledge, and without established trust, set up tent clinics in locations that were not convenient to the local community (for example, with poor access to transport and communication technologies) and were not as successful in engaging community people for timely health outcomes. Rhonda and Donna positioned themselves as partners with the AMS, and took the lead, which was critical to success. However, for other agencies, *coming in, doing to* and *without adequate consultation* led to significant delays in achieving outcomes. In this case, where timeliness was critical, a clinical yarning as a model of care was ideally suited and aligned with community expectations in response to a critical community health threat.

Relationships and trust were established. Rhonda's first patient for vaccination was one of the oldest community Elders in the town. Sitting with Auntie, listening to her and holding space for her to raise her fears and discuss risks, she could come to a consensus on an agreed way forward. She had her vaccination, and Rhonda thanked her for her courage and leadership. Rhonda and Donna had a plan to encourage others to come for vaccinations. And Mob did – in one week they vaccinated over 600 people in a small town of less than 3000 population.

REFLECTION

1. Referring to the clinical yarning cycle in Table 5.1, can you map the stages of the cycle within Rhonda's narrative about her clinical experience in an Aboriginal community impacted by COVID-19?

2. Imagine you are the health practitioner sitting with the Auntie in this case study. Discuss with your learning peers about any strategies you might use to draw close, listen deeply and hold space for a client such as her.

3. What struck you most profoundly about the case study story? How might you describe it as a determinant of health?

Cultural responsiveness in practice

Being culturally responsive is a legitimate decolonising methodology that enhances cultural safety, creates opportunities for reciprocal relationships to develop and provides options for well-being to flourish through self-worth and personal recognition.

Decolonising can be a confronting concept for some. It is difficult to think of oneself as 'colonising' anyone in the historical sense, but it is important to break down exactly what is meant here. 'Colonising' is the act of imposing power over another through force, weight of numbers, dispossession, system bias, privilege and/or discrimination. 'Decolonising' is the thoughtful undoing of those disempowering elements in a relationship. Whose preferred way of 'doing' is privileged in an encounter between a client and a nurse, for example? A nurse may want a client to 'comply' with a recommended treatment. The client may not want to for any number of reasons. How this is navigated will determine whether or not it is a colonising experience for the client.

How do we progress in developing the degree of cross-cultural competencies required by PHC workers to execute cultural responsiveness? The Indigenous Allied Health Association (IAHA) (2015, p. 7) captures the ideas of respectful engagement, reciprocity, safety, spirituality and culture in its *Cultural Responsiveness in Action: An IAHA Framework* to highlight how practical strategies can build cultural safety using strengths-based and action-oriented approaches. This framework provides guidance about the knowledge and skills required to be culturally responsive.

It lists six key capabilities:

1. Respect for the centrality of culture
2. Self-awareness
3. Proactivity
4. Inclusive engagement
5. Leadership
6. Responsibility and accountability.

This set of capabilities relates to First Nations health care and well-being, including:

- having *knowledge of culture*
- integrating *holistic* and *inclusive* views of health and well-being
- adopting a *rights-based culturally responsive approach*
- recognising *leadership, strength, resilience,* and *self-determination*

- understanding the unique professional and cultural perspectives of First Nations Australians
- acknowledging the *diversity of individuals, families, and communities*
- undertaking rigorous *education, evidence-based practice* and *research.*

Reciprocity: genuine care through shared learning

Reciprocity is foundational to 'wise practice' where knowledge is drawn from different people around the PHC worker. This is also when cultural humility (having critical self-awareness, and reflexivity) continues to develop. Reciprocity involves a shared responsibility to resources and obligations in which we are all bound by when working in and with community (National Health and Medical Research Council, 2018). By joining other individuals to facilitate a safe space, knowledge can be renamed in a conscious act of claiming stories from the past and naming stories from the present, to deliberately reclaim heritage. The process of comparing different truths, perspectives and realities can result in powerful engagement for those involved. This reclamation of heritage by sharing stories is undertaken through a profound and essential decolonising lens (Muller, 2010; 2014), which also has the capacity for healing. It is essential that for these wise behaviours to occur, health care workers must engage in decolonising behaviours alongside First Nations; acknowledging and critiquing their own lack of cultural awareness and competence, their power and privilege, as well as any prejudice that could contribute to the marginalisation, stereotyping, isolation and lack of determination for their Indigenous/First Nations people.

Quite simply, wise practice incorporates a way of working alongside First Nations that is considered more culturally relevant and inclusive of First Nations' *thinking, being and doing,* as well as being responsive to First Nations' knowledge systems (Blackstock, 2008).

Safety in culture: truth telling and truth listening; more than a micro-skill

The Bathurst Wiradyuri Elders in Australia shared their understanding of yarning as providing the means for 'truth telling' (verbal communication with the Elders in June 2021), and this sentiment was added to in verbal communication with a Bundjalung Goenpul Woman academic (July 2022), that essential to yarning was the commitment to 'truth listening'. These tenets form the safe boundaries for yarning to occur. Work undertaken by Māori nurse educator Dianne Wepa resulted in the extension and recognition of *cultural safety* (Wepa, 2015) in nurse education. This was raised at a significant *hui* (meeting/gathering) in 1988, and then expanded to encompass critical components of practice including:

- not blaming or passing judgement on a client's current situation
- examining one's own realities, and personal attitudes.

The underlying message overall, especially with regard to health care, suggests that an understanding of one's own culture is a beginning step towards cultural safety, and that reflection is not only a key principle of cultural safety but also a requisite competency in nursing, midwifery and a number of other health professions (Taylor & Guerin, 2019).

In practice, there has to be no outward blame or judgement made on the part of the PHC worker towards First Nations individuals or their families in respect to their current medical situation. Instead, there must be knowledge, respect and quiet contemplation from the professional to understand situations.

For example, anecdotal evidence suggests that 'when people have to pay more for their prescriptions they sometimes stop not only "non-essential" medicines, but also medicines for serious and potentially life-threatening illnesses such as hypertension, hyperlipidaemia, depression, osteoporosis, prevention of stroke, asthma, and diabetes' (New Zealand Medical Association, 2012, p. 78). Individuals may well be able to afford medication and medical treatment, either by themselves or through the intervention of their children. For example, many Māori families created family trust funds from the rewards of *Te Tiriti ō Waitangi* claims or from monetary royalties from land and kiwi fruit orchard shares that most Māori have in the community. However, the burden of ongoing grief and loss, and the onset of several illnesses, often produces flippancy towards taking medication or having regular health check-ups.

Spirituality: the 'head and the heart' together

Pastoral and cultural support are integral factors in contributing to the spiritual well-being of Māori and other First Nations. For example, Aotearoa's New Zealand's Māori Health Strategy, *He Korowai Oranga* (Ministry of Health, 2014) sets the overarching framework that guides the government and the overall health sector to achieve the best health outcomes for Māori. Māori views on health are framed by a comprehensive approach that encompasses four key elements: *wairua* (spiritual), *hinengaro* (head – psychological), *tinana* (body – physical) and *whānau* (extended family) (Capital, Coast and Hutt Valley, 2024, p. 5). These elements are similar to those in *He Korowai Oranga*: *mauri ora* (healthy individuals), *whānau ora* (healthy families) and *wai ora* (healthy environments) (Ministry of Health, 2014). Included in the responsibility for implementing strategies to achieve those elements are some 20 district health boards (DHBs). Alongside the formal management and delivery of their services is the opportunity to also access *Rongoā Māori* traditional healing as practised in a Māori culturally responsive context. The Ministry of Health (2019) currently funds some 20 rongoā providers throughout Aotearoa New Zealand to help provide Māori spiritual well-being through *mirimiri* (massage), *karakia* (pastoral support) and *whitiwhiti kōrero* (cultural support).

The principle of *karakia* (blessing or prayer) is an 'essential element in protecting and maintaining wairua, hinengaro, tinana and well-being of whānau – particularly in a hospital setting' (Capital, Coast and Hutt Valley, 2024, p. 9). These similar tenets for working with Māori are encapsulated in every health board's practice in Aotearoa New Zealand. However, First Nations Australians may struggle to recognise the same self-determination principles required for their care. It is an ongoing project that requires acknowledgement of historical injustices captured in the colonisation of First Nations continuing intergenerational grief and loss around the Stolen Generations (Muller, 2014), and racism and Whiteness behaviours towards Indigenous peoples (Mlcek 2014; Walter, Taylor & Habibis, 2013).

There is little doubt that Māori views on health can be acknowledged through the way that spirituality and sacredness are understood. The Capital, Coast and Hutt Valley (2024, p. 6) also advises that, in some instances, behaviour and practices that are not consistent with Māori beliefs and values can cause distress, and result in a loss of engagement in health care services by Māori. How to approach and touch *kaumātua* (Elder) patients, for example, is embedded in a deep cultural understanding of the sacredness between the mind and the body. This is because Māori rituals of care involve a complex system of *tapu* (sacred/forbidden/restricted) and *noa* (free from *tapu*/unrestricted) that forms the basis of order and disorder, of safe and unsafe practice. These considerations are still deeply relevant in today's health and medical environment. To engage in practices that are counter to upholding *tapu and noa regimes* can offend and diminish *wairua* (spirituality).

The role of the community nurse in PHC and health promotion

The community nurse is in a unique position to establish meaningful relationships with First Nations communities. First Nations utilise health services but their experiences of these services and the individuals within them can impact their future health-seeking behaviours. There can be no denying that encounters with nurses and other health professionals have not always been positive for First Nations. Historically, nurses have been at the forefront of implementing sometimes harmful policies and procedures. PHC offers a chance to challenge the status quo and enter meaningful and therapeutic relationships such as the work undertaken by the Inala clinic.

While PHC provides a template for a more equitable, accessible and effective way of working, the focus on clinical and curative services should focus on robust and ongoing community engagement and intersectoral partnerships that are crucial to best practice health promotion (Durey et al., 2016; Sivertsen et al., 2022).

Further, recognising that intergenerational trauma has had a detrimental impact on First Nations' health disparity in general and continues to do so with child removal from families being an ongoing concern in many communities (Ward & Wilson, 2022). Social and emotional well-being continues to be measured using the deficit discourse, including a count of completed suicide (Ward & Wilson, 2022). Meanwhile, stigma and identity continue to contribute to experiences of racism for many people, and we know racism leads to poorer health outcomes in general (Wilson & Waqanaviti, 2021). It is important to recognise that Indigeneity is not a skin colour, and that asking clients about their cultural identity, rather than making assumptions, is an important aspect of holistic health and social care. Treatment planning, particularly aimed at social and emotional well-being outcomes, can be improved and tailored for First Nations by asking questions such as:

- Are you living on or off Country?
- Are you new to this location? If so, how does that affect how you are feeling?
- Do you know your First Nations family?
- Did you grow up knowing you were a First Nations person? (Doyle, Hungerford, & Clearly, 2017).

Access to PHC is complex and better understood as being part of a 'framework synthesis' (Davy et al., 2016). From one such framework about access and accessibility, for example, Levesque, Harris and Russell (2013) highlight a critical appraisal of the situation whereby First Nations Australians may be able to overcome barriers to access. Importantly, the onus of responsibility should not be on the client but instead on the approach and accountability of the nurse and/or health practitioner in consultation with local communities (Biles & Biles, 2019). For example, if we look at the framework by Levesque and colleagues (2013) (Figure 5.1), within stage two of five stages it seeks to understand how people can obtain access and accessibility to PHC. Consider how you could adapt, modify and change your practice/approach to ensure it is acceptable to end users. What steps would you need to take to ensure the acceptability by end users?

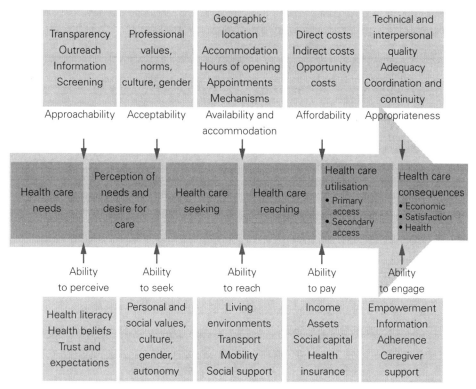

Figure 5.1   A conceptual framework of access to health care
Source: Levesque et al. (2013).

On the other hand, health professionals need to be aware of their role in contributing to the *accessibility* for Indigenous peoples seeking PHC. In Figure 5.1, five dimensions of accessibility are identified, as noted at the beginning of this chapter:

1. Approachability
2. Acceptability
3. Availability and accommodation
4. Affordability
5. Appropriateness.

As part of the framework, five corresponding abilities – to perceive, seek, reach, pay and engage – are employed to identify the dimensions of accessibility to generate access to PHC. These abilities occur in the following stages (Davy et al., 2016):

- Stage one is about people's ability *to perceive* a need to seek care, and whether a health care service is known to be available and approachable.
- Stage two focuses on the ability of people *to seek out* appropriate and acceptable services when needed. The acceptability of a service is an important consideration to match with the social and cultural values and behaviours that relate to how communities' function.
- Stage three relates to the ease with which individuals are encouraged and accommodated *to reach* or obtain available services when needed, especially in a timely manner.

- Stage four increases the accessibility of PHC through the extent to which services are affordable, and the degree to which users can *pay* for these.
- Stage five involves not only the ability of the individual user *to engage* with the PHC that is available, but also to provide appropriate services that meet the overall needs of communities.

Conclusion

In urban areas, where the highest numbers of First Nations Australians live, access to health care is still problematic, which reinforces the need for First Nations PHC services right across the country. Nurses, within or outside of community-controlled organisations, can improve the acceptability and accessibility of their service through adhering to key PHC principles such as:

- working in partnership with clients and communities
- reflecting on own culture and its impact on others
- facilitating change, not imposing it
- working intersectionally
- being proactive in researching and learning about First Nations cultures and histories
- engaging in decolonising practice.

Australia and Aotearoa New Zealand, as well as Indigenous peoples all around the world, are still dealing with the legacy of their respective pasts in terms of the health disparities between First Nations and non-Indigenous peoples, especially after ongoing colonial as well as imperialist impositions by others. However, community health nurses can have a significant impact for positive change through opening themselves to First Nations' ways of *thinking, being and doing*. There is an opportunity for genuine partnership and PHC is a valuable mechanism for ensuring culturally safe and responsive health care practice.

CRITICAL THINKING ACTIVITIES

1. Compare the way that holding different world views to the First Nations clients in your care could affect the outcomes of any engagement that you undertake within different situations. What information and understanding about those differences could contribute in a positive way? What could be some negative impacts within the care encounter?
2. How does the role of a PHC nurse differ in a First Nations health context, if at all?
3. How can PHC create a space where First Nations definitions of health can be privileged?

FURTHER READING

Durie, M. (2006). *Measures of Māori wellbeing.* New Zealand Treasury Guest Lecture Series, 2006. www.treasury.govt.nz/publications/media-speeches/guestlectures/pdfs/tgls-durie.pdf

Ministry of Health. (n.d.). *Māori health Hauora Māori.* New Zealand Government. www.health.govt .nz/our-work/populations/maori-health/maori-health-models

Phillips, B., Daniels, J., Woodward, A., et al. (2017). Mortality trends in Australian Aboriginal peoples and New Zealand Maori. *Population Health Metrics, 15*(25), 1–12. https://pophealthmetrics. biomedcentral.com/articles/10.1186/s12963-017-0140-6

Schultz, R., Abbott, T., Yamaguchi, J. & Cairney, S. (2018). Indigenous land management as primary health care: Qualitative analysis from the Interplay research project in remote Australia. *BMC Health Services Research, 18*, 960.

REFERENCES

Australian Institute of Health and Welfare (AIHW). (2023). *Stronger evidence, better decisions, improved health and welfare.* Australian Government. www.aihw.gov.au/

Bessarab, D. & Ng'andu, B. (2010). Yarning about yarning as a legitimate method in indigenous research. *International Journal of Critical Indigenous Studies, 3*(1), 37–50.

Biles, B., & Biles, J. (Eds.) (2019). *Aboriginal and Torres Strait Islander peoples' health & wellbeing.* (1st ed.) Oxford University Press.

Biles, J. (2017). *Undergraduate nursing and Indigenous Australian cultural competence: The lived experience of students.* [Doctoral Thesis, Charles Sturt University]. Charles Sturt University.

Blackstock, C. (2008). *The Breath of Life: A First Nations Alternative to Western Social Theories.* University of Kwa Zulu Natal. http://ccs.ukzn.ac.za/files/South%20Africa%20%5BCompatibility%20Mode%5D.pdf

Bulloch, H., Fogarty, W. & Bellchambers, K. (2019). *Aboriginal health and wellbeing services.* Lowitja Institute, Australian National University.

Butler, T., Gall, A., Garvey, G., et al. (2022). A comprehensive review of optimal approaches to co-design in health with First Nations Australians. *International Journal of Environmental Research and Public Health 2022, 19*, 16166. https//doi.org/10.3390/ijerph1923116166

Burke, A.W., Welch, S., Power, T., Lucas, C. & Moles, R.J. (2022). Clinical yarning with Aboriginal and/or Torres Strait Islander peoples – A systematic scoping review of its use and impacts. *Systematic Reviews, 11*(1). https://doi.org/10.1186/s13643-022-02008-0

Capital, Coast and Hutt Valley. (2024). *Māori health.* Capital & Coast District Health Board. www.ccdhb.org.nz/our-services/a-to-z-of-our-services/maori-health/

Charles Sturt University (CSU). (2016). *Citation for 'Yindyamarra Winhanganha'.* www.csu.edu.au

Davy, C., Harfield, S., McArthur, A., Munn, Z. & Brown, A. (2016). Access to primary health care services for Indigenous peoples: A framework synthesis. *International Journal for Equity in Health, 15*(163), 1–9. https://doi.org/10.1186/s12939-016-0450-5

Dominelli, L. (2010). *Social Work in a Globalizing World.* Polity Press.

Doyle, K., Hungerford, C. & Clearly, M (2017) Study of intra-racial exclusion within Australian Indigenous communities using eco-maps. *International Journal of Mental Health Nursing, 26*, 129–41.

Durey, A., McEvoy, S., Swift-Otero, V., et al. (2016). Improving healthcare for Aboriginal Australians through effective engagement between community and health services. *BMC Health Services Research, 16*, 1–13.

Gordon-Burns, D. & Campbell, L. (2014). *Inakitia rawatia hei kakano mō apōpō: Students encounter with bicultural commitment, Childhood Education, 90*(1), 20–8. https://doi.org/10.1080/00094056.2014.872506

Haggerty, J., Roberge, D., Levesque, J-F., et al. (2014). An exploration of rural-urban differences in healthcare-seeking trajectories: Implications for measures of accessibility. *Health Place 2014, 28*, 92–8.

Harfield, S., Davy, C., McArthur, A., et al. (2018). Characteristics of Indigenous primary health care service delivery models: A systematic scoping review. *Global Health, 12*(2018). https://doi.org/10.1186/s12992-018-0332-2

Indigenous Allied Health Association (IAHA). (2015). *Cultural Responsiveness in Action: An IAHA Framework.* https://iaha.com.au/wp-content/uploads/2020/08/IAHA_Cultural-Responsiveness_2019_FINAL_V5.pdf

Kana'iaupuni, S. & Malone, N. (2006). This land is my land: The role of place in native Hawaiian identity. In J. Frazier & E. Tetty-Fio (eds), *Race, Ethnicity and Place in a Changing America* (pp. 291–305). Global Press.

Levesque, J.F., Harris, M.F. & Russell, G. (2013). Patient-centred access to health care: Conceptualising access at the interface of health systems and populations. *International Journal of Equity Health*, *12*(18), 16–28. https://doi.org/10.1186/1475-9276-12-18

The Lowitja Institute (Australia's National Institute for Aboriginal and Torres Strait Islander Health Research). (2014). *Culture is Key: Towards Cultural Determinants-Driven Health Policy*. www.lowitja.org.au/resource/culture-is-key-towards-cultural-determinants-driven-health-policy/

Martin, K. (2003). Ways of knowing, being and doing: A theoretical framework and methods for Indigenous and Indigenist research. *Journal of Australian Studies*, *27*(6), 203–14.

McGough, S., Wynaden, D., Gower, S., Duggan, R. & Wilson, R. (2022). There is no health without cultural safety: Why cultural safety matters. *Contemporary Nurse*, *58*(1), 1–15. https://doi.org/10.1080/10376178.2022.2027254

Ministry for Culture and Heritage. (2005). *Te Ara – The Encyclopedia of New Zealand*. New Zealand Government. www.teara.govt.nz/en

Ministry of Health. (2023). *Māori health models – Te Wheke*. New Zealand Government. www.health.govt.nz/our-work/populations/maori-health/maori-health-models/maori-health-models-te-wheke

——— (2014). *The Guide to He Korowai Oranga – Māori Health Strategy*. New Zealand Government. www.health.govt.nz/publication/guide-he-korowai-oranga-maori-health-strategy

——— (2019). Rongoā Māori. Retrieved from www.health.govt.nz/our-work/populations/maori-health/rongoa-maori-traditional-maori-healing

Mlcek, S. (2011). Competing knowledges in lifelong education. *International Journal of Lifelong Education*, *30*(6), 815–29.

——— (2014). Are we doing enough to develop cross-cultural competencies for social work? *British Journal of Social Work*, *44*(7), 1984–2003. https://doi.org/10.1093/bjsw/bct044

Muller, L. (2010). *Indigenous Australian Social Health theory [PhD thesis]*. James Cook University, Townsville, Queensland.

——— (2014). *A Theory for Indigenous Australian Social Work and Health*. Allen & Unwin.

National Health and Medical Research Council. (2018). *The Australian Code for the Responsible Conduct of Research*. Australian Research Council and Universities Australia.

National Indigenous Australians Agency. (n.d.). *Indigenous advancement strategy*. Australian Government. www.indigenous.gov.au/indigenous-advancement-strategy

New Zealand Medical Association. (2012). Increasing prescription part charges will increase health inequalities in New Zealand. *New Zealand Medical Journal*, *125*(1355), 78–80. www.otago.ac.nz/wellington/otago034549.pdf

Percival, N., O'Donaghue, L., Lin, V., Tsey, K. & Baillie, R. (2016). Improving health promotion using quality improvement techniques in Australian Indigenous primary health care. *Frontiers in Public Health*, *4*(53), 1–16. www.ncbi.nlm.nih.gov/pmc/articles/PMC4812048/

Phillips, B., Daniels, J., Woodward, A., et al. (2017). Mortality trends in Australian aboriginal peoples and New Zealand Māori. *Population Health Metrics*, *15*, 1–12.

Rigby, W. & Jeeawody, B. (2014). Indigenous health nursing. In D. Guzys & E. Petrie (eds), *An Introduction to Community and Primary Health Care* (pp. 282–92). Cambridge University Press.

Sivertsen, N., Deverix, J., Gregoric, C. et al. (2022). A call for culture-centred care: exploring health workers' perspectives of positive care experiences and culturally responsive care provision to Aboriginal women and their infants in mainstream health in South Australia. *Health Res Policy Sys*, *20*, 132. https://doi.org/10.1186/s12961-022-00936-w

Smith, L.T. (2000). Kaupapa Māori research. In M. Battiste (ed.), *Reclaiming Indigenous Voice and Vision* (pp. 225–47). UBC Press.

——— (2012). *Decolonizing Methodologies. Research and Indigenous Peoples* (2nd ed.). Zed Books and University of Otago Press.

Taranaki District Health Board. (2014). *Patient and Family/Whanau-Centred Care Framework 2014–2017*. www.tdhb.org.nz/misc/documents/2014-Patient-Family-Whanau-Centred-Care.pdf

Taylor, K. & Guerin, P. (2019). *Health Care and Indigenous Australians: Cultural Safety in Practice* (3rd ed.). Macmillan.

Ungunmerr-Baumann, M.R. (2015). *Dadirri*. www.dadirri.org.au/wp-content/uploads/2015/03/Dadirri-Inner-Deep-Listening-M-R-Ungunmerr-Bauman-Refl1.pdf

Walter, M., Taylor, S. & Habibis, D. (2013). Australian social work is white. In B. Bennett, S. Green, S. Gilbert & D. Bessarab (eds), *Our Voices: Aboriginal and Torres Strait Islander Social Work* (pp. 230–44). Palgrave Macmillan.

Ward, K. & Wilson, R.L. (2022) The social and emotional well-being (SEWB) of First Nations Australians. In N. Proctor, R.L. Wilson, H. Hamer, D. McGarry & M. Loughhead (eds), *Mental Health: A person-centred approach* (3rd ed., pp. 61–80). Cambridge University Press.

Wepa, D. (2015). *Cultural Safety in Aotearoa New Zealand* (2nd ed.). Cambridge University Press.

Wilson, R.L. & Waqanaviti, K. (2021). Emotional and social well-being for First Nations people in the mental health context. In Best & Fredericks (eds), *Yatdjulgin: Aboriginal and Torres Strait Islander Nursing and Midwifery Care* (pp. 281–306). Cambridge University Press.

Wingard, B., Johnson, C. & Drahm-Butler (eds). (2015). *Aboriginal Nnarrative Practice: Honouring Storylines of Pride, Strength and Creativity.* Dulwich Centre.

6

Intersectional and gendered approaches to health and well-being

Kath Peters, Lauretta Luck and Ruth Mursa
With acknowledgement to Rhonda Brown and
Stéphane Bouchoucha

LEARNING OBJECTIVES

At the completion of this chapter, you should be able to:

- explain gender and its relationship to health.
- describe gendered social determinants of health (SDH).
- identify major health concerns for women, men and sexually and gender-diverse people.
- describe the impact of domestic and family violence.
- identify challenges engaging in health care for women, men and sexually and gender-diverse people.
- identify implications for person-centred care.

Introduction

Sex – a set of biological attributes including chromosomes, gene expression, hormone levels and functions, and reproductive/sexual anatomy. Sex is usually categorised as female or male, but there are variations that comprise sex and the way attributes are expressed (Canadian Institutes of Health Research (CIHR), 2023).

Sex and gender have a significant relationship to health and health outcomes for women, men, and sexually and gender-diverse people (World Health Organization (WHO), 2024a). **Sex** relates to biological attributes, whether born female or male, while gender identity 'refers to a person's deeply felt, internal and individual experience of gender, which may or may not correspond to the person's physiology or designated sex at birth' (WHO, 2024a). Biological characteristics expose women and men to different health risks and health conditions. **Gender** also exposes people to different health risks, and **gender inequity** impacts their potential to achieve health and well-being.

Health is not simply a biological phenomenon. It is influenced by social, cultural, psychological and historical factors which impact an individual's health and health outcomes

(WHO, 2024b). Biological characteristics related to sex are often categorised as either female or male, but variation exists in biological attributes and the concept of sex (CIHR, 2023). For example, **intersex** people are born with sex characteristics that do not fit within the binary notions of female or male bodies, which may be visible at birth or not apparent until puberty (Australian Institute of Family Studies, 2022). Gender is political and hierarchical, and this results in inequities that intersect with other forms of discrimination, which is called intersectionality. Gender diversity exists within many cultures, and there are many ways people may identify and express their gender (WHO, 2024a). These include, but are not limited to, **transgender**, **gender-diverse** and **non-binary**. Transgender and gender-diverse individuals face additional challenges related to their affirmed gender being acknowledged and needing to access health services related to their physical characteristics. This chapter focuses on biological and sociocultural factors that impact the health of women, men and sexually and gender-diverse people and how health professionals, such as nurses, working in community and primary health care (PHC) settings, can mitigate health disparities and inequities.

SDH: the impacts of gender

SDH are the non-medical factors that influence health outcomes and are conditions in which people are born, live, work and age. The SDH include factors such as income, education, work, housing, social inclusion and health care (WHO, 2024b).

Gender norms, roles and relations, together with inequality and inequity, affect the lives of all people throughout the world. The impact of gender, like other SDH, can be cumulative across the life course and shape all aspects of a person's health and well-being. A person's gender influences their vulnerabilities and susceptibility to illness, access to health care, water, hygiene and sanitation, as well as their experiences of crisis and emergency situations (WHO, 2021). When gender inequity intersects with other SDH, the experience of discrimination, health risks and lack of access to health resources are compounded (WHO, 2021).

Gender inequality disproportionally affects women, heightened by limited access to finances, a lack of decision-making autonomy and discriminatory attitudes of health care providers, impacting their ability to access health care and critical services (WHO, 2021). Women globally face issues of gender inequality in the workplace, as well as being underpaid and undervalued in child care and work around the home (Klasen, 2020). Gender norms and stereotypes for gender-diverse people exacerbate discrimination in health care and in society resulting in poorer health outcomes (Blondeel et al., 2018). Men are not immune to the impact of gender on health, as men are more likely to engage in high-risk behaviours, including the overconsumption of alcohol (Fetherston & Craike, 2020), and are less likely to engage with health care services compared to women (Mursa, Patterson & Halcomb, 2022). Health disparities between people can be understood by considering gender indicators that measure gender equality and, in particular, the realities of the lives of all people in relation to their role in society, community and family (United Nations Economic Commission for Europe (UNECE), 2015) (see Figure 6.1).

Gender – 'the socially constructed roles, behaviours, expressions and identities of girls, boys, women, men, and gender-diverse people. It influences how people perceive themselves and each other, how they act and interact, and the distribution of power and resources in society. Gender identity is not confined to a binary (girl/woman, boy/man) nor is it static; it exists along a continuum and can change over time' (CIHR, 2023).

Gender inequity – unfair allocation of resources, programs, decision making and opportunities for women, men and gender-diverse people.

Intersex – is a broad term that is used to describe individuals who have 'anatomical, chromosomal and hormonal characteristics that differ from medical and conventional understanding of male and female' (Child Family Community Australia, 2022, p. 2). There are many different underlying variations that may become apparent over the individual's life.

Transgender – Transgender or trans is an umbrella term encompassing individuals whose gender identity differs from their sex assigned at birth. There are a number of ways trans people may express their preferred gender identity such as a trans man or trans women, Sistergirl, Brotherboy, non-binary, genderqueer, gender fluid – and this is not an exhaustive list. Trans individuals' sexual orientation may be fluid and trans people may identify as lesbian, gay, heterosexual, bisexual, asexual, or pansexual.

Gender-diverse – an umbrella term to describe people whose gender, experience or expression of gender is different to the sex they were prescribed at birth (ACON, 2019).

Non-binary – an umbrella term describing a person whose gender identity is not female or male (ACON, 2019).

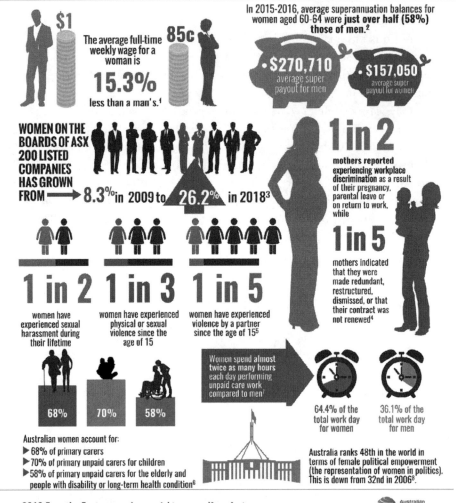

Figure 6.1   Gender indicators

Source: Australian Human Rights Commission (2018).

REFLECTION

Consider how gender inequality highlighted in these indicators might affect women's health. What national programs are you aware of that redress gender inequality?

Major health concerns for people

Men's health concerns

Globally, females have a life expectancy of five years longer than males (WHO, 2021). In Aotearoa New Zealand, males live to an average of 80.0 years (Stats NZ, 2021), and in

Australia, 81.3 years (Australian Institute of Health and Welfare (AIHW), 2023b). The leading cause of death of males in Australia and Aotearoa New Zealand is heart disease (AIHW, 2023b; Ministry of Health, 2018) (Figure 6.2).

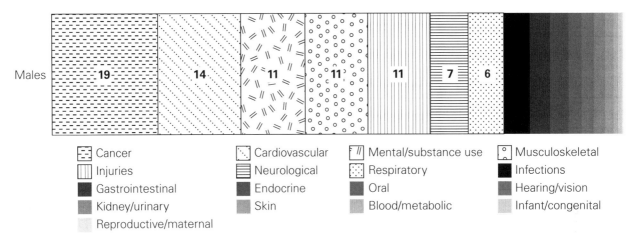

Males   19   14   11   11   11   7   6

- Cancer
- Injuries
- Gastrointestinal
- Kidney/urinary
- Reproductive/maternal
- Cardiovascular
- Neurological
- Endocrine
- Skin
- Mental/substance use
- Respiratory
- Oral
- Blood/metabolic
- Musculoskeletal
- Infections
- Hearing/vision
- Infant/congenital

Figure 6.2   The leading causes of ill health and death (per cent DALY) by disease group in males 2022
Source: AIHW (2022).

Approximately 74 per cent of all deaths globally are attributed to chronic health conditions (WHO, 2023), with 49 per cent of Australian males having one or more chronic conditions (AIHW, 2023b). Being overweight is a well-established risk factor for many chronic health conditions, including hypertension, cardiovascular disease, diabetes, osteoarthritis and obstructive sleep apnoea (AIHW, 2023b; Ministry of Health, 2024).

Aotearoa New Zealand has the third highest rate of adult obesity in the Organization for Economic Cooperation and Development (OECD), with one in three adults being obese (Ministry of Health, 2024). In Australia, 75 per cent of men are classified as being overweight or obese (AIHW, 2022). Overweight and obesity is the second leading cause of ill health and premature deaths in males (AIHW, 2023b).

Three in five males in Australia, rate their health as excellent or very good (AIHW, 2023a). Despite the figure, males are more likely to engage in risky health behaviours, including high alcohol consumption, poor dietary choices, physical inactivity and smoking. Smoking is the leading preventable cause of ill health and premature deaths and is responsible for 9.2 per cent of the total disease burden in Australia (AIHW, 2023b). Excess alcohol consumption, sexual health risks, violence and low health literacy are some other factors that influence men's health, with a higher incidence of males reporting worse health status. These factors, combined with lower levels of accessing health services, result in higher levels of ischaemic heart disease, type 2 diabetes, anxiety and depression, lung cancer, stroke, chronic obstructive pulmonary disease, prostate, and colorectal cancers, self-inflicted injuries and suicide (AIHW, 2023b).

Suicide is another leading cause of death for males in Australia and Aotearoa New Zealand. Males are around three times more likely to die as a result of suicide compared to females in Australia and more than twice as likely to die by suicide than females in Aotearoa New Zealand (Australian Bureau of Statistics (ABS), 2021a; Coronial Services of New

Zealand, 2022). The *National Men's Health Strategy 2020–2030* (Department of Health, 2019) outlines Australia's national approach to improving the health of men and boys, highlighting five priority issues to address the country's health disparities. These are:

1. Mental health and well-being
2. Chronic health conditions
3. Sexual and reproductive health
4. Injuries and risk-taking behaviour
5. Healthy aging.

The strategy also highlights nine key population groups with worse reported health outcomes, including males who are:

- Indigenous
- living in rural and remote areas
- socially isolated
- veterans
- in the criminal justice system
- from cultural and linguistically diverse backgrounds
- socio-economically disadvantaged
- living with a disability
- members of the LGBTQIA+ community.

The strategy aims to empower and support males to optimise their health and well-being, build an evidence base for the future and strengthen health services capacity to provide quality age-appropriate management (Department of Health, 2019).

Globally, there has been an increased awareness of the health challenges faced by men. However, the health of men remains a concern and highlights the need for ongoing research and gender-specific health policies implemented to improve the health of all (Xiao et al., 2022).

Women's health concerns

Women in Australia and Aotearoa New Zealand comprise around 50 per cent of their respective populations (AIHW, 2023a; Stats NZ, 2023). Around 14 per cent of Australian females are living in poverty with an estimated 54 000 being homeless in 2021. This is an increase of over 10 per cent from 2016, compared to an increase of only 1.6 per cent for men (AIHW, 2023a). Women account for around 50 per cent of the homeless population in Aotearoa New Zealand and younger, Māori women who are single parents are disproportionately represented.

Women in Aotearoa New Zealand and Australia are financially disadvantaged, earning lower wages than men. While the gender pay gap in Australia is estimated at 16 per cent (ABS 2024), in Aotearoa New Zealand it has been steadily decreasing since 1998 to 8.6 per cent in 2023 (Ministry for Women, 2023). Financial disadvantage for women is important because, when compared to the general population, socio-economically disadvantaged women have poorer health outcomes (AIHW, 2023a). Some 56 per cent of Australian females have one or more chronic conditions, including arthritis, asthma, back problems, cancer, chronic obstructive pulmonary disease, diabetes, heart, stroke and vascular disease, chronic kidney disease, osteoporosis and mental health concerns and 34 per cent of the disease burden for women is preventable (AIHW, 2023a).

Cardiovascular disease and breast cancer are leading causes of ill health and death in Australian and Aotearoa New Zealand women (AIHW, 2023a; Royal Australian and New Zealand College of Obstetricians and Gynaecologists (RANZCOG), 2023). Obesity is a common health issue in both countries, affecting 30 per cent of women (AIHW, 2024b; RANZCOG, 2023). This is concerning as overweight and obesity increase the risk of cardiovascular disease, type 2 diabetes, chronic kidney disease, cancers, musculoskeletal conditions, dementia and asthma (AIHW, 2023a). Musculoskeletal disorders, including osteoporosis and arthritis, account for 16 per cent of the disease burden in women in Australia, and around half of the women in Aotearoa New Zealand over 60 years of age have osteoporosis (AIHW, 2023a; RANZCOG, 2023). Women are more likely than men to experience mental health concerns (AIHW, 2022; RANZCOG, 2023) with 45 per cent of women in Australia aged 16 and over reporting they have had a mental health disorder at some time in their life (AIHW, 2022).

Due to their sex and gender, women experience substantial disadvantage and discrimination across their lifespan. The health outcomes of women are influenced by multiple sociocultural factors, including unequal power relationships and gender inequality, where men often have greater access to education and financial opportunities (WHO, 2024a). Women are at higher risk of experiencing domestic and family violence, including sexual violence (RANZCOG, 2023; WHO, 2024a). Further barriers to the good health of women include the focus on their sexual and reproductive health at the expense of their broader health needs due to women's biological role in childbearing and how they are socialised to prioritise motherhood (Mello et al., 2019).

Women have traditionally been under-represented in research, which has led to a lack of knowledge regarding gender-specific conditions, for example, reproductive health issues such as endometriosis. Due to this lack of understanding, there are substantial delays for women to be diagnosed with this condition (Cromeens et al., 2021). Additionally, limited gender-specific research means there is a lack of knowledge and understanding about differences in how men and women experience disease and respond to treatment (RANZCOG, 2023). This is particularly evident with cardiovascular disease, where women are underdiagnosed and undertreated, more likely to receive inappropriate treatment for myocardial infarction (Department of Health, 2018) and more likely to die after cardiac surgery, cardiac arrest and sustaining severe burns (Modra et al., 2022). There is also limited knowledge about the intersectionality of women's health and how women from diverse backgrounds experience health and health concerns (RANZCOG, 2023). Contributing to a lack of knowledge about women's health is the lack of funding for women's health research and the stigma that surrounds some women's health concerns, such as menstrual disorders and menopause. The *National Women's Health Strategy 2020–2030* identified that further research and education about menstrual health and menstrual disorders are necessary to improve health and well-being outcomes for women (Department of Health, 2018).

Health concerns for LGBTQIA+ people

The acronym LGBTQIA+ identifies diverse sexuality and gender orientations and refers to **lesbian**, bisexual, **gay**, transgender, **queer/questioning**, intersex, asexual and + to recognise

Lesbian – a term describing a woman who is sexually and romantically attracted to other individuals who also identify as women.

Gay – a term describing a man who is sexually and romantically attracted to other individuals who also identify as men. Sometimes the term 'gay' can be used as an umbrella term that is inclusive of lesbians and gay men.

Queer/questioning – a broad term to include and embrace all sexual and gender-diverse identities. It can also be used by people when other terms related to sexuality or gender identity do not fit with their identity. 'Questioning' is a term describing a person who is exploring or questioning their sexuality or gender. They do not want labels applied to how they experience their sexual or gender identity.

other terms that people may use to describe their body, sexuality and gender diversity such as non-binary, pansexual and gender fluid. This is not an exhaustive list, and individuals' bodies, gender and sexuality can change over time. The SDH have some nuanced differences for LGBTQIA+ individuals and negative interactions with health care providers can, at times, lead to poor health outcomes. The LGBTQIA+ community have additional health burdens beyond those of men and women.

LGBTQIA+ individuals generally report having lower self-rated health than the general population, and over half have one or more health conditions (Hill et al., 2020) (Figure 6.3). LGBTQIA+ people have a higher burden of health conditions such as sexually transmitted

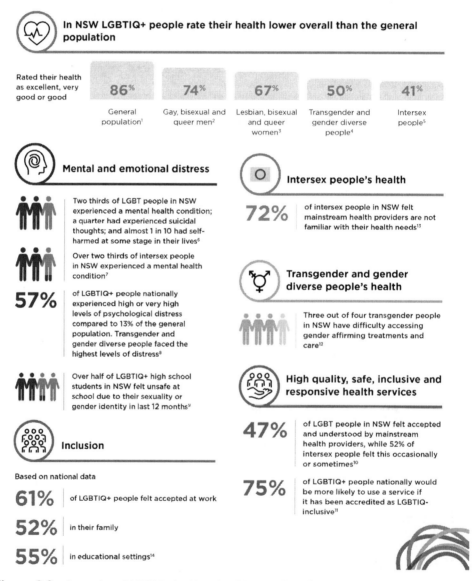

Figure 6.3   A snapshot of LGBTIQ+ health and well-being in New South Wales and Australia
Source: Reproduced by permission, NSW Health © 2024.

infection and Human Immunodeficiency Virus (HIV), and they are more likely to smoke and consume excessive amounts of alcohol (Hill et al., 2020).

More than half the LGBTQIA+ individuals report higher emotional and psychological distress and a higher prevalence of mental health diagnoses, in particular depression and anxiety, than the general population (Hill et al., 2020; Veale et al., 2019). Mental ill health is increased for LGBTQIA+ individuals who experience discrimination and have multiple marginalities (Dickson & Betts, 2018; Swan et al., 2023). LGBTQIA+ communities in Australia and Aotearoa New Zealand have a higher risk of suicidality and self-harm than the general population, and trans people are at significantly greater risk of taking their own lives (Dickson & Betts, 2018; Hill et al., 2020; Marchi et al., 2022). Precursors to the high risk of suicidal ideation attempted suicide and self-harm for trans people include transphobia, desiring gender-affirming surgery, discrimination, stigmatisation, marginalisation and violence (Loo et al., 2021; Veale et al., 2019; Zwickl et al., 2021).

Domestic and family violence

Domestic and family violence can affect all people regardless of age, ethnicity and gender; however, women and children are over-represented (AIHW, 2024a). Although men are less likely to experience domestic and family violence, they may find it difficult to access support and/or be stigmatised when they do. Violence against women is defined as 'any act of gender-based violence that results in, or is likely to result in, physical, sexual, or mental harm or suffering to women, including threats of such acts, coercion or arbitrary deprivation of liberty, whether occurring in public or in private life' (UN Women Australia, 2020). Domestic violence is not limited to physical violence and can also include economic, psychological, emotional, verbal and sexual abuse, controlling behaviour, stalking and technology-facilitated abuse (UN Women Australia, 2020).

One in three women globally has experienced physical and/or sexual violence in their lifetime, with most of this violence being perpetrated by their intimate partners (Figure 6.4). Intimate partner violence has serious consequences for women, negatively impacting their mental, physical, social, psychological and financial well-being (WHO, 2021). In Australia, 23 per cent of women aged 15 or over have experienced physical or sexual abuse by an intimate partner, compared to 7.8 per cent of men. Additionally, 16.9 per cent of women and 5.5 per cent of men were physically or sexually abused before the age of 15 and one woman is killed every 9 days by a partner (AIHW, 2024a; UN Women Australia, 2020). In Aotearoa New Zealand in 2018, 4.2 per cent of women aged 15–49 years reported they had experienced physical and/or sexual intimate partner violence in the past 12 months and on average, 9 women die at the hands of a current or ex-partner annually (Family Violence Death Review Committee, 2021).

As domestic and family violence contributes substantially to the disease burden for women in Australia and Aotearoa New Zealand, nurses in community settings need to be able to identify patients at-risk. In addition to screening for domestic and family violence, health professionals in PHC settings require knowledge about available resources and referral pathways to adequately support women and ensure their safety (Usanov et al., 2023).

How common is family, domestic and sexual violence?

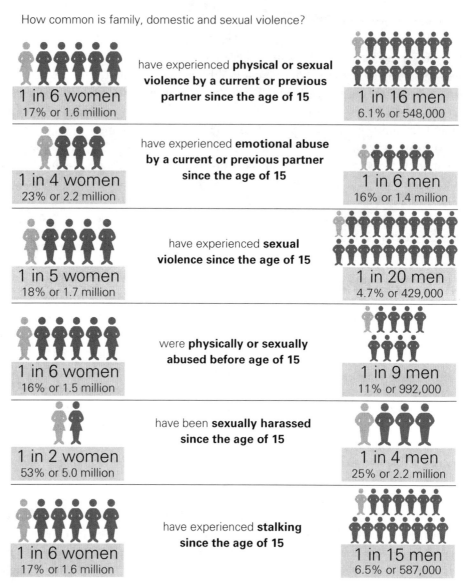

Figure 6.4   The prevalence of family, domestic and sexual violence
Source: Australian Institute of Health and Welfare (2019).

Challenges engaging in health care

Challenges for men

Men are less likely to seek advice from health professionals and use health care services than women (Sharp et al., 2022). They have shorter consultations and attend medical appointments with health care professionals when a condition or illness is in its later stages (Yousaf, Grunfeld & Hunter, 2015). When health advice is delayed, it reduces the opportunity for early diagnosis and intervention, which can significantly impact illness trajectory and prognosis (Yousaf et al., 2015). Men can find general practice unwelcoming and unaccommodating for their health care needs (Mursa et al., 2022).

Commonly reported barriers preventing men from accessing effective health care include individual, health system, structural and cultural issues (Macdonald et al., 2022). Individual barriers include issues pertaining to masculinity, self-resilience and the outward perception of being in control and strong. The reluctance in admitting to ill health or needing to seek advice from a health professional was associated with a perception of male strength and stoicism (Rice et al., 2020). Similarly, delaying seeking health advice and downplaying concerns of physical or emotional symptoms are not uncommon in males, and the motivation to finally seek advice comes when symptoms are severe and the condition is beyond the point of early intervention (Macdonald et al., 2022; Yousaf et al., 2015). Fear of a diagnosis, required treatment and mortality impact men's health care engagement (Macdonald et al., 2022), as might the need to share the intimate nature of a health concern or undergo a physical examination (Saab, Landers & Hegarty, 2017).

Health system barriers impact health care engagement for men and include issues in relation to access and availability of health care providers, particularly evident in smaller or rural, regional or remote communities (Macdonald et al., 2022). Relationships with health care providers are crucial, with communication and trust paramount in building therapeutic relationships and supporting sustained engagement (Davy et al., 2016). Health care providers' skills in questioning and delivering care, together with their knowledge or lack of understanding around the specific needs of men, impact engagement. The detrimental effects of stigma and feeling judged by health care providers can negatively impact help-seeking and deter men from disclosing symptoms such as depression and/or suicidal ideation (Mackenzie et al., 2019). Services that fail to provide information on the health care needs of men impact their sense of inclusion, (McCabe et al., 2016) and the promotion of male health literacy (Whitehead et al., 2020).

There are a number of structural barriers that negatively impact health care engagement for men including limited accessible appointments and minimal availability of consultations outside of traditional working hours, ultimately making timely access difficult (Ashley et al., 2020).

Cultural barriers that negatively impact health care engagement for men include issues such as culturally unsafe services, a lack of cultural knowledge, stigma, discrimination and language (Macdonald et al., 2022). Masculinity and culture are richly interwoven, and this can have a profound impact on help-seeking and engagement in health care for men, particularly around mental health concerns (Gough & Novikova, 2020). When engagement with health services and health care providers who fail to consider cultural values, norms and beliefs, trust is lost and future help-seeking and engagement is detrimentally impacted (Canuto et al., 2019).

CASE STUDY 6.1

Richard is a 42-year-old tradesman who works as a Fly-in Fly-out (FIFO) worker for a big mining company interstate. Richard is married and has three children under 15. When he is not working, he lives with his family in rural Victoria. His roster is a 'four weeks on, two weeks off' pattern. By necessity, Richard's wife is a stay-at-home parent.

Richard has become increasingly preoccupied with the future of his employment at the mine as there have been rumours that the company might be laying off workers soon. Richard is concerned that he might not be able to find another job to support his family.

> ## CASE STUDY 6.1 Continued
>
> Lately, Richard has been finding it difficult to get up and attend his shifts and has become less interested in socialising after work, although he finds that having a few drinks when not on duty helps him with his anxiety. His work colleagues have commented that he does not seem like his usual self. His wife has also expressed concern that he seems to drink a lot when off duty.
>
> Recently, an information session was organised at the mine by the local clinic nurses for R U OK? Day. Richard has been wondering if he should discuss his concerns with a nurse, but he is not sure what to do, does not want anybody to know and thinks he should be able to sort out his own problems.
>
> ### REFLECTION
> 1. What are the biological and psychosocial factors that could have an impact on Richard's health and his willingness to seek help?
> 2. What other information might be needed for the PHC nurse to be able to design interventions for Richard?
> 3. What support could you put in place for Richard?

Challenges for women

Women experience significant challenges engaging in health care due to the limited availability of services, which has resulted in 26 per cent of women waiting longer than they want for an appointment with a GP (ABS, 2021b; RANZCOG, 2023). Gender inequality in society is also responsible for women not being able to access care. The gender pay gap may mean that women are unable to afford transportation to or access affordable health care. Therefore, they either delay or do not seek health care advice and delay/avoid filling prescriptions for essential medications, which can result in poor health outcomes (ABS, 2021b).

Low health literacy provides a substantial challenge for women engaging with health care services. Health literacy is defined as 'the ability of a health seeker to find, access and make decisions about health content without relying on others to navigate or interpret it' (Bartlett et al., 2022, pp. 584–5), and lower levels of health literacy results in poor health outcomes. Women who are socio-economically disadvantaged and have lower levels of education have been found to have lower health literacy (Hosking et al., 2018). Low health literacy has also been found in women who are older and have lifestyle risk factors for chronic disease (Hosking et al., 2018), as well as culturally diverse women (Bartlett et al., 2022), which provides unique challenges to engaging with health care services.

The existence of gender bias in health care has resulted in women's concerns not being taken seriously, with over one in three women reporting their health concerns have been dismissed by a GP. This has deterred women from accessing care and has been responsible for a failure to thoroughly investigate symptoms, resulting in delays in diagnosis and access to timely and appropriate care (RANZCOG, 2023). Although gender bias affects all women, some experience additional types of discrimination for example based on their race, ethnicity or disability. Discrimination can result in women not feeling safe when accessing health services and acts as a barrier to future access (RANZCOG, 2023).

Women experiencing mental health concerns and trauma from sexual or domestic violence face multiple barriers to engaging with health care providers. They can experience stigma and shame, and often have a mistrust of health care systems and providers (de Boer et al., 2022). They also have poor access to trauma-informed care and specialised services are costly and not sustainable (de Boer et al., 2022).

Geographic location and cultural and language barriers can be substantial challenges for women in seeking help and receiving appropriate care. Women living in rural, regional and remote areas experience challenges due to inadequate services, limited availability of health care professionals and less access to gender-specific health care (RANZCOG, 2023). Cultural and language barriers to effective health care exist for women who are from Indigenous, migrant or refugee populations. Language difficulties can result in a lack of knowledge and awareness of health concerns. Further, women have reported their inability to make appointments and express their health concerns due to a lack of English proficiency (Kim, 2021). Difficulties with language can also limit communication between women and their health care providers, which prevents rapport building and may lead to mistrust in health services (Kim, 2021). Cultural barriers to engaging in health care can also include cultural norms and beliefs that do not align with evidence and treatment options provided by health services (Ndwiga et al., 2023). Therefore, to ensure that women receive appropriate care, it is imperative that nurses understand the nuances of culture and provide culturally tailored advice to promote positive health outcomes for women from all backgrounds (Ndwiga et al., 2023).

Challenges for gender-diverse people

Accessing health care services can be complicated for LGBTQIA+ people because of the heteronormative systems that pathologise body, sexual, and gender identities (Hill et al., 2021). It is illegal in Australia and Aotearoa New Zealand to discriminate against people on the grounds of their sexual orientation or gender identity (Government of Australia, 2022; Human Rights Commission, n.d.). Some of the barriers LGBTQIA+ people experience when accessing health care include the clinicians' lack of knowledge heteronormative health care services, stigmatisation, persistent exposure to discrimination and concerns about being disrespected (Hill et al., 2021; New South Wales Health, 2022; Veale et al., 2019).

Care for LGBTQIA+ people's mental health and emotional distress is paramount. While there has been a positive and increasing focus on everyone's mental health, LGBTQIA+ people have been shown to have high needs for mental health care and suicide prevention services (Dickson & Betts, 2018; Hill et al., 2020; Veale et al., 2019). PHC providers are a common source of professional care and can support and assist by including mental health questions in their interactions with LGBTQIA+ clients (McNair & Bush, 2016). Having contact details of culturally safe mental health care services for referrals assists clients in accessing professional support (Lucas et al., 2023).

Institutions and service providers can support LGBTQIA+ individuals when seeking PHC by using culturally safe, person-centred strategies. Historically, most health-related documents have been restrictive regarding the pronouns they use on forms. The use of pronouns is important for the LGBTQIA+ community, with some individuals preferring not to use the binary she/her or he/him but rather they/them or some other combination. Changing current practices by changing the language used on admission and assessment forms such as adding she/her he/him 'they/them' and 'prefer to write myself' with respect to the preferred pronouns, improves cultural safety for LGBTQIA+ clients (Loo et al., 2021).

Patients have identified that disclosure of sexual orientation and gender identity are beneficial to individualised care, however, they report concerns about the risk of bias and discrimination (Maragh-Bass et al., 2017). In contrast, providers report feeling uncomfortable asking questions about sexual orientation and were concerned about causing offence, but only a minority of LGBTQIA+ people report they would be offended. However, research shows that only 51 per cent of older lesbians and 64 per cent of older gay men felt comfortable disclosing their sexuality (Lyons et al., 2021). Internalised homophobia and lower connection to the LGBTQIA+ community led to older gay and lesbian people not feeling comfortable disclosing their sexual identity to their health care provider.

It is important not to assume bodily, sexual or gender identity based on the person's appearance, style of dress or tone of voice. Many important health care issues related to biological characteristics can be missed if assumptions are made and the client is not included in their health care choices. Therefore, pertinent health care screening, considering the natal body of the person is important. For example, an older trans man who has not had gender-affirming surgery may still need cervical screening. Failing to engage the trans man in his care may lead to poor health outcomes. Ensuring the physical health assessment includes information about the person's natal body as well as relevant information about the person's gender identity will improve health outcomes for trans, non-binary and gender-diverse people.

As more transgender, gender non-binary and gender-diverse youth self-identify, there is a growing need to offer safe and appropriate information and support for gender-affirming care (Lane et al., 2021). Gender-affirming care is particularly essential when the person's expressed or experienced gender does not align with their assigned sex (Lane et al., 2021). Gender-affirming therapy can improve quality of life, self-esteem, body satisfaction and social functioning, mitigate distress and decrease poor mental health outcomes. There are, however, barriers to people accessing hormones, medications, advice, referrals and mental health care plans (Strauss et al., 2022). The process of undertaking gender-affirming therapy can be interminable and very expensive, and this may impact the person's ability to access these services (Lane et al., 2021). Staff knowledge and attitudes towards gender diversity can be suboptimal, where trans, non-binary and gender-diverse people report needing to educate providers about the experience of being gender-diverse (Cosio et al., 2022; Strauss et al., 2022). Other barriers include disorganised and uncoordinated care, referrals being lost, miscommunication between services and needing to see multiple PHC providers to obtain timely and supportive care. PHC providers need knowledge related to monitoring and administering hormonal interventions and have appropriate referral pathways for trans, non-binary and gender-diverse people for gender-affirming therapies (Loo et al., 2021).

PHC services can provide culturally safe and inclusive care, promoting psychological safety by:

- asking about preferred pronouns and the person's preferred name and updating their medical records (Strauss et al., 2022).
- supporting LGBTQIA+ people's visibility by not making cis-heteronormative assumptions.
- providing education and training about the LGBTQIA+ community and their health needs (Loo et al., 2021).
- displaying positive LGBTQIA+ related imagery such as rainbow flags or LGBTQIA+ health-related literature in the waiting areas (Lucas et al., 2023).
- providing access to gender-neutral bathrooms and spaces (Cosio et al., 2022).

CASE STUDY 6.2

Peter is a 65-year-old self-identified gay man in a loving relationship with his long-time partner Aata. Peter has been seeing his regular GP for over 20 years. His GP, however, has told him that she is retiring so he needs to find another GP. He feels concerned about this. He knows he will need to do 'the usual' things. Peter's experience is that if he mentions he has a partner, health practitioners usually assume it is a woman, and it is up to him to correct this assumption. He knows that typically following his 'coming out', there is usually a small silence that often feels awkward. He has always felt this is the moment when the practitioner considers Peter's sexual preference. Depending on the GP's response, Peter knows he will either feel comfortable or will decide to find another GP. As the nurse, you will be seeing Peter before he meets the new GP.

REFLECTION

1. Why do you think Peter is hesitant to meet a new GP?
2. How can you help create a safe practice environment so that Peter feels comfortable disclosing his sexuality?
3. Do you think there are any particular health concerns that you might need to be aware of with Peter's health?

Implications for person-centred practice

Gender stereotypes, role modelling, social norms and unconscious and conscious bias contribute to gender inequity (VicHealth, 2017). Unconscious or implicit bias refers to attitudes people may not be aware of. However, these alter perceptions, affect information processing, behaviours and interactions with others, and decision making (Marcelin et al., 2019). Conscious or explicit bias stems from discriminatory values, is more targeted and can lead to abuse (Persaud, 2019). Neither form of bias is acceptable in health care. Gender bias, whether unconscious or conscious, results in unequal access to care or inadequate or inappropriate treatment, which perpetuates health disparities (Marcelin et al., 2019). Restrictive gender norms and gender bias affect everybody – men, women and sexually and gender-diverse people. Nurses working in PHC settings need to reflect on their own biases to prevent them from harming those seeking health care (Marcelin et al., 2019). PHC nurses may require additional training and education focusing on diversity and inclusion, incorporating understanding and self-reflection of unconscious and gender bias (Persaud, 2019).

Nurses working in PHC settings require an understanding of how gender intersects with other societal oppressions, including social class, ethnicity and sexual orientation, which also impact health and access to health care (Alexander et al., 2017). Additionally, they must be aware of vulnerable populations who may experience various forms of discrimination, isolation, social exclusion, income inequity and interpersonal violence. Nurses in PHC have a role in social justice and advocacy by raising awareness and contributing to public debates about how privilege and disadvantage are created and sustained in society and challenging the status quo to disrupt gender norms in health systems (Alexander et al., 2017; Hay et al., 2019).

> ## REFLECTION
>
> Conscious and unconscious bias directed by health professionals towards the LGBTQIA+ community can adversely affect health outcomes. Reflect on your own biases and think about how you would manage these in interactions with people in PHC settings.

Conclusion

Women, men and sexually and gender-diverse people may require different approaches in health care delivery. Health disparities between people exist due to their biological characteristics, different social positions, gender-specific roles and socialisation shaped by their cultural context. An understanding of the impact of biology and gender, and how they intersect with other SDH of health is important for PHC providers to be effective in assessing needs and planning interventions. Nurses play an important role in promoting access to care and breaking down barriers around stigma. As such, nurses need to consider the impact that their practice has on those seeking health care.

CRITICAL THINKING ACTIVITIES

1. How can PHC nurses improve health outcomes for all people using a PHC approach?
2. What strategies could you implement to provide sensitive and person-centred care?
3. What further education and training do you require to deliver culturally competent and gender-sensitive care in the PHC setting?

FURTHER READING

Department of Families, Fairness and Housing (2023). *LGBTIQA+ Inclusive Language Guide*. State Government of Victoria. www.vic.gov.au/inclusive-language-guide

Fanslow, J.L. & McIntosh, T. (2023). *Key findings and policy and practice implications from He Koiora Matapopore. The 2019 New Zealand Family Violence Study*. University of Auckland. https://hdl .handle.net/2292/64262

Healthy Male. (2023). Resources and tools. www.healthymale.org.au/resources-tools

REFERENCES

ACON. (2019). *A language guide: Trans and gender diverse inclusion*. www.acon.org.au/wp-content/ uploads/2019/07/TGD_Language-Guide.pdf

Alexander, I., Johnson-Mallard, V., Kostas-Polston, E., et al. (eds). (2017). *Women's Health Care in Advanced Practice Nursing* (2nd ed.). Springer Publishing Company.

Ashley, C., Halcomb, E., McInnes, S., et al. (2020). Middle-aged Australians' perceptions of support to reduce lifestyle risk factors: A qualitative study. *Australian Journal of Primary Health, 26*(4), 313. https://doi.org/10.1071/PY20030

Australian Bureau of Statistics (ABS). (2021a). *Patient Experiences in Australia: Summary of Findings*. www.abs.gov.au/statistics/health/causes-death/causes-death-australia/latest-release#cite-window1

—— (2021b). *Patient experiences in Australia: Summary of findings*. www.abs.gov.au/statistics/health/health-services/patient-experiences/2020-21#data-downloads

—— (2024). *Average weekly earnings, Australia*. www.abs.gov.au/statistics/labour/earnings-and-working-conditions/average-weekly-earnings-australia/latest-release#:~:text=Estimates%20for%20average%20weekly%20ordinary%20time%20earnings%20for,For%20females%20were%20%20%241%2C897.70%20%20%28public%29%2C%20and%20%20%241%2C605.30%20%20%28private%29

Australian Human Rights Commission (AHRC). (2018). *Face the facts: Gender equality 2018*. https://humanrights.gov.au/sites/default/files/2018_Face_the_Facts_Gender_Equality.pdf

Australian Institute of Health and Welfare (AIHW). (2019). *The health of Australia's males*. Australian Government. Retrieved from https://www.aihw.gov.au/reports/men-women/male-health

—— (2022). *Australia's health 2022: In brief*. Australian Government. www.aihw.gov.au/reports/australias-health/australias-health-2022-in-brief

—— (2023a). *The health of Australia's females*. Australian Government. www.aihw.gov.au/reports/men-women/female-health/contents/about

—— (2023b). *The health of Australia's males*. Australian Government. www.aihw.gov.au/reports/men-women/male-health

—— (2024a). *Family, domestic and sexual violence*. Australian Government. https://www.aihw.gov.au/reports/domestic-violence/family-domestic-and-sexual-violence#common

—— (2024b). *Overweight and obesity*, Australian Government. www.aihw.gov.au/reports/overweight-obesity/overweight-and-obesity/contents/about

Australian Institute of Family Studies. (2022). *LBGTIQA+ glossary of common terms*. https://aifs.gov.au/resources/resource-sheets/lgbtiqa-glossary-common-terms

Bartlett, R., Robinson, T., Anand, J., et al. (2022). Empathy and journey mapping the healthcare experience: A community-based participatory approach to exploring women's access to primary health services within Melbourne's Arabic-speaking refugee communities. *Ethnicity & Health*, *27*(3), 584–600.

Blondeel, K., de Vasconcelos, S., García-Moreno, C., et al. (2018). Violence motivated by perception of sexual orientation and gender identity: A systematic review. *Bulletin of the World Health Organization*, *96*(1), 29–41E. https://doi.org/10.2471/BLT.17.197251

Canadian Institutes of Health Research (CIHR). (2023). *What is gender? What is sex?* Government of Canada. https://cihr-irsc.gc.ca/e/48642.html

Canuto, K., Harfield, S., Wittert, G., et al. (2019). Listen, understand, collaborate: Developing innovative strategies to improve health service utilisation by Aboriginal and Torres Strait Islander men. *Australian and New Zealand Journal of Public Health*, *43*(4), 307–9. https://doi.org/10.1111/1753-6405.12922

Coronial Services of New Zealand. (2022). *Suicide*. New Zealand Government. https://coronialservices.justice.govt.nz/suicide/suicide-statistics/

Cosio, I., Goldman, L., MacKenzie, M., et al. (2022). Gender-affirming primary care. *BC Medical Journal*, *61*(1), 20–2.

Cromeens, M.G, Carey, E.T, Robinson, WR., et al. (2021). Timing, delays and pathways to diagnosis of endometriosis: a scoping review protocol. *BMJ Open* 2021, *11*, e049390. https://doi.org/10.1136/bmjopen-2021-049390

Davy, C., Cass, A., Brady, J., et al. (2016). Facilitating engagement through strong relationships between primary healthcare and Aboriginal and Torres Strait Islander peoples. *Australian and New Zealand Journal of Public Health*, *40*(6), 535–41. https://doi.org/10.1111/1753-6405.12553

de Boer, K., Arnold, C., Mackelprang, J, et al. (2022). Barriers and facilitators to treatment seeking and engagement amongst women with complex trauma histories. *Health and Social Care in the Community*, *30*, e4303–e4310.

Department of Health. (2018). *National Women's Health Strategy 2020–2030*. Commonwealth of Australia. www.health.gov.au/sites/default/files/documents/2021/05/national-women-s-health-strategy-2020-2030_0.pdf

———— (2019). *National Men's Health Strategy 2020–2030*. Commonwealth of Australia. www.health .gov.au/resources/publications/national-mens-health-strategy-2020-2030?language=en

Dickson, S. & Betts, D. (2018). *All Right? An Exploration of Wellbeing in the Ōtautahi LGBTIQA+ Community*. Flipside Consulting. https://legacy.allright.org.nz/media/documents/LGBTQIA_Wellbeing_Report_-_FINAL_post.pdf

Family Violence Death Review Committee. (2021). Intimate partner violence deaths in Aotearoa New Zealand. Health, Quality and Safety Commission, New Zealand. www.hqsc.govt.nz/assets/Our-work/Mortality-review-committee/FVDRC/Publications-resources/Supplementary_detail_IPV_2021.pdf

Fetherston, H. & Craike, M. (2020). *Australia's Gender Health Tracker*. Mitchell Institute Victoria University. www.vu.edu.au/sites/default/files/australias-gender-health-tracker-2020.pdf

Gough, B. & Novikova, I. (2020). *Mental health, men and culture: How do sociocultural constructions of masculinities relate to men's mental health help-seeking behaviour in the WHO European Region?* World Health Organization. https://apps.who.int/iris/handle/10665/332974

Government of Australia. (2022). *Act No.4, Sex Discrimination Act 1984*. Government of Australia. www.legislation.gov.au/Details/C2023C00003

Hay, K., McDougal, L., Percival, V., et al. (2019). Disrupting gender norms in health systems: making the case for change. *The Lancet, 393*(10190), 2535–49.

Hill, A.O., Bourne, A., McNair, R., et al. (2020). *Private Lives 3: The Health and Wellbeing of LBGTIQ People in Australia*. (ARCSHS Monograph Series no. 122.) Australian Research Centre in Sex, Health and Society, La Trobe University.

Hill, A.O., Lyons, A., Jones, J., et al. (2021). *Writing Themselves in 4: The Health and Wellbeing of LBGTIQA+ young people in Australia*. (National Report, Monograph Series no. 124.) Australian Research Centre in Sex, Health and Society, La Trobe University.

Hosking, S., Brennan-Olsen, S., Beauchamp, A., et al. (2018). Health literacy in a population-based sample of Australian women: A cross-sectional profile of the Geelong Osteoporosis study. *BMC Public Health, 18*(876), 18:876. https://doi.org/10.1186/s12889-018-5751-8

Human Rights Commission. (n.d.). *What is unlawful discrimination*. https://tikatangata.org.nz/human-rights-in-aotearoa/what-is-unlawful-discrimination

Kim, S.K. (2021). Beyond language: Motivators and barriers to breast cancer screening among Korean-speaking women in Sydney Metropolitan, Australia. *Health Promotion Journal of Australia, 33*(2), 412–25. https://doi.org/10.1002/hpja.507

Klasen, S. (2020). From 'MeToo' to Boko Haram: A survey of levels and trends of gender inequality in the world. *World Development*, 128, 104862. https://doi.org/10.1016/j.worlddev.2019.104862

Lane, J., McCarthy, C., Dart, G., et al. (2021). Establishing a province-wide referral network to improve access to gender-affirming primary healthcare services. *The Nurse Practitioner, 46*(8), 39–43.

Loo, S., Almazan, A.N., Vedilago, V., et al. (2021). Understanding community member and health care professional perspectives on gender-affirming care – A qualitative study. *PloS ONE, 16*(8), e0255568.

Lucas, J.J., Afrouz, R., Brown, A.D., et al. (2023). When primary healthcare meets queerstory: Community-based system dynamics influencing regional/rural LGBTQ+ people's access to quality primary healthcare in Australia. *BMC Public Health, 23*(1), 387.

Lyons, A., Alba, B., Waling, A., et al. (2021). Comfort among older lesbian and gay people in disclosing their sexual orientation to health and aged care services. *Journal of Applied Gerontology, 40*(2), 132–41.

Macdonald, J.A., Mansour, K.A., Wynter, K., et al. (2022). *Men's and boys' barriers to health system access: A literature review*. Prepared for the Australian Government Department of Health and Aged Care, Canberra.

Mackenzie, C.S., Visperas, A., Ogrodniczuk, J.S., et al. (2019). Age and sex differences in self-stigma and public stigma concerning depression and suicide in men. *Stigma and Health, 4*(2), 233–41. https://doi.org/10.1037/sah0000138

Marcelin, J.R., Siraj, D.S., Victor, R., et al. (2019). The impact of unconscious bias in healthcare: How to recognize and mitigate it. *Journal of Infectious Diseases, 220*: S62–S73. https://doi .org/10.1093/infdis/jiz214

Maragh-Bass, A.C., Torain, M., Adler, R., et al. (2017). Risks, benefits, and importance of collecting sexual orientation and gender identity data in healthcare settings: A multi-method analysis of patient and provider perspectives. *LGBT Health, 4*(2), 141–52.

Marchi, M., Arcolin, E., Fiore, G., et al. (2022). Self-harm and suicidality among LGBTIQ people: A systematic review and meta-analysis. *International Review of Psychiatry, 34*(3–4), 240–56. https://doi.org/10.1080/09540261.2022.2053070

McCabe, M.P., Mellor, D., Ricciardelli, L.A., et al. (2016). Ecological model of Australian Indigenous men's health. *American Journal of Men's Health, 10*(6), NP63–NP70. https://doi .org/10.1177/1557988315583086

McNair, R.P. & Bush, R. (2016). Mental health help seeking patterns and associations among Australian same sex attracted women, trans and gender diverse people: A survey-based study. *BMC Psychiatry, 16*, 1–16.

Mello, S., Tan, A.S.L., Sanders-Jackson, A., et al. (2019). Gender stereotypes and preconception health: Men's and women's expectations of responsibility and intentions to engage in preventive behaviors. *Maternal & Child Health Journal, 23*(4), 459–69.

Ministry for Women (2023). *The gender pay gap.* New Zealand Government. https://women.govt.nz/ women-and-work/gender-pay-gap

Ministry of Health. (2018). *Major causes of death.* New Zealand Government. www.health.govt.nz/ our-work/populations/maori-health/tatau-kahukura-maori-health-statistics/nga-mana-hauora-tutohu-health-status-indicators/major

——— (2024). *Obesity.* New Zealand Government. www.health.govt.nz/our-work/diseases-and-conditions/obesity

Modra, L., Higgins, A., Pilcher, D., et al. (2022). Sex differences in mortality of ICU patients according to diagnosis-related sex balance. *American Journal of Respiratory Critical Care Medicine, 206*(11), 1353–60.

Mursa, R., Patterson, C. & Halcomb, E. (2022). Men's help-seeking and engagement with general practice: An integrative review. *Journal of Advanced Nursing, 78*(7). https://doi.org/10.1111/jan.15240

Ndwiga, D., McBride, K., Thompson, R., et al. (2023). "We are competing with culture" the chasm between healthcare professionals and Australian Samoan women in the prevention and management of gestational diabetes mellitus. *Australian Journal of Advanced Nursing, 40*(2), 5–14. www.ajan.com.au/index.php/AJAN/article/view/591/version/576

New South Wales Ministry of Health. (2022). *NSW LGBTIQ+ Health Strategy 2022–2027.* NSW Government. www.health.nsw.gov.au/lgbtiq-health/Pages/lgbtiq-health-strategy.aspx

——— (2024). *The Impact of Stigma and Discrimination on Health and Wellbeing.* NSW Government. www.health.nsw.gov.au/lgbtiq-health/Publications/lgbtiq-health-strategy.pdf

Persaud, S. (2019). Addressing unconscious bias: A nurse leader's role. *Nursing Administration Quarterly, 43*(2), 130–7. https://doi.org/10.1097/naq.0000000000000348

Rice, S.M., Oliffe, J.L., Kealy, D., et al. (2020). Men's help-seeking for depression: Attitudinal and structural barriers in symptomatic men. *Journal of Primary Care & Community Health, 11*, 2150132720921686. https://doi.org/http://dx.doi.org/10.1177/2150132720921686

Royal Australian and New Zealand College of Obstetricians and Gynaecologists (RANZCOG). (2023). *Aotearoa New Zealand Women's Health Strategy.* https://ranzcog.edu.au/wp-content/uploads/2023/03/RANZCOG-Womens-Health-Strategy-Submission-2023-03-20.pdf

Saab, M.M., Landers, M. & Hegarty, J. (2017). Exploring awareness and help-seeking intentions for testicular symptoms among heterosexual, gay, and bisexual men in Ireland: A qualitative descriptive study. *International Journal of Nursing Studies, 67*, 41–50. https://doi.org/10.1016/j.ijnurstu.2016.11.016

Sharp, P., Bottorff, J.L., Rice, S., et al. (2022). "People say men don't talk, well that's bullshit": A focus group study exploring challenges and opportunities for men's mental health promotion. *PloS ONE, 17*(1), e0261997–e0261997. https://doi.org/10.1371/journal.pone.0261997

Stats NZ. (2021). *Growth in life expectancy slows*. New Zealand Government www.stats.govt.nz/news/growth-in-life-expectancy-slows/

—— (2023). *National population estimates: At June 2023*. New Zealand Government. www.stats.govt.nz/information-releases/national-population-estimates-at-30-june-2023/

Strauss, P., Winter, S., Waters, Z., et al. (2022). Perspectives of trans and gender diverse young people accessing primary care and gender-affirming medical services: Findings from trans pathways. *International Journal of Transgender Health, 23*(3), 295–307.

Swan, J., Phillips, T.M., Sanders, T., et al. (2023). Mental health and quality of life outcomes of gender-affirming surgery: A systematic literature review. *Journal of Gay & Lesbian Mental Health, 27*(1), 2–45.

United Nations Economic Commission for Europe (UNECE). (2015). *Indicators of Gender Equality*. www.unece.org/fileadmin/DAM/stats/publications/2015/ECE_CES_37_WEB.pdf

UN Women Australia. (2020). *Types of violence against women and girls*. https://unwomen.org.au/types-of-violence-against-women-and-girls/

Usanov, C., Keedle, H., Peters, K., et al. (2023) Exploration of barriers to screening for domestic violence in the perinatal period using an ecological framework. *Journal of Advanced Nursing, 79*(4), 1437–50.

Veale, J., Byrne, J.L., Tan, K.K., et al. (2019). *Counting Ourselves: The Health and Wellbeing of Trans and Non-binary People in Aotearoa New Zealand*. Transgender Health Research Lab.

Victorian Health Promotion Foundation (VicHealth). (2017). *Gender Equality, Health and Wellbeing Strategy 2017–19*. VicHealth. www.vichealth.vic.gov.au/-/media/ResourceCentre/PublicationsandResources/General/Gender-equality-health-wellbeing_strategy_2017-19.pdf?la=en&hash=E6D063A18B5FE1EF434C76040FE41DCB96DDABE9

Whitehead, M., Ng Chok, H., Whitehead, C., et al. (2020). Men's health promotion in waiting rooms: An observational study. *European Journal of Public Health, 30*(Supplement_5). https://doi.org/10.1093/eurpub/ckaa166.360

World Health Organization (WHO). (2021). *Gender and health*. www.who.int/news-room/questions-and-answers/item/gender-and-health

—— (2023). *Noncommunicable diseases*. www.who.int/news-room/fact-sheets/detail/noncommunicable-diseases

—— (2024a). *Gender and health*. www.who.int/health-topics/gender#tab=tab_1

—— (2024b.). *Social determinants of health*. www.who.int/health-topics/social-determinants-of-health#tab=tab_1

Xiao, H., Doolan-Noble, F., Liu, L., et al. (2022). Men's health research in New Zealand: A scoping review. *International Journal of Men's Social and Community Health, 5*(SP1), 1–28. https://doi.org/10.22374/ijmsch.v5iSP1.67

Yousaf, O., Grunfeld, E.A. & Hunter, M.S. (2015). A systematic review of the factors associated with delays in medical and psychological help-seeking among men. *Health Psychology Review, 9*(2), 264–76. https://doi.org/10.1080/17437199.2013.840954

Zwickl, S., Wong, A.F.Q., Dowers, E., et al. (2021). Factors associated with suicide attempts among Australian transgender adults. *BMC Psychiatry, 21*(1), 81. https://doi.org/10.1186/s12888-021-03084-7

A lifespan- and settings-based approach to mental health promotion[1]

7

Dean Whitehead

LEARNING OBJECTIVES

At the completion of this chapter, you should be able to:

- determine the context of mental health promotion.
- distinguish between the concepts of mental health and mental health wellness and well-being against mental illness, disease and disability.
- understand how both lifespan and health-promoting settings, along their continuum, influence mental health promotion in primary health care (PHC).

Introduction

In the 'classic' sense, health professionals often view the health of individuals from a three-part *biopsychosocial* model of health. In this case, the 'psych' part relates directly to **'mental health'**. However, it is important to resist the temptation to separate this part from the bio and social aspects of the well-established model. Instead, it is best to view all parts of the established model as equally important and interrelated to each other. For instance, it is difficult to maintain good mental health and well-being if we lack either good social or 'bio' (physical) health. Traditionally, however, health professionals have tended to focus on the physical health component of the biopsychosocial model, especially those working in acute hospital/clinic environments. From a PHC perspective, the 'social' (community development-focused) aspect is supposed to be the most dominant part of the model. It is from this position that Arango and colleagues (2018, p. 591) state:

> Gaps between knowledge, policy, and practice need to be bridged. Future steps should emphasise mental health promotion, and improvement of early detection and interventions in clinical settings, schools, and the community, with essential support from society and policy makers.

Mental health – the health of people regarding their psychological and emotional health.

---

1   This chapter is based on the following article: Whitehead, D. (2011). Before the cradle and beyond the grave: A lifespan/settings-based framework for health promotion. *Journal of Clinical Nursing, 20*(15–16), 2183–94.

Unfortunately, and mostly due to a lack of understanding and negative stereotypes, mental health (psych) is often the least represented of the three model components. Furthermore, mental health is often viewed by health professionals in the context of illness, disease and/or disability and often as the domain of specific mental health specialists. The reality is, though, that all health professionals should be actively engaged in mental health promotion and particularly at the 'preventative' PHC level, in effect, 'refocusing upstream'. Where this is not happening, Calloway (2007) has asked the question of mental health promotion: 'Is nursing dropping the ball?' To address the criticism of 'dropping the ball', Lahti and colleagues (2018) identify that postgraduate nurses need further education and training related to lifespan issues in mental health promotion at the preventative level.

There are many known perceived 'taboos' and stigmas attached to mental illness that further education, training, research, management and resourcing would go a long way to address. Informed awareness-raising is key. The intention of this chapter is to dispel those stereotypes and myths. In doing so, it explores how best to overcome these barriers and view mental health in the context of something we all live with – and 'can live well with'. The focus is on positive mental health, wellness and well-being, and the role of all health practitioners in promoting and achieving this in the PHC setting.

Defining mental health promotion

Mental health wellness and well-being – the acknowledgement that mental health is more than just the absence of mental illness, disease or disabilities – but a broader positive state of health.

Mental health wellness and well-being are states in which individuals work through their potential to cope with normal life stresses. Mental illness occurs when individuals become emotionally and psychologically overwhelmed and are unable to cope with the demands of everyday life. This is a common state for many and presents a significant health burden for both individuals and communities. Almost half (7.3 million) of Australian adults experience a mental health-related condition at some point in their lives (Department of Health and Aged Care, 2020). One-quarter of Australians experience a mental health disorder per year with anxiety disorders being the most common (Department of Health, 2020). The figures are similar for the Aotearoa New Zealand population – 47 per cent of Aotearoa New Zealand adults will experience a mental health disorder in their lifetime and one in five experience a mental health issue per year (Ministry of Health, 2019). In terms of mental health service provision, in Aotearoa New Zealand, 154 752 individuals were seen by mental health and addiction services between 2012 and 2013 (Ministry of Health, 2016). The relatively recent passing of the COVID-19 pandemic has significantly exacerbated and increased the current figures due to the negative influences of issues such as forced social isolation (Botha, Butterworth & Wilkins, 2022; Zhao et al., 2022). How an altered mental health state presents itself and for how long depends on many factors including personal resilience, self-efficacy, support mechanisms (social and professional), age, gender, culture and socio-economic status.

Mental health promotion – the promotion of the social, psychological and emotional well-being of individuals within and aligned to their communities – and outside of them.

At an individual level, **mental health promotion** focuses on increasing resilience and capacity to avoid or overcome a negative mental health state (Arango et al., 2018). It seeks to do so through fostering the development of positive personal skills and enhancing self-esteem. At a wider community level, it seeks to develop healthy environments that further promote individual and collective esteem. This is mainly achieved through developing and supporting inclusive social networks. Here, the important role of 'social' health as it impacts mental health is directly witnessed. At a wider structural, economic and political level, mental health promotion is directly influenced by public health policy processes that address mental health and well-being through promoting equity and inclusion, and reducing discrimination and stigmatisation (Kalra et al., 2012). If we list some of the more common reasons, in society, for mental 'illness', it is easier to see where discrimination might stem from and understand how certain 'marginalised' populations are at increased risk of mental ill health:

- homelessness
- low levels of education, low-status occupations and low incomes
- unemployment
- criminality
- social disadvantage
- discrimination (based on race, gender, religion, etc.).

Incorporating mental health promotion, prevention and early intervention improves mental health for all (especially within the highlighted marginalised populations) and reduces the prevalence and impact of mental health disorders across all populations. It ideally needs to occur beyond traditional acute health care systems and services and, instead, in PHC sectors that directly impact the daily lives of individuals and communities. These include housing, education, employment, welfare and justice. As Wand (2011, p. 131) critically states:

> The indication is that a broader public health approach that addresses social and environmental factors related to mental health and well-being is required. Mainstream mental health services, however, continue to operate in relative isolation, allocating the greatest proportion of funding and resources to the treatment of mental health illness and disorder.

Related to this is the 'conceptual' confusion that occurs between mental health promotion and mental health illness. In their concept analysis of mental health promotion, Tamminen and colleagues (2016, p. 177) state:

> a common feature has been the rather puzzling use of the term 'mental health' to describe matters related to mental ill health, causing confusion regarding the relationship between mental health and mental illness. Such differing definitions make it difficult to comprehend what mental health promotion is and what it constitutes.

To overcome the stated conceptual dilemmas, mental health promotion should aim to maximise the ability of children, youth, adults and older people to realise their mental health potential, cope with normal stresses of life and meaningfully participate with and be included in their communities (Walsh, Sheridan & Barry, 2023; Westrupp et al., 2023). Assisting this process are mainstream mental health promotion programs that have received national attention such as destigmatisation and awareness-raising campaigns that target whole communities (Walsh et al., 2023). These incorporate national organisations such as R U OK?, which is an Australian not-for-profit suicide prevention organisation (www.ruok.org.au) and the Aotearoa New Zealand Like Minds, Like Mine organisation campaigning against mental illness discrimination (www.likeminds.org.nz).

REFLECTION

One of the biggest challenges to mental health promotion for nurses in the PHC setting is the misconception that these services are serviced and implemented by specialist mental health nurses. Separating mental health from biophysical and social community roles is problematic. Mental health spans all ages and all populations in all settings. It does not just refer to people accessing specific mental health services (Verhaeghe et al., 2011; Wang et al., 2022).

Mental health care is the business of all health professionals and part of an inherent role and function for all.

Where do you think this misconception that mental health issues are exclusively serviced and implemented by specialist mental health nurses arises from?

A lifespan- and settings-based approach

Most people live busy lives. Most work and play in busy communities both professionally and socially. Innovations, particularly technological advances (such as social media), have made our lives even more hectic. Many people struggle with increasing day-to-day demands and hectic schedules. It is perhaps unsurprising that many people feel that they are not able to manage these demands or cope as well as they would like or compared to others around them. Such pressures inevitably impact a person's capacity to engage with and perform social and professional tasks – eventually impacting on their personal health (Povlsen & Borup, 2011). An inability to cope can often lead to mental health problems (Lahti et al., 2018). Individuals with mental health disorders often struggle to incorporate mental health promotion lifestyle activities into their lives, especially physical activity and a healthy diet (Verhaeghe et al., 2011). Furthermore, due to the previously highlighted nature and lack of understanding and awareness of mental health issues throughout communities, mental health 'disorders' are far more likely to be ignored, concealed and/or misunderstood than both physical and social health issues. That said, physical, social and mental health problems commonly accompany each other (Snelling, 2024). People with chronic condition physical comorbidities, such as diabetes and heart disease, often have accompanying mental health issues due to the physical and/or social limitations that their conditions may impose. The opposite can also be witnessed, such as when people with mental health issues may neglect their physical and social health and/or be more at risk of adopting or exacerbating lifestyle behaviours (use of alcohol and drugs) that lead to an increased risk of physical ill health.

The pressures and demands of society and community affect most people and they have the potential to adversely affect the health status of anyone at any time in any given place. With this in mind, it is useful that we acknowledge and view a person's (and a community's) overall health status from both a 'mental health lifespan' (from cradle to grave) and a 'mental health settings-based' perspective. What this view typifies is the notion that 'Health promotion takes place in "settings" – environments where people learn, work, play and love' (Hesman, 2007, p. 175). In turn, this helps us to understand, appreciate and predict the 'cause-and-effect' dynamics of PHC and health promotion problems rooted in systems of processes, structure and meaning (Whitehead, 2011).

Figure 7.1 illustrates the health-promoting lifespan continuum and its key stages as it relates to various settings (places and spaces) (Whitehead, 2011). The continuum associates and links related settings along a 'timeline' sequence that is commonly experienced by people as they progress through their lifespan. The two more peripheral 'outer continuums' acknowledge 'potential' health-related settings and settings that may or may not make up the 'normal' sequence of an individual's lifespan and unique health journey (Whitehead, 2011). Highlighting and linking up these continuums acknowledges the fact that 'people's lives straddle settings' (Dooris, 2004, p. 58). Dooris (2004) precedes this by stating that 'quite apart from the fact that one setting can learn from another, it is clear that in relation to health-related topics, an issue impacting on health in one setting frequently has its origin or solution in another' (p. 58). For instance, a strong evidence base informs us that children who are bullied earlier on in their lives are at high risk of low self-esteem and mental illness later in life (Weare & Nind, 2011). Therefore, rather than a focus on reacting to and treating adults for existing mental health problems, a far more effective strategy is to target school children at a much earlier stage (in the school setting) and put in place preventative anti-bullying and self-efficacy strategies with the intention that fewer adults will experience mental health issues later on in life (Dressler-Hawke & Whitehead, 2009).

While the lifespan/setting continuum is useful to adopt, there also must be a realisation that not all of us and our clients share the same health journey. Part of the consideration for viewing mental health promotion this way is to individualise it to each person dealt with using the continuum as a 'reference point' (Whitehead, 2011). For instance, not all clients will go to university, be unemployed, encounter a prison setting or be churchgoers. That is why the lower 'strand' of the continuum is separated out. However, what we do know is that those who suffer from mental illness are more likely to encounter unemployment and/or imprisonment, especially if their condition is related to factors such as illicit drug use and/or alcohol abuse which may, in turn, be directly related to an increased exposure to criminal behaviours and activities such as domestic violence (Whitehead, 2011).

REFLECTION

There is a tendency to view certain members of the population to be most at risk of mental health problems, especially those who are vulnerable and/or on the 'fringes of society'. While there is a relationship, we should not generalise too much. In a modern era where people are hurried, time-poor and often stressed (especially due to the demands of increasing technology and media communication – see Chapter 13), any member of a community faces real mental health challenges at any time. What do you think are the main mental health challenges that potentially affect everyone today?

In direct relation to the Figure 7.1 lifespan/setting continuum, each of the stages along the inner continuums are now discussed (along with additional stages not mentioned in the figure).

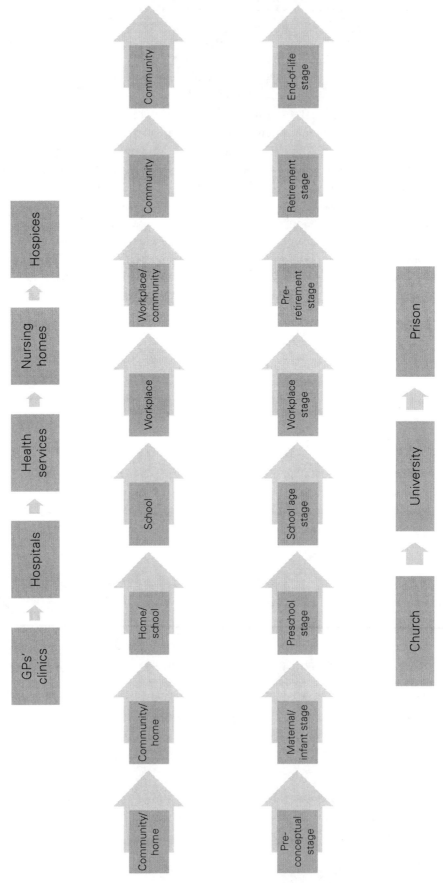

Figure 7.1 The lifespan/setting continuum

Source: Whitehead (2011).

Preconceptual, maternal and infant stage

These are important stages of any individual's health development and likely indicators of future mental health status. In these phases, Schmied and colleagues' (2013) review of Australian- and Aotearoa New Zealand-based maternal mental health longitudinal studies states that health promotion communities view access to effective preconceptual/prenatal care as a major public health solution to the reduction of health disparities in birth outcomes and related mental health issues. Seimyr, Welles-Nystrom and Nissen (2013) stress that nurses and midwives in the PHC setting should work in partnership with women and families and other agencies to facilitate decisions about care that mothers require prior to and after the birth of their children, and further identify that mental health promotion strategies should focus on young mothers from socially disadvantaged groups who are most at risk of developing mental illness and are more likely to have a pre-existing history of mental illness (Whitehead, 2011). Lasater and colleagues (2021) highlight the need for effective integration of mental health into maternal health care in the rural setting – where disadvantage and inequity are often more visible. Similarly, Domian and colleagues (2010) highlight the active mental health promotion role of public health nurses working with disadvantaged mothers in their My Baby and Me comprehensive parenting intervention program. This type of intervention is at the heart of current public health policy around childbirth and child care, where the emphasis has moved from targeted individual behavioural-change strategy to addressing inequalities and divisions within society (Fisher & Baum, 2010; Whitehead, 2011). That said, there is also a need to target individual health behaviour as well. Woolhouse and colleagues' (2014) Australian study identifies a close link between poor physical health and maternal depression in the first 12 months post-partum. Alderdice, McNeill and Lynn's (2013) systematic review of maternal mental health and well-being interventions highlights the need for further research including midwifery-led models of care in the prevention of post-partum depression, psychological and psychosocial interventions for treating post-partum depression and facilitation/coordination of parent training programs.

Preschool stage

The concept of health-promoting schools (HPS) is one of the more visible in the nursing and general PHC and mental health promotion literature (Weare & Nind, 2011; Whitehead, 2011). However, the notion of earlier lifespan health-promoting preschools, day-care education or kindergartens is not as well established as later school stages (Dressler-Hawke, Whitehead & Coad, 2009). A few isolated studies have sought to overcome this. For instance, McKey and Huntington (2004) discuss the implications for nursing in child health practice related to the topical and relevant issue of preschool childhood obesity that is closely linked to bullying and its negative mental health impact. Perrin and Alasker (2006) subsequently provide novel findings that help to put in place early learning anti-bullying strategies. They investigated varying bullying behaviours of children at the level of preschool kindergarten and their associated later links to various negative mental health states throughout the lifespan. The outcomes were especially linked to how children fared from a mental health perspective when they moved into later school settings. Essex and colleagues (2009) recommend universal targeted public mental health screening for children from kindergarten through to Year 5. Dodd and colleagues (2023) highlight the significant changes in preschoolers' mental health symptoms over the COVID-19 period.

CASE STUDY 7.1

Lauren was born with Down syndrome and manages well with most daily activities of living. She is a happy child with a close and supportive family network. Lauren will be starting her local primary school in six months time. Lauren and her parents' preference is for 'main schooling'. However, they are a little apprehensive about the potential challenges that mainstream integration may bring, especially relating to mental health.

REFLECTION

1. As Lauren's main PHC support health professional, what information could you offer to Lauren and her parents to reassure them that clear support policies and resources are in place?
2. If any issues came to light while attending school, such as bullying, what type of support services and strategies would you like to see in place?
3. Outside the school support environment, what other local community services might be available to assist Lauren and her family?

School age stage

The school setting is seen as one of the most important health-related growth and front-line defence areas for PHC and mental health promotion interventions (Weare & Nind, 2011). The prevalence of mental disorders among children and adolescents is a known global problem. Schools have therefore been positioned at the forefront of promoting positive mental health and well-being as a front-line preventative measure (O'Reilly et al., 2018). It is seen as imperative that health professional disciplines and services intervene at the early stages of the lifespan continuum in actively promoting healthy mental health strategies that school children will then take with them into their young and middle adult lives and beyond (Stallard et al., 2015; Svedberg 2011; Whitehead, 2011). Specific groups – such as PHC nurses, school nurses and health and community public health nurses – are often active in this setting but their public mental health role has been reported as being limited more towards a medical model of health care provision (Whitehead, 2006b). Hoskote and colleagues (2023) have reviewed the 'evolution' of the school nurses' role in adolescent mental health. There are some exceptions though. Mäenpää, Paavilainen and Åstedt-Kurki (2007) reported their school nurse-led project involving Finnish sixth graders. Twenty-two sixth graders (aged 11–12 years) were participants in their study. The findings suggested that pupils 'thrived', and their mental health benefited, where individual counselling and coping skills were reinforced alongside mental health education interaction with the family unit (Hoskote et al., 2023; Whitehead, 2011). In Stallard and colleagues' (2007) study, school nurses were trained to deliver an evidence-based emotional health cognitive behaviour therapy (CBT) program (called FRIENDS) to 106 non-referred children aged 9–10 years attending three schools with known high rates of emotional and behavioural problems in deprived areas. The CBT program ran over 10 sessions. The study found that three months after completing FRIENDS, anxiety had significantly decreased and self-esteem increased in most participants (Stallard et al., 2007). Children with the most severe emotional problems benefited most from the program. This study was followed up by a later randomised control study with similar results (Stallard et al., 2015). It did not involve school nurses this time but trained 'school leaders'. The study was unable to identify which group was the most effective. Similarly, Whitley and colleagues (2018) identify that mental health literacy is an essential component of school's curriculum reform and that educators are best placed to deliver it. It is suggested here that this would be a good place and opportunity for nurses to be engaged in the delivery and support of such programs. Interestingly, Weare (2015) raises another issue worth considering and relates this issue to the 'workplace stage' of the continuum. She argues that, in promoting mental health promotion in schools, we should start with the mental health and well-being of teachers themselves. Topically, Ancheta and colleagues (2020) highlight that lesbian, gay, bisexual, transgender and queer/questioning (LGBTQIA+) adolescents are more likely to report suicidality and worse mental health than their heterosexual peers – highlighting the need for targeting of specific youth groups.

Programs, out of school, yet supporting them, are another essential consideration in this part of the lifespan continuum. A good example is Vella and colleagues' (2018) Ahead of the Game program. The authors state the well-established fact that young, adolescent males are a high-need group who are more sceptical towards accessing mental health services – an attitude reflective of a perceived/actual 'man up' culture. The aim of the Ahead of the Game program is to 'test the effectiveness of a multi-component, community-sport based program targeting prevention, promotion, and early intervention for mental health among adolescent males' (Vella et al., 2018, p. 390).

Higher education stage

Universities and other higher education settings are not always going to figure in the lives of all clients. However, greater numbers of individuals are accessing this setting as a 'routine' follow-on to post-secondary school education (Dooris, 2009; Whitehead, 2011). Nursing has been slow to establish itself in this setting and, where it has, it is often limited to the mental health promotion of nursing students enrolled in 'demanding' educational and clinical roles rather than the wider university population. For example, Timmins and colleagues' (2011) study surveyed student stressors associated with nursing programs across two universities and the commonly occurring negative impact on their mental health status. Whitehead (2004), however, stresses the wider role of the health-promoting university and nursing students in raising awareness of mental health promotion that students can then promote in clinical practice with their clients. These students can also become active in specific mental health well-being events that are often promoted in Australasian universities. In 2016, R U OK? Day and the Australia and New Zealand universities' Mental Health Day involved 26 universities. In 2016, the mental health university day 2016 focused on:

- 'resilience' and how it can be developed and/or strengthened in order that we better deal with life's stressors.
- the promotion of resources that students and staff can access and use in the development and strengthening of resilience.

Lahti and colleagues (2018) report their eMenthe mental health promotion study that investigated postgraduate mental health students in the university setting and identified that they needed further education on mental health issues and how they relate to and impact the lifespan journey of individuals and communities at large. Reverté-Villarroya (2021) and colleagues have investigated the influence of COVID-19 on the mental health of final-year nursing students as they look to enter the workforce comparing the situation before and during the pandemic.

Workplace stage

The health-promoting workplace is fast gaining pace as one of the more important mental health promotion settings (Cancelliere et al., 2011; Czabala, Charzynska & Mroziak, 2011). Mental health disorders account for the most common reason for long-term sickness absence (Henderson et al., 2011). The setting holds a unique place where the health and well-being of workers inevitably impact the mental health of individuals within the workplace setting, their families, the local community and society at large (Barkway, 2006; Whitehead, 2006c). Subsequently, and in line with the public health and PHC commitments of health service organisations, the extension of a positive healthy culture in the workplace is the potential influence on the health of immediate and wider family groups of health employees (Russell, Anstey & Wells, 2015; Whitehead, 2011). In reporting their two Canadian workplace mental health promotion programs Road to Mental Readiness for First Responders (R2MR) and The Working Mind (TWM), Dobson and colleagues (2018, p. 370) identify that many workplaces have structurally embedded stressors that increase the risk of mental health problems. They frame the solution as follows:

> When issues related to lost productivity, increased disability rates, and the indirect costs associated with hiring and training replacement employees are also considered, employers are well advised to promote optimal mental health – which means building structures and a cultural environment that are supportive of mental health in the workplace.

It is already established that mental health promotion programs offered in the workplace setting have a positive effect on rates and levels of depression and anxiety symptoms (Martin, Sanderson & Cocker, 2009). They also serve to help overcome the problem of 'presenteeism'. This is where individuals are 'present' at work but have the incapacity to function or cope well (Cancelliere et al., 2011, Henderson et al., 2011; Whitehead, 2006c). Studies have shown that mental health promotion programs and interventions seem to be the most effective. These include stress management programs; individual CBT; healthy lifestyle interventions, such as healthy canteens; and specific interventions, such as stress inoculation training (Czabala et al., 2011; Henderson et al., 2011). Screening programs are sometimes recommended but the evidence suggests that they are mostly inconclusive about positive mental health outcomes (Henderson et al., 2011). It is worth noting that Badu and colleagues (2020) have explored workplace stress and resilience in the Australian nursing workforce.

Within the workplace stage are the detention, unemployment, and welfare stages. While these stages represent adults that are not currently working or in the workplace, they most appropriately sit here because they most likely begin/occur during the adult 'working life' stage of the continuum.

Detention stage

The link between work, socio-demographic status, healthy aging and well-being is well-established (Fisher & Baum, 2010). It is not to suggest here that people who are unemployed or receiving welfare will go to prison. However, there are established links between long-term unemployment, low income, geographical location and race that correlate to a higher incidence of criminality and penal incarceration in these sections of society encountered by nurses (Fraser, Gatherer & Hayton, 2009; Whitehead, 2011). It is also well established that prison populations often have one of the highest rates of mental illness (Rybacka & Brooke, 2023). In turn, this is known to have an adverse mental health effect on prison-based nurses (Goddard et al., 2019). Establishing mental health promotion strategies within the prison setting is notably difficult as its context often works counter to the health-promoting principles of negotiation, autonomy, empowerment and self-determination – much as there is also a tension between 'custody' and 'care' (Powell et al., 2010; Whitehead, 2006a). Jordan (2011, p. 1061) states that 'the aims of imprisonment could be typified as punishment, deterrence, reform, and public protection'. However, nurses and other health professionals working in the prison setting have a growing PHC role. Their priorities are to address the immediate social and mental health needs of their clients – improving their individual health status (mainly related to drug and alcohol rehabilitation) and preventing reoffending – as well as protecting the wider community (Fraser et al., 2009; Jordan, 2011; Powell et al., 2010; Rybacka & Brooke, 2023).

Unemployment and welfare stage

Whether dealing with prison-based or unemployed clients, much of the health promotion work within this stage involves nurses from various disciplines introducing or reorientating affected individuals to mental health programs that rehabilitate them to become active and productive members of their local community workforce (Whitehead, 2011). Rose and Thompson (2012) describe their community mental health development program in a high-unemployment deprived Sydney community. Their mental health intervention is at three levels: people (promoting individual capabilities), space (enabling environmental infrastructure) and place (developing 'soft' infrastructure). They advocate the targeting of traditionally complex social groups, such as unemployed clients, into health-promoting community empowerment and advocacy schemes (Whitehead, 2011). This mirrors the sentiments of Hollederer (2019) who suggests that established relationships between unemployment and health highlight a specific need for mental health promotion interventions that consider the diversity of those who are unemployed (i.e. short-term, long-term, skilled, unskilled) and their different individual needs. The potential role for nurses in formulating and implementing mental health promotion programs in various settings with people who are unemployed has been highlighted (Harris et al., 2009). They advocate the use of CBT programs. Martin, Keswick and LeVeck (2010) describe their nurse-developed Welfare-to-Wellness-to-Work health promotion program. It provided a holistic self-esteem peer-support program promoting participants to learn about and change their mental health behaviour that, subsequently, would improve their ability to return to the workforce with its associated mental health benefits. Virgolino and colleagues (2022) conducted a systematic review of the association between unemployment and mental health.

Pre-retirement stage

This stage has not been well researched and has only more recently been accepted as an actual stage on the lifespan continuum (Yeung, 2013). This is even though the need to promote healthy active aging is well recognised in offsetting the impact of an aging population on national resources and in ensuring a high quality of life in older age (Adams & Rau, 2011). Secker and colleagues (2004) refer to this stage as the 'midlife' part of the lifespan continuum. They report their evaluation of a national pre-retirement health initiative in England. Their findings indicated that health improvement services could be effectively targeted at people in midlife, and that service settings and style played an important part in the engagement of this usually neglected client group (Whitehead, 2011) – especially as they are known to be particularly at risk of mental health deterioration as they enter this 'vulnerable' stage of the lifespan moving from active professional engagement through to retirement (Kalra et al., 2012). Handley and colleagues (2021) have identified that the health and well-being of individuals both in the workplace and those fully retired are generally better compared to those in the pre-retirement stages of life. Against the backdrop demographic of the 'baby boomer' generation of the early 1960s, this generation is in or nearing this stage which most commonly falls within the midlife/pre-retirement age of 55–65 years (Oksanen et al., 2011). Friis and colleagues (2007) highlight the influence on health, mental health and lifestyle of early retirement among a cohort of Danish nurses. From a settings-based point of view, most mental health promotion activity around pre-retirement is likely to occur either in the workplace or, from a social point of view, within the local community. It may also include, as part of or separate to, settings such as health-promoting churches (Peterson, Atwood & Yates, 2002). Wherever it occurs, Yeung (2013) identifies that planning for retirement involves four main areas: financial, physical health, social health and psychological health.

Retirement stage

Where pre-retirement ends, and actual retirement begins, is an important stage in the health status of individuals and their closest ones. Olesen, Butterworth and Rodgers' (2012) longitudinal population survey found a high risk of poor mental health following retirement particularly, among males. De Vaus and colleagues (2007) reported on their prospective longitudinal Healthy Retirement Project study. They found that retiring gradually allows for clients to make preparatory changes to their current and future lifestyles. They suggest that health care policies and work practices that promote control of retirement decisions for clients will enhance their overall well-being later in life. When actual retirement occurs, mental health promotion is of considerable importance for retirees for sustaining a productive and healthy societal role and function. It is a significant area for health care workers responsible for drafting policies and programs to consider when helping to improve health and wellness in older adults (Kalra et al., 2012; Whitehead, 2011). For instance, Bekhet and Zauszniewski (2012) and Luo and colleagues (2012) advocate intervention programs that are designed to prevent or reduce loneliness in older retired adults. Although the age of retirement can vary significantly between individuals, professions and countries, the general rule is that this age group commences around the 65-year-old mark (Yeung, 2013; Whitehead, 2011).

Kennedy (2006) identifies that health-promoting environments found in some naturally occurring retirement communities may be a low-cost community-based means of sustaining both the mental health and well-being of older people. He reports on the efforts to link biomedical and psychosocial services within naturally occurring retirement communities which assist seniors age in their own homes. Similarly, Sharda, Daniel and White (2019) highlight the importance of clinicians monitoring levels of mental health promotion prevention in this population and of addressing mental health within the context of cognitive and physical-related social determinants of health. The desired outcomes were optimal mental health and independence relevant to and mutually desired by both health and social service providers. Wilson and Palha (2007) conducted a qualitative review of the literature related to mental health promotion of adults at the age of retirement. Four themes emerged from the analysis of this literature:

1. The considerable effect of retirement on retiring individuals and thus the need for support for more positive retirements
2. Identifying and overcoming barriers to health promotion at retirement
3. Evaluating the methods by which mental health promotion is introduced for positive and long-term change
4. Describing the short- and long-term benefits of mental health promotion at retirement.

In their study, Hitt and colleagues (1999) identified that most centenarians enjoyed a healthy and independent lifespan usually right up to a rapid terminal decline. Their 'compression of mortality paradigm', rather than the more commonly held view of 'the older people get the sicker they become' reported the more positive view that 'the older an individual gets the healthier they have been'.

End-of-life stage

Rosenberg and Yates (2010, p. 201) suggest that mental health promotion and palliative care may appear as 'conceptually incongruent fields'. Similarly, Kellehear (2008, p. 139) stresses that health promotion and palliative care can appear, at first glance, as both contradictory and strange companions; with dying patients there is no room for preventative advice. However, he goes on to highlight that palliative care is closely related to health promotion as its premise is based on holistic and humanistic therapeutic care. In this sense, the role of the nurse is to develop personal skills for clients, develop participatory relationships, educate and inform clients and families, offer mental health and death education, offer social support, and strengthen community action and community participation. Rosenberg and Yates (2010) propose that end-of-life palliative care is, after all, very amenable to the application of mental health promotion practice especially for the wider family. Richardson (2002) mirrors much of this sentiment aligned with the role of community-based palliative care nurses. In turn, they have been able to offer a previously absent definition for mental health promotion in nursing-based palliation. Both Berg and Sarvimäki (2003) and Whitehead (2003) also highlighted the importance and place of wider existential components of health promotion that can be linked to this stage. In this context, clients draw on existential forces to either help overcome adversity or give strength in facing a peaceful death. For dying patients, existential strength can offer hope, and, for some, mental health fulfilment. Fulfilment, in this case, may relate to the previously mentioned notion of faith-related or transcendental beliefs around potential 'afterlife' considerations. From a settings-based perspective, this stage of the lifespan continuum could potentially involve settings such as mental health-promoting nursing homes and mental health-promoting hospices (Richardson, 2002). Jang and colleagues (2022) stress the unmet mental health needs of palliative patients with non-cancer diseases.

The potential 'other' settings

It may not always be prudent to refer to all the recognised health promotion settings from the point of view of a mental health promotion lifespan continuum. For instance, despite their important place in nursing, direct health care-related settings – such as acute health-promoting hospitals (Whitehead, 2005), GPs' clinics, nursing and rest homes, and hospices – are not really addressed in this chapter because they are not always a natural part of a person's health journey. However, they are represented in Figure 7.1 (Whitehead, 2011).

It is often difficult to predict when mental health episodes will occur (Walsh et al., 2023). When they do, they tend to be short term and are not usually the most desirable situations for the implementation of mental health promotion and PHC initiatives (Russell et al., 2015). Instead, it is probably more appropriate to consider chronic illness and disability events in the context of social models of community intervention that promote recovery, rehabilitation and self-management of clients. These inevitably include mental health promotion interventions (Rose & Thompson, 2012).

CASE STUDY 7.2

Phyllis is a full-time carer for her husband, Bob, who has advanced dementia. She has fulfilled this demanding role for the last five years with Bob's own cognitive mental health recently rapidly deteriorating. As part of the recognised 'caregiver' burden that affects many carers with family members who require full-time support with daily activities, Phyllis has become more socially isolated and depressed. Her immediate family lives overseas, so she has little contact with them. She has noticed that she is more frequently turning to alcohol to help her cope better and has recently been prescribed antidepressants by her GP.

The role of the caregiver of a person with dementia is known to be stressful; particularly if the caregiver is an unsalaried family member. Depressive symptoms, anxiety, stress, the inability to cope, frustration, anger, guilt and role conflict are common issues that arise from what is often termed 'caregiver burden'. Secondary stressors are known to be related to personal 'overload' due to excessive work schedules, relationship deprivation in terms of lack of intimacy and caregiver activities, family conflict, balancing job and caregiving duties, economic strain and restricted social life. Supporting this, caregivers have been described by Reinhard and colleagues (2008) as 'hidden patients themselves with serious adverse physical and mental health consequences from their demanding work as caregivers and reduced attention to their own healthcare'. To confront these stressors, coping strategies in the form of both self-management and health care assistance are essential.

REFLECTION
1. What do you feel are Phyllis' immediate health care needs? What type of community-based mental health 'services' might be available to support her?
2. Do you know of any PHC voluntary support groups that exist in your community that could complement other health services for someone like Phyllis? If not, perform an online search and note what you uncover.
3. Beyond Phyllis' immediate mental health needs, what type of mental health wellness and well-being strategies could also be promoted? Think particularly about strategies and advice for self-help and self-management to prevent further mental health deterioration.

Conclusion

It is well known that vast numbers of people in Australia and Aotearoa New Zealand will experience mental health problems as a 'natural' part of their health journey across their lifespan and across a variety of different settings. Many mental health services exist to assist individuals, groups, families and populations when this occurs. However, evidence suggests that preventative approaches to mental health promotion – particularly at the PHC level – present a more effective strategy. This is particularly so when we use frameworks to guide us such as the lifespan/setting framework identified in this chapter (Whitehead, 2011). From a mental health promotion perspective, it highlights the factors that influence the mental health of individuals and communities across time, space and place and how they are closely interrelated. It also highlights that mental health promotion is complex and diverse. The more proactive mental health illness prevention and mental wellness and well-being promotion interventions are, the better for everyone in society and health care. Effective intervention and implementation of preventative strategy from an early age is also strongly encouraged to target maternal and infant settings, schools, school children and growing families. PHC nurses are well placed to champion, lead and action such programs across a range of settings and across the lifespan.

CRITICAL THINKING ACTIVITIES

1. Are there certain points on the lifespan continuum where you think individuals may be more vulnerable to mental health problems? Are there certain 'settings' where you think this might be the same? Are there certain points on the lifespan continuum where you think individuals may be best able to experience mental health wellness and well-being? Are there certain 'settings' where you think this might be the same? Are there certain settings and points on the lifespan where PHC nurses are best positioned to focus their resources and activities?

2. Targeting individuals in terms of preventative mental health promotion interventions early in life is known to be an effective strategy in promoting and maintaining positive mental health later in life. What do you think is the 'optimum' age to target and why? What do you think are the current mental health promotion priorities for your specified age group?

3. Mental health problems occur most often in certain vulnerable (and often disadvantaged) community members. The solution seems to lie in what many refer to as 'focusing upstream'. What do you think is meant by this term and what does it involve? If you are not sure, search online using the term.

FURTHER READING

Health Promotion Agency (New Zealand). (n.d.). *Mental health.* www.hpa.org.nz/programme/mental-health

Ministry of Health. (n.d.). *Mental health and addiction.* New Zealand Government. www.health.govt.nz/regulation-legislation/mental-health-and-addiction

Taylor and Francis. (n.d.). *International Journal of Mental Health Promotion.* https://www.tandfonline.com/journals/rijm20

VicHealth. (n.d.). *Prevention and promotion.* Victorian Government. www.health.vic.gov.au/mental-health/prevention-and-promotion

World Health Organization (WHO). (2022). *Mental health: Strengthening our response.* www.who.int/news-room/fact-sheets/detail/mental-health-strengthening-our-response

REFERENCES

Adams, G.A. & Rau, B.L. (2011). Putting off tomorrow to do what you want today: Planning for retirement. *American Psychologist, 66,* 180–92.

Alderdice, F., McNeill, J. & Lynn, F. (2013). A systematic review of systematic reviews of interventions to improve maternal mental health and well-being. *Midwifery, 29,* 389–99.

Ancheta A.J., Bruzzese J.-M. & Hughes T.L. (2020). The impact of positive school climate on suicidality and mental health among LGBTQ adolescents: A systematic review. *The Journal of School Nursing, 37*(2), 75–86. https://doi.org/10.1177/1059840520970847

Arango, C., Díaz-Caneja, C.M., McGorry, P.D., et al. (2018). Preventive strategies for mental health. *The Lancet Psychiatry, 5*(7), 591–604.

Badu, E., O'Brien, A.P., Mitchell, R., et al. (2020). Workplace stress and resilience in the Australian nursing workforce: A comprehensive integrative review. *International Journal of Mental Health Nursing, 29*(1), 5–34. https://doi.org/10.1111/inm.12662

Barkway, P. (2006). Creating supportive environments for mental health promotion in the workplace. *Contemporary Nurse, 21,* 131–41.

Bekhet, A.K. & Zauszniewski, J.A. (2012). Mental health of elders in retirement communities: Is loneliness a key factor? *Archives of Psychiatric Nursing, 26,* 214–24.

Berg, G.V. & Sarvimäki, A. (2003). A holistic-existential approach to health promotion. *Scandinavian Journal of Caring Sciences, 17,* 384–91.

Botha, F., Butterworth, P. & Wilkins, R. (2022). Evaluating how mental health changed in Australia through the COVID-19 pandemic: Findings from the '*Taking the Pulse of the Nation*' (TTPN) survey. *International Journal of Environmental Research and Public Health, 19*(1), 558. https://doi.org/10.3390/ijerph19010558

Calloway, S. (2007). Mental health promotion: Is nursing dropping the ball? *Journal of Professional Nursing, 23,* 105–9.

Cancelliere, C., Cassidy, D.J., Ammendolia, C. & Cote, P. (2011). Are workplace health promotion progams effective at improving presenteeism in workers? A systematic review and best evidence synthesis of the literature. *BMC Public Health, 11*(395).

Czabala, C., Charzynska, K. & Mroziak, B. (2011). Psychosocial interventions in workplace mental health promotion: An overview. *Health Promotion International, 26,* i70–i84.

De Vaus, D., Wells, Y., Kendig, H. & Quine, S. (2007). Does gradual retirement have better outcomes than abrupt retirement? Results from an Australian panel study. *Ageing & Society, 27,* 667–82.

Department of Health and Aged Care. (2020). *Mental health.* Commonwealth of Australia. https://www.health.gov.au/topics/mental-health-and-suicide-prevention

Dobson, K.S., Szeto, A., Knaak, S., et al. (2018). Mental health initiatives in the workplace: Models, methods and results from the Mental Health Commission of Canada. *World Psychiatry: Official Journal of the World Psychiatric Association (WPA), 17*(3), 370–1. https://doi.org/10.1002/wps.20574

Dodd, H., Skripkauskaite, S., Shum, A., Waite, P. & Lawrence, P. (2023). Changes in UK pre-Schooler's mental health symptoms over the first year of the Covid-19 pandemic: Data from Co-SPYCE study. *European Psychiatry, 66*(S1), S121–S121. https://doi.org/10.1192/j.eurpsy.2023.321

Domian, E.W., Baggett, K.M., Carta, J.J., Mitchell, S. & Larson, E. (2010). Factors influencing mothers' abilities to engage in a comprehensive parenting intervention program. *Public Health Nursing, 27,* 399–407.

Dooris, M. (2004). Joining up settings for health: A valuable investment for strategic partnership? *Critical Public Health*, *14*(1), 49–61.

——— (2009). Holistic and sustainable health improvement: The contribution of the settings-based approach to health promotion. *Perspectives in Public Health*, *129*, 29–36.

Dressler-Hawke, E. & Whitehead, D. (2009). The Behavioral Ecological Model as a framework for school-based anti-bullying health promotion interventions. *Journal of School Nursing, 25*, 195–204.

Dressler-Hawke, E., Whitehead, D. & Coad, J. (2009). What are New Zealand children eating at school? A content analyses of 'consumed versus unconsumed' food groups in a lunch-box survey. *Health Education Journal, 68*, 3–13.

Essex, M.J., Kraemer, H.C., Slattery, M.J., et al. (2009). Screening for childhood mental health problems: Outcomes and early identification. *The Journal of Child Psychology and Psychiatry, 50*, 562–70.

Fisher, M. & Baum, F. (2010). The social determinants of mental health: Implications for research and health promotion. *Australian and New Zealand Journal of Psychiatry, 44*, 1057–63.

Fraser, A., Gatherer, A. & Hayton, P. (2009). Mental health in prisons: Great difficulties but there are opportunities. *Public Health, 123*, 410–14.

Friis, K., Ekholm, O., Hundrup, Y.A., Obel, E.B. & Gronbaek, M. (2007). Influence of health, lifestyle, working conditions, and sociodemography on early retirement among nurses: The Danish Nurses Cohort Study. *Scandinavian Journal of Public Health, 35*, 23–30.

Goddard, D., de Vries, K., McIntosh, T., Theodosius, C. (2019). Prison nurses' professional identity. *Journal of Forensic Nursing, 15*(3), 163–71. https://doi.org/10.1097/jfn.0000000000000239

Handley, T.E., Lewin, T.J., Butterworth, P. et al. (2021). Employment and retirement impacts on health and wellbeing among a sample of rural Australians. *BMC Public Health, 21*(888). https://doi.org/10.1186/s12889-021-10876-9

Harris, E., Rose, V., Ritchie, J. & Harris, N. (2009). Labour market initiatives: Potential settings for improving the health of people who are unemployed. *Health Promotion Journal of Australia, 20*, 214–20.

Henderson, M., Harvey, S.B., Overland, S., Mykletun, A. & Hotopf, M. (2011). Work and common psychiatric disorders. *Journal of the Royal Society of Medicine, 104*, 198–207.

Hesman, A. (2007). Creating supportive environments for health. In J. Wills (ed.), *Promoting Health: Vital Notes for Nurses* (pp. 175–93). Blackwell Publishing.

Hitt, R., Young-Xu, Y., Silvr, M. & Peris, T. (1999). Centenarians: The older you get, the healthier you have been. *The Lancet, 354*(9197), 652.

Hollederer, A. (2019). Health promotion and prevention among the unemployed: A systematic review. *Health Promotion International, 34*(6), 1078–96. https://doi.org/10.1093/heapro/day069

Hoskote, A.R., Croce, E. & Johnson, K.E. (2023). The evolution of the role of U.S. school nurses in adolescent mental health at the individual, community, and systems level: An integrative review. *The Journal of School Nursing. 39*(1), 51–71. https://doi.org/10.1177/10598405211068120

Jang, H., Lee, K., Kim, S. et al. (2022). Unmet needs in palliative care for patients with common non-cancer diseases: A cross-sectional study. *BMC Palliative Care, 21*(151). https://doi.org/10.1186/s12904-022-01040-0

Jordan, M. (2011). The prison setting as a place of enforced residence, its mental health effects, and the mental healthcare implications. *Health & Place, 17*, 1061–6.

Kalra, G., Chrisodoulou, G., Jenkins, R., et al. (2012). Mental health promotion: Guidance and strategies. *European Psychiatry, 27*, 81–186.

Kellehear, A. (2008). Health promotion in palliative care. In G. Mitchell (ed.), *Palliative Care: A Patient-Centred Approach* (pp. 139–56). Radcliffe Publishing.

Kennedy, G.J. (2006). Naturally occurring retirement communities: An expanding opportunity for health promotion and disease prevention. *Primary Psychiatry, 13*, 33–5.

Lahti, M., Ellilä, H., Jormfeldt, H., et al. (2018). The required knowledge for lifespan mental health promotion and prevention for Master's level mental health nurse education – the eMenthe project. *International Journal of Health Promotion and Education, 56*(3), 143–54. https://doi .org/10.1080/14635240.2018.1431953

Lasater, M.E., Murray, S.M., Keita, M., et al. (2021). Integrating mental health into maternal health care in rural Mali: A qualitative study. *Journal of Midwifery & Women's Health, 66*: 233–9. https://doi.org/10.1111/jmwh.13184

Luo, Y., Hawkley, L.C., Waite, L.J. & Cacioppo, J.T. (2012). Loneliness, health and mortality in old age: A national longitudinal study. *Social Science & Medicine, 74*, 907–14.

Mäenpää, T., Paavilainen, E. & Åstedt-Kurki, P. (2007). Cooperation with school nurses described by Finnish sixth-graders. *International Journal of Nursing Practice, 13*, 304–9.

Martin, A., Sanderson, K. & Cocker, F. (2009). Meta-analysis of the effects of health promotion intervention in the workplace on depression and anxiety symptoms. *Scandinavian Journal of Work, Environment & Health, 35*, 7–18.

Martin, C.T., Keswick, J.L. & LeVeck, P. (2010). A welfare-to-wellness-to-work program. *Journal of Community Health Nursing, 27*, 146–59.

McKey, A. & Huntington, A. (2004). Obesity in pre-school children: Issues and challenges for community based child health nurses. *Contemporary Nurse, 18*, 145–51.

Ministry of Health. (2016). *Mental Health and Addiction: Service Use 2012/2013*. New Zealand Government

——— (2019). *Mental health work at the ministry*. New Zealand Government.

Oksanen, T., Vahtera, J., Westerlund, H., et al. (2011). Is retirement beneficial for mental health? Antidepressant use before and after retirement. *Epidemiology, 22*, 553–9.

Olesen, S.C., Butterworth, P. & Rodgers, B. (2012). Is poor mental health a risk factor for retirement? Findings from a longitudinal population survey. *Social Psychiatry and Psychiatric Epidemiology, 47*, 735–44.

O'Reilly, M., Svirydzenka, N., Adams, S. & Dogra, N. (2018). Review of mental health promotion interventions in schools. *Social Psychiatry and Psychiatric Epidemiology, 53*(7), 647–62.

Perrin, S. & Alasker, P.D. (2006). Social behaviour and peer relationships of victims, bully-victims, and bullies in kindergarten. *Journal of Child Psychology and Psychiatry, 47*, 45–57.

Peterson, J., Atwood, J.R. & Yates, B. (2002). Key elements for church-based health promotion programs: Outcome-based literature review. *Public Health Nursing, 19*, 401–11.

Povlsen, L. & Borup, I.K. (2011). Holism in nursing and health promotion: Distinct or related perspectives? A literature review. *Scandinavian Journal of Caring Sciences, 25*, 798–805.

Powell, J., Harris, F., Condon, L. & Kemple, T. (2010). Nursing care of prisoners: Staff views and experiences. *Journal of Advanced Nursing, 66*, 1257–65.

Reinhard, S.C., Given, B., Petlick, N. & Bemis, A. (2008). Supporting family caregivers in providing care. In R.G. Hughes (ed.), *Patient Safety and Quality: An Evidence-Based Handbook for Nurses* (pp. 341–62). Agency for Healthcare Research and Quality.

Reverté-Villarroya, S., Ortega, L., Lavedán, A., et al. (2021). The influence of COVID-19 on the mental health of final-year nursing students: Comparing the situation before and during the pandemic. *International Journal of Mental Health Nursing, 30*, 694–702. https://doi .org/10.1111/inm.12827

Richardson, J. (2002). Health promotion in palliative care: The patients' perception of therapeutic interaction with the palliative nurse in the primary care setting. *Journal of Advanced Nursing, 40*, 432–40.

Rose, V.K. & Thompson, L.M. (2012). Space, place and people: A community development approach to mental health promotion in a disadvantaged community. *Community Development Journal, 47*, 604–11.

Rosenberg, J.P. & Yates, P.M. (2010). Health promotion in palliative care: The case for conceptual congruence. *Critical Public Health, 20*, 201–10.

Russell, L.M., Anstey, M.H.R. & Wells, S. (2015). Hospitals should be exemplars of healthy workplaces. *The Medical Journal of Australia, 202*, 424–6.

Rybacka, M. & Brooke, J. (2023). Mental health care in prison. In J. Brooke (ed.), *Nursing in Prison* (pp. 109–33). Springer. https://doi.org/10.1007/978-3-031-30663-1_5

Schmied, V., Johnson, M., Naidoo, N., et al. (2013). Maternal mental health in Australia and New Zealand: A review of longitudinal studies. *Women and Birth, 26*, 167–78.

Secker, J., Bowers, H., Webb, D. & Llanes, M. (2004). Theories of change: What works in improving health in mid-life? *Health Education Research, 20*, 392–401.

Seimyr, L., Welles-Nystrom, B. & Nissen, E. (2013). A history of mental health problems may predict maternal distress in women postpartum. *Midwifery, 29*, 122–31.

Sharda N., Daniel K. & White H. (2019). The principles of disease and disability prevention and health promotion with increasing age. In P. Coll (ed.), *Healthy Aging*. Springer.

Snelling, A. (2024). *Introduction to Health Promotion* (2nd ed.). John Wiley & Sons.

Stallard, P., Simpson, N., Anderson, S., Hibbert, S. & Osborn, C. (2007). The FRIENDS Emotional Health Programme: Findings from a school-based project. *Child and Adolescent Mental Health, 12*, 32–7.

Stallard, P., Skryabina, E., Taylor G., et al. (2015). A cluster randomised controlled trial comparing the effectiveness and cost-effectiveness of a school-based cognitive–behavioural therapy programme (FRIENDS) in the reduction of anxiety and improvement in mood in children aged 9/10 years. *Public Health Research, 3*(14).

Svedberg, P. (2011). In what direction should we go to promote health in mental health care? *International Journal of Qualitative Studies in Health and Well-Being, 6*, 1–5.

Tamminen, N., Solin, P., Barry, M.M., et al. (2016). A systematic concept analysis of health promotion. *International Journal of Mental Health Promotion, 18*, 177–98.

Timmins, F., Corroon, A.M., Byrne, G. & Mooney, B. (2011). The challenge of contemporary nurse education programmes. Perceived stressors of nursing students: Mental health and related lifestyle issues. *Journal of Psychiatric and Mental Health Nursing, 18*, 758–66.

Vella, S.A., Swann, C., Batterham, M., et al. (2018). Ahead of the game protocol: A multicomponent, community sport-based program targeting prevention, promotion and early intervention for mental health among adolescent males. *BMC Public Health, 18*(1), 390. https://doi.org/10.1186/s12889-018-5319-7

Verhaeghe, N., De Maeseneer, J., Maes, L., Van Heeringen, C. & Annemans, L. (2011). Perceptions of mental health nurses and patients about health promotion in mental health care: A literature review. *Journal of Psychiatric and Mental Health Nursing, 18*, 487–92.

Virgolino, A., Costa, J., Santos, O., et al. (2022) Lost in transition: a systematic review of the association between unemployment and mental health. *Journal of Mental Health, 31*(3), 432–44. https://doi.org/10.1080/09638237.2021.2022615

Walsh, O., Sheridan, A. & Barry, M.M. (2023). The process of developing a mental health promotion plan for the Irish health service, *Advances in Mental Health, 21*(2), 115–28. https://doi.org/10.1080/18387357.2022.2161402

Wand, T. (2011). Real mental health promotion practice requires a reorientation of nursing education, practice and research. *Journal of Psychiatric and Mental Health Nursing, 18*, 131–8.

Wang, S., Huang, X., Hu, T., et al. (2022). The times, they are a-changin': Tracking shifts in mental health signals from early phase to later phase of the COVID-19 pandemic in Australia. *BMJ Global Health, 7*(1), e007081. https://doi.org/10.1136/bmjgh-2021-007081

Weare, K. (2015). Child and adolescent mental health in schools. *Child and Adolescent Mental Health, 20*(2), e6–e8.

Weare, K. & Nind, M. (2011). Mental health promotion and problem prevention in schools: What does the evidence say? *Health Promotion International, 26*(Suppl.1), i29–i69.

Westrupp, E.M., Bennett, C., Berkowitz, T., et al. (2023). Child, parent, and family mental health and functioning in Australia during COVID-19: comparison to pre-pandemic data. *European Child & Adolescent Psychiatry, 32*, 317–30. https://doi.org/10.1007/s00787-021-01861-z

Whitehead, D. (2003). Beyond the metaphysical: Health-promoting existential mechanisms and their impact on the health status of clients. *Journal of Clinical Nursing, 12,* 678–88.

———— (2004). Health Promoting Universities (HPU): The role and function of nursing. *Nurse Education Today, 24,* 466–72.

———— (2005). Health Promoting Hospitals (HPH): The role and function of nursing. *Journal of Clinical Nursing, 14,* 20–7.

———— (2006a). Health Promoting Prisons (HPP) and the imperative for nursing. *International Journal of Nursing Studies, 43,* 123–31.

———— (2006b). The Health Promoting School (HPS): What role for nursing? *Journal of Clinical Nursing, 15,* 264–71.

———— (2006c). Workplace health promotion: The role and responsibilities of nursing managers. *Journal of Nursing Management, 14,* 59–68.

———— (2011). Before the cradle and beyond the grave: A lifespan/settings-based framework for health promotion. *Journal of Clinical Nursing, 20*(15–16), 2183–94.

Whitley, J., Smith, J.D., Vaillancourt, T. & Neufeld, J. (2018). Promoting mental health literacy among educators: A critical aspect of school-based prevention and intervention. In A. Leschied, D. Saklofske & G. Flett (eds), *Handbook of School-Based Mental Health Promotion. The Springer Series on Human Exceptionality.* Springer.

Wilson, D.M. & Palha, P. (2007). A systematic review of published research articles on health promotion at retirement. *Journal of Nursing Scholarship, 39,* 330–7.

Woolhouse, H., Gartland, D., Perlen, S., Donath, S. & Brown, S.J. (2014). Physical health after childbirth and maternal depression in the first 12 months post partum: Results of an Australian nulliparous pregnancy cohort study. *Midwifery, 30,* 378–84.

Yeung, D.I. (2013). Is pre-retirement planning always good? An exploratory study of retirement adjustment among Hong Kong Chinese retirees. *Aging & Mental Health, 17,* 386–93.

Zhao, Y., Leach, L.S., Walsh, E. et al. (2022). COVID-19 and mental health in Australia – a scoping review. *BMC Public Health, 22,* 1200. https://doi.org/10.1186/s12889-022-13527-9

Rural health nursing

8

Melissa Hanson, Maryanne Podham and Judith Anderson
With acknowledgement to Diana Guzys, Sandi Grieve
and Eileen Petrie

LEARNING OBJECTIVES

At the completion of this chapter, you should be able to:

- understand what makes a community 'rural'.
- describe the barriers to health care in rural communities.
- discuss how health care is delivered in rural areas.
- understand the role of Fly-in Fly-out (FIFO) services in Australia and Aotearoa New Zealand.
- describe how collaboration with rural communities could be approached.

Introduction

Nurses work in a wide variety of settings, and this includes a wide variety of communities. In Australia and Aotearoa New Zealand, many of these communities are rural and require nurses to have a broad general range of skills to meet the diversity of needs that their clients present with. Rural health nurses (RHNs) may be sole practitioners, providing health care on their own or as part of a small team that sometimes may include doctors (Australian Institute of Health and Welfare (AIHW), 2022; New Zealand Health Workforce Advisory Board, 2022). An increased scope of practice and greater reliance on collaboration, **interdisciplinary** and **transdisciplinary** practice is common (LaMothe et al., 2021).

Nurses who practise in remote areas, such as those employed by the Royal Flying Doctor Service (RFDS) of Australia, with Indigenous communities, in isolated towns or sometimes as part of the FIFO medical services provided by mining companies and other organisations, are known as remote area nurses (RANs). The emphasis of discussion in this chapter is more generally on RHNs with the acknowledgement that RANs face similar issues that are exacerbated by community size and composition, environmental challenges, greater geographical isolation and increased difficulty in accessing resources (Whiteing, Barr & Rossi, 2021).

There has been an increased emphasis on primary health care (PHC), rather than the traditional focus on acute care service delivery in hospitals evident in rural areas, to better address the inequities in access and outcomes for rural and remote residents (Department of

Interdisciplinary – a collaborative and coordinated partnership approach for providing services to achieve a common goal that supports shared decision-making between health care disciplines.

Transdisciplinary – an interdisciplinary team whose members have developed sufficient trust and mutual confidence resulting in the blurring of disciplinary-specific boundaries, the overlapping of expertise and the sharing of professional functions.

Health and Aged Care, 2021b; New Zealand Minister of Health, 2023a). However, barriers in relation to funding arrangements, resources and educational opportunities must also be recognised. The lack of access to other health care providers and the generalist role that RHNs have necessitates an increased emphasis on promoting health and well-being (Griffiths & Smith, 2020; Smith et al., 2022).

RHNs usually provide PHC for the community as well as delivering primary care, requiring clinical skills associated with rehabilitation, emergency and subacute care nursing. The complexity of rural nursing requires the nurse to provide generalist and specialist services in geographical and professional isolation (Harper et al., 2021). The likelihood of providing care to individuals who may be friends, neighbours and associates increases the complexity of practice (Whiteing et al., 2021). Despite the wide range of challenges faced in rural health nursing, it provides practitioners with an opportunity to undertake truly **holistic nursing** and can lead to a great sense of job satisfaction (Blay et al., 2022).

> **Holistic nursing –** nursing practice that focuses on promoting health and wellness, assisting healing, preventing or alleviating suffering, and is conscious of the interrelationship of human beings, events and the environment.

Defining 'rural'

Rural and remote areas have comparatively smaller populations, which are more highly dispersed and in more isolated areas than the metropolitan cities. In order to illustrate the definitions of 'regional', 'rural' and 'remote', the Australian Statistical Geography Standard Remoteness Structure (Australian Bureau of Statistics (ABS), 2021) defines rurality and remoteness based on road distances that people must travel to access services. There are five classes of relative remoteness:

1. Major cities
2. Inner regional
3. Outer regional
4. Remote
5. Very remote.

In Aotearoa New Zealand, the geographic classification for health categorises communities based on their population size and drive time to the edge of an urban area. It has a total of five categories; two are urban and three are rural:

1. Urban 1 (major urban)
2. Urban 2
3. Rural 1
4. Rural 2
5. Rural 3 (small, larger drive time) (Whitehead, 2022).

The health of rural communities

According to the AIHW, approximately 28 per cent of the Australian population reside in areas classified as rural and/or remote (AIHW, 2023). Similarly, in Aotearoa New Zealand, approximately 19 per cent of the population lives in rural areas (New Zealand Minister of Health, 2023c). The health of this population is impacted by several considerations including distance to and from, availability and appropriateness, affordability, and accessibility of health care services (Leach, Gunn & Muyambi, 2022). These considerations are further impacted by person factors such as health literacy, health behaviours, health beliefs and trust in providers (Leach, Gunn & Muyambi, 2022) particularly those outside the community of residence, thus often leading to unmet health care needs.

As a result of these disparities, there is a greater burden of disease in rural areas, particularly coronary heart disease, type 2 diabetes, chronic kidney disease, lung conditions, mental health and self-inflicted injuries (National Rural Health Alliance, 2021).

Barriers to health care in rural areas

The barriers to health care access in regional, rural and remote Australia are multi-factorial, such as widespread workforce and staffing challenges; a lack of resources; limited ambulance and GP services; a lack of availability of oncology treatments, palliative and specialist care; the distance to travel to available services; and even the weather. It is, however, important to consider that these challenges are not uniform, as access and service are highly varied between towns and states. There is a lack of specialists to fulfil the required health care services which results in people often having to travel to neighbouring towns or metropolitan cities. This creates problems due to the transport issues in isolated rural and remote communities (AIHW, 2022; Victorian Auditor-General's Office, 2018). Regional, rural and remote areas can be heavily reliant on internationally trained nurses and doctors (AIHW, 2022), who are often attracted by enhanced opportunities for permanent residency (Ung et al., 2024). Remote areas, in particular, often have transient workforces (McCullough et al., 2022), however, attachment to the community that a person lives in is also a retention factor. People who have a social bond with and feel part of a community are more likely to stay in that community long term. Although this in itself may create issues of possible burn-out when health care workers are required to care for people that they have a strong bond to, it is also likely to keep them in the community (Beccaria et al., 2021).

The provision of primary care services to rural and remote populations is an important consideration for improving access to health care. This PHC approach is flexible, encouraging practitioners to accept others, including their beliefs, and to take their life circumstances into account in order to care for people who have a broad range of health issues and contexts. This approach is important because it considers social justice, equity and community consultation and empowerment as part of its methodology of health. This is a sustainable approach that meets the needs of rural communities when community partnerships are fostered and encouraged and the service is flexible to the evolving health of the community (Bourke, Dunbar & Murakami-Gold, 2021; Gilbert et al., 2020).

Delivery of rural health

Nurses and midwives constitute the largest group of health providers in the rural and remote workforce, and many communities are dependent on nurse-led services (Australian College of Nursing, 2018; Department of Health and Aged Care, 2023b). This is especially important when considering the challenges surrounding recruitment and retention of the health workforce in rural and remote areas, such as a lack of medical specialists and a heavy reliance on a FIFO or locum workforce. Nurses are often the first point of contact for consumers in the health care system, provide the most hands-on care and sometimes are the only health care workers that health care consumers will see. As such, nurses are intrinsic to the successful delivery of health care for rural and remote communities and supporting the people who live in them.

Communities in rural and remote areas rely heavily on nurses with broad generalist skills and experience as well as advanced practice skills, including nurse practitioners. It is important to consider that the more remotely a nurse lives and works, the greater the generalist nature of their work (Australian College of Nursing, 2018). This generalist role enables rural and remote communities to be provided with much-needed flexibility in the provision of health care through the sharing of staff across the boundaries of care provision, especially in those isolated rural communities where it is difficult to recruit and retain specialists (Gilbert et al., 2020; Victorian Auditor-General's Office, 2018). As such, the contribution of nurses to lead and shape the delivery of health care in these areas has helped to improve health care outcomes, drive innovation and helped nurses to work autonomously and to the full extent of their scope of practice.

Although some perspectives of rural and remote nursing seem negative, it is worth noting that many nurses enjoy this work. They like the relative autonomy of working independently, or even alone (although this is more common in remote areas) and have greater career opportunities than nurses working in metropolitan areas. Even though there is a requirement for a broad scope of practice, this comes with a diversity of work and many nurses embrace this challenge and opportunity to extend their skills and be useful members of their community. Community members often embrace their health care staff, making them feel welcome and valued within and outside working hours, although FIFO staff are not able to accept this type of hospitality to the same extent as those nurses who are embedded in their communities. Many nurses also value the greater opportunities they feel exist in rural and remote practice to work in multidisciplinary teams (Ryan, de Klerk & Green, 2024).

Rural and remote health care is delivered by nurses in conjunction with the multidisciplinary team through health promotion, disease prevention and identification, and early intervention. Community-based services such as GP clinics, multipurpose services (MPS) and community health centres are present in rural and remote areas to provide PHC, acute and emergency care, and sometimes even specialist services. These multifaceted service delivery centres are designed to best support the needs of isolated rural and remote communities by offering flexible health care services targeted to individual communities and their populations.

Multidisciplinary teams in rural and remote areas often include Māori and Aboriginal and Torres Strait Islander health workers and practitioners. These workers can assist in bridging gaps between Indigenous patients and health care workers such as nurses (Drummond, 2021; Tipene-Leach, 2021). These health workers and practitioners also assist in advocating for their clients to work towards more holistic models of health care and to incorporate traditional treatment options within the care being provided. They assist in creating a more welcoming environment in health care settings and often empower their clients to ask more questions, leading to them being better informed and advocating for them to participate more actively in decision-making about their health (Gott et al., 2023; Tipene-Leach, 2021). In some situations, these health workers and practitioners lead, manage and co-design programs that can increase the trust of the community in the services being offered and thereby increase access to and use of those services (Arriero et al., 2023; Naren et al., 2021).

MPS

The MPS model is an integrated care model designed to address the health needs of small rural and remote communities. They integrate acute care, PHC, aged care and other health care services such as health improvement and prevention programs as appropriate to the community. They acknowledge the unique nature of these rural and remote communities and provide the flexibility necessary to meet those community needs, improving community access to such services (Colman, 2021; Gilbert et al., 2020; Victorian Auditor-General's Office, 2018). The model has been particularly well adapted to aged care services but could be effectively extended to meet the needs of younger people within the community too. They frequently combine aged care and acute services such as an emergency department (ED) and inpatient ward, as well as other ambulatory services such as walk-in antenatal clinics, immunisation clinics, wound care and mental health services, with an aim to meet current and future needs, and to address and improve rural and remote population health outcomes.

Aged care services

The inequities that prevail in other rural and remote health care also affect aged care services in those areas. Elderly people in Australia are less likely than other members of the population to live in metropolitan areas, so aged care is a particular issue in rural and remote areas. However, as remoteness increases, the proportion of these people who use aged care facilities (especially residential aged care) decreases (Colman, 2021; Pagone & Briggs, 2021). Rural and remote areas also frequently lack infrastructure that assists elderly people, such as public transport. Most people would prefer to age in their own homes, however in rural and remote areas, the distances between people requiring services then increases creating additional costs for the health care provider (Colman, 2021). As financial resources are often allocated per person/patient, the smaller a community is, the less funding they can attract, creating issues related to economies of scale. The MPS program described earlier is an attempt to address such issues, in particular, by including an aged care component (Colman, 2021; Pagone & Briggs, 2021). In Australia, access to aged care is controlled by the Commonwealth aged care assessment process requiring an external assessment in order to change eligibility for different services, in contrast with Aotearoa New Zealand where a care provider can manage such transitions (Gilbert et al., 2020).

Mental health services

As with other health issues, mental health in rural and remote areas is affected by geographical issues, lack of infrastructure and the difficulty in attracting and retaining suitably qualified staff. These issues contribute to poorer mental health outcomes for people living in these areas (Fitzpatrick et al., 2021; Matta et al., 2021). One significant mental health issue in rural and remote communities relates to suicide. Suicide rates in rural and remote areas are higher than in metropolitan areas and most have previously been diagnosed with mental illnesses. Several factors have been identified that may contribute towards this issue, including socio-economic disparities, higher alcohol consumption, limited access to services, stoicism and poor health literacy (Fitzpatrick et al., 2021). PHC has a large role to play in preventing mental health issues. In rural and remote areas, generalist community health nurses and nurse practitioners, either in generalist or specialist mental health roles, are a significant part of the workforce to address this issue (Blay et al., 2022; Department of Health and Aged Care, 2021b).

Remote area nursing

You can see from the earlier discussion of the classification of areas, that it is common to consider driving times as an important aspect of whether a community is a rural or a remote location. Naturally, this is related to access to health care services. Communities that are classified as remote have significant challenges in this regard. Even from a primary health care perspective, this can mean reduced access to fresh, healthy food, as well as other goods and services that are essential for healthy living, e.g. refrigeration, phone services, exposure to extreme temperatures. From an emergency care perspective, it can mean significant delays to receiving definitive treatment, not only due to distance, but also due to a lack of specialists and infrastructure, for example, blood banks and imaging services. Some benefits are noted when helicopter or fixed-wing retrieval services are utilised, but these resources can also be limited in number or are unable to operate in poor weather conditions (Morgan & Calleja, 2020).

Nursing in remote areas often involves the nurse being the first point of call in a community that frequently does not have other health care providers. For this reason, scope of practice may extend beyond the usual duties, including taking X-rays, responding to emergencies or dispensing medications. This isolated work environment can lead to a need to provide emergency coverage 24 hours a day and generally working autonomously. For many remote area nurses, particularly when they begin working in these areas, this can be a great concern as they are often extending their practice significantly (McCullough et al., 2022).

The role of nurse practitioners in rural and remote areas

Rural and remote nurses frequently work to the extent of their scope of practice. Limited other health care workers in these areas make this a necessity in order to meet the needs of the communities they work in (Fedele & Dragon, 2023; Jennings, Lowe & Tori, 2021). Particularly in rural and remote areas, health services rely on visiting medical officers but face significant issues staffing these positions (Jennings et al., 2021). Nurse practitioners, through their extended scope of practice, are able to meet these needs more effectively, for example, by prescribing medication (Chiarella, Currie & Wand, 2020; Fedele & Dragon, 2023; Jennings et al., 2021; McCullough et al., 2022) and ordering radiology or pathology tests (McCullough et al., 2022). Many countries, including Australia, introduced nurse practitioners in response to the need for advanced practice nurses in rural and remote areas. However, the percentage of nurse practitioners working in remote areas continues to be low (McCullough et al., 2022) despite the significant opportunity for expanded scope of practice in these areas (Ryan et al., 2024). Some health services are now using a nurse practitioner locum service for on-call or on-site care to supplement rural health care (Jennings et al., 2021). The role of nurse practitioners continues to develop and change and there is more potential for them to work more effectively in the future, as recognition for their work as independent practitioners increases (Chiarella et al., 2020). A study undertaken in 2021 found that Australians in general were still fairly limited in their knowledge and understanding of the nurse practitioner role but were positive about their willingness to utilise such services (Dwyer, Craswell & Browne, 2021).

In rural and remote aged care, specialists in psycho-geriatrics are filling gaps within the aged care system to improve accessibility to assessment and after-hours advice in an area with limited resources (Fedele & Dragon, 2023). Similarly, nurse practitioners working in PHC in rural and remote areas are often the first people who are contacted for a variety of conditions. This often includes answering questions, for example, about skin conditions, where new technologies may place them at the front-end of diagnosis with the assistance of digital platforms, and being the person who delivers care as part of the multidisciplinary health team in acute and home settings (Adelson & Eckert, 2020).

FIFO services

Since 1928, the RFDS has been synonymous with the support of the health and well-being of people living in rural and remote areas of Australia. What began as an experiment by Reverend John Flynn, the RFDS today provides medical treatment on the ground in weekly clinics staffed by doctors and nurses and 24-hour emergency evacuations of injured and unwell individuals who require transfer to metropolitan medical services (RFDS, 2023).

In Aotearoa New Zealand, the New Zealand Flying Doctor Service was established 26 years ago to support the provision of medical care to remote and isolated areas of the South Island. Similarly, to the RFDS, this service operates 24 hours a day, 7 days a week and services include transfer of critically ill people, neonatal and pediatric care, organ and blood deliveries and equipment to individuals and health services (New Zealand Flying Doctor Service, 2024).

Both services work alongside other state- and territory-based services that provide aeromedical transport and services to people in areas outside the metropolitan footprint. The nurses' roles as FIFO workers vary depending on the service that they work for and the location. Although these roles involve short-term contact between the community and the health care worker, which inhibits the ability to develop solid relationships with health care consumers and other health care providers, they fill a gap that would otherwise be unmet. Mobile health care involves the transportation of individuals who require non-urgent medical care, such as medical appointments, rehabilitation and transfer between hospitals (RFDS, 2023). Outreach services, also known as Drive In, Drive Out, involve the provision of health care to rural and remote communities and use a combination of telehealth consultations along with primary health care clinics that offer a range of services including immunisation, health check-ups, the management of chronic conditions, such as cardiovascular illnesses, and lifestyle issues, such as mental health and well-being considerations (RFDS, 2024). Consultation between a doctor and nurse can occur via telehealth, where subjective assessments (McPherson & Nahon, 2021) and phone orders for interventions, such as immunisations, can be provided. Outreach services can operate out of a clinic, bus or community setting and provide multidiscipline health care options for rural and remote communities with the aim of developing sustainable and culturally safe models of care for all community members (Jacups & Kinchin, 2021).

CASE STUDY 8.1

Tessa grew up in a larger regional town in New South Wales and attended university there where she completed a bachelor of nursing degree. Tessa has accepted a postgraduate position as a registered nurse in a small rural town with a population of 25 000. The town is serviced by a multipurpose centre that includes a doctor's surgery, which operates 4 days a week, and a 15-bed inpatient hospital, which includes two emergency beds. There are also weekly visits from a physiotherapist, chiropractor and dentist. Tessa has completed placements in multipurpose centres during her course and has some understanding of telehealth and the impacts of reduced access and availability to services including health care.

REFLECTION
1. What challenges could Tessa encounter in her first month of practice in this facility?
2. What challenges could Tessa encounter in her first month living in the town?
3. Identify strategies that Tessa could self-initiate to ensure her success as a clinician and community member.
4. Tessa is keen to advance her practice as a rural clinician. What strategies could she consider?

Collaboration with local communities

Health inequities are greater in rural communities. Due to the isolation in some of these communities and small population numbers, health care needs to be adapted to empower individuals, focus on primary health care and utilise more generalist health care providers (Harper et al., 2021). This increases the need to collaborate with community members to a greater extent than is required in metropolitan areas. In Australia, this includes rural communities and people of Aboriginal and Torres Strait Islander (Department of Health and Aged Care, 2021b; Deravin, Francis & Anderson, 2018; Griffiths & Smith, 2020) and Māori backgrounds (Harding et al., 2021; New Zealand Minister of Health, 2023a). In some rural communities of Australia and Aotearoa New Zealand, this also needs to value cultural well-being (Department of Health and Aged Care, 2021b; New Zealand Minister of Health, 2023a), which is particularly supported by First Nations peoples, such as Aboriginal, Torres Strait Islander and Māori peoples (Cox et al., 2022; Deravin, Anderson & Mahara, 2021; Morey et al., 2023).

REFLECTION

Consider the social determinants of health and identify how these may influence the health of rural communities for better or worse. What differences in social determinants may be responsible for the variations in health behaviours and outcomes observed across rural communities?

Collaboration and co-design

Collaboration and co-design of projects with a wide range of community groups is seen to be beneficial to promote healthy living overall and to ensure a holistic approach to health care, particularly in relation to the prevention of chronic conditions. This includes neighbourhood, cultural and social groups, workplaces, schools and government and non-government organisations (Department of Health, 2021b; New Zealand Minister of Health, 2023a). Engaging with such organisations allows nurses to assist a wider range of people and support them in addressing their own needs.

When collaborating and co-designing projects with community groups, it is important that the community groups firstly need to be heard and engaged in discussion; only then can action be taken together and decision-making shared (Bateman et al., 2022; Harding et al., 2021; Morey et al., 2023). It is also important to note that healthy relationships involve shared power, and this is the primary principle of co-design (Wall et al., 2022). If entering a community, it is generally wise to find out what has been done previously, who is already linked with health care who can provide advice and to locate some 'guides' – people from the respective community who are interested in helping with the new project and can provide guidance on how the initial consultation should take place. Different communities will function in different ways. Some will have senior representatives who can provide advice on who should be approached and how that should take place (Bateman et al., 2022).

Trust

Trust is not easy to establish. It takes a significant amount of time to build genuine relationships (Wall et al., 2022). If members of a health service have already developed trust with a community, then those people may be of assistance to develop new projects. However, it is important not to take advantage of such trust as it can easily be lost and then may affect several projects. Consultation is important in order to ensure that projects will meet the unique requirements of each community, but not lead people to think that all needs can be met, as there is often limited funding available (Bateman et al., 2022; Harding et al., 2021). In Aotearoa New Zealand, a research project into barriers for the co-design of community projects found that mismanaged expectations were the greatest barrier (Harding et al., 2021). Harding and colleagues identified that the term 'co-design' was often applied to lure people into working with teams, but the expected participation was not achievable within the project and raised expectations that were unable to be met both in design and output. Such mismanaged expectations damaged the trust that had been built within the community for the existing projects and possibly for future ones (Harding et al., 2021). When possible, fostering self-determination and community autonomy can empower communities to address issues themselves creating much better outcomes than those that are imposed upon them (Cox et al., 2022; Kelly et al., 2022).

When working with First Nations peoples, cultural safety is an important concept. It is not necessarily something that can be learned at one point in time. Most cultures change over time, and how they are perceived may even vary between individuals within the same culture. So, it is important to keep an open mind and continue learning about the variety of cultures we are exposed to. For a variety of reasons, it is preferable that health care is provided by health care professionals from the same cultural group as the people receiving the care, so supporting these professionals in their careers is also important (Biles et al., 2021; Kelly et al., 2022).

CASE STUDY 8.2

Jane is the local physiotherapist in your small rural town. At a multidisciplinary team meeting, she mentions how one of her clients had an embarrassing experience. Bob had a stroke approximately 12 months ago and she has been helping him with his walking, which has been improving slowly. He was in the local shopping centre with his wife when a young shop assistant asked him to leave as she had assumed that he had been drinking. A security guard was called when Bob refused to leave and commented on Bob's slurred speech and unsteady gait. Jane points out that Bob is from an Aboriginal background and feels that this also contributed to the response that he had received.

With the rest of the team, you brainstorm what can be done to assist some clients and how they can be accepted within the local shopping area. You arrange to meet the shopping centre's management team, and they agree that some education would be useful for staff working there. They also mention that some older patrons have difficulty negotiating the centre during busy times of the day and were wondering if some additional shopping hours would be appreciated by the elderly and perhaps people with a disability.

Together, you organise a trial of late-night shopping during the Christmas period, specifically targeted at the elderly and people with a disability. The local bus service agrees to run an extra bus that will stop at the local nursing homes, and each of the shops in the shopping centre agrees to provide at least one additional staff member during this time to assist people who may otherwise have difficulty with their shopping. Staff members of the shopping centre attend an education and awareness-raising session, and Bob is one of the speakers, telling people about his situation and how embarrassed he felt. Afterwards, the young shop assistant seeks him out and apologises for the incident.

REFLECTION

1. Are there any potential ethical issues for the nurse in becoming involved in this type of community engagement?
2. Is asking Bob to be a speaker in an education session an appropriate nursing action?
3. Although this intervention may have gone some way in addressing discrimination against people with a disability, it did not specifically address racial discrimination. What do you think could be done to tackle this issue?

REFLECTION

Consider why you would want to work in a rural or remote community.

1. What would you find attractive about this type of work?
2. What barriers do you think you would need to overcome?

Conclusion

Although RHNs face considerable challenges and need to be a specialist across a wide range of areas, there are also many benefits. RHNs are generally held in very high esteem by the community in which they work. Having a close knowledge of clients can lead to a greater capacity for holism. Having a greater understanding of home life and family dynamics in a very small community can mean that the nurse can be more effective when providing care. Many rural nurses have amazing experiences with First Nations when they understand their culture and work with them collaboratively. Genuinely knowing clients through inevitable social contact can lead to genuine caring, as opposed to the more generic caring that occurs in other environments. This can lead to the potential for RHNs to be significantly affected by the health outcomes of their patients.

CRITICAL THINKING ACTIVITIES

1. How do you think that someone new to an area could find key members of a First Nations community to guide them in a health promotion project?
2. What are the potential consequences for rural communities that do not have access to health care services?
3. What self-care strategies might RHNs engage in to prevent 'burn out' from their role?
4. How could RHNs manage their role and the ambiguity of professional boundaries?

FURTHER READING

Bateman, S., Arnold-Chamney, M., Jesudason, S., et al. (2022). Real ways of working together: Co-creating meaningful Aboriginal community consultations to advance kidney care. *Australian and New Zealand Journal of Public Health*, *46*(5), 614–21. https://doi.org/10.1111/1753-6405.13280

Harding, T., Oetzel, J.G., Foote, J. & Hepi, M. (2021). Perceptions of co-designing health promotion interventions with Indigenous communities in New Zealand. *Health Promotion International*, *36*(4), 964–75. https://doi.org/10.1093/heapro/daaa128

Smith, J.A., Canuto, K., Canuto, K., et al. (2022). Advancing health promotion in rural and remote Australia: Strategies for change. *Health Promotion Journal of Australia*, *33*(1), 3–6. https://doi.org/10.1002/hpja.569

REFERENCES

Adelson, P. & Eckert, M. (2020). Skin cancer in regional, rural and remote Australia; opportunities for service improvement through technological advances and interdisciplinary care. *Australian Journal of Advanced Nursing*, *37*(2), 25–30. https://doi.org/10.37464/2020.372.74

Arriero, I.M., Lalovic, A., Flicker, L., et al. (2023). Co-design of an Aboriginal health practitioner-led dementia prevention program (DAMPAA) using a theory of change framework. *Alzheimer's & Dementia*, *19*(S8). https://doi.org/10.1002/alz.065352

Australian Bureau of Statistics (ABS). (2021). *Remoteness structure*. www.abs.gov.au/statistics/standards/australian-statistical-geography-standard-asgs-edition-3/jul2021-jun2026/remoteness-structure

Australian College of Nursing. (2018). *Improving health outcomes in rural and remote Australia: Optimising the contribution of nurses*. www.acn.edu.au/wp-content/uploads/position-statement-discussion-paper-improving-health-outcomes-rural-remote-australia.pdf

Australian Institute of Health and Welfare (AIHW). (2022). *Health workforce*. Australian Government. www.aihw.gov.au/reports/workforce/health-workforce

——— (2023). *Rural and remote health*. Australian Government. www.aihw.gov.au/reports/rural-remote-australians/rural-and-remote-health

Bateman, S., Arnold-Chamney, M., Jesudason, S., et al. (2022). Real ways of working together: Co-creating meaningful Aboriginal community consultations to advance kidney care. *Australian and New Zealand Journal of Public Health, 46*(5), 614–21. https://doi.org/10.1111/1753-6405.13280

Beccaria, L., McIlveen, P., Fein, E.C., et al. (2021). Importance of attachment to place in growing a sustainable Australian rural health workforce: A rapid review. *The Australian Journal of Rural Health, 29*(5), 620–42. https://doi.org/10.1111/ajr.12799

Biles, J., Deravin, L., Seaman, C.E., et al. (2021). Learnings from a mentoring project to support Aboriginal and Torres Strait Islander nurses and midwives to remain in the workforce. *Contemporary Nurse: A Journal for the Australian Nursing Profession, 57*(5), 327–37. https://doi.org/10.1080/10376178.2021.1991412

Blay, N., Sousa, M.S., Rowles, M. & Murray-Parahi, P. (2022). The community nurse in Australia. Who are they? A rapid systematic review. *Journal of Nursing Management, 30*(1), 154–68. https://doi.org/10.1111/jonm.13493

Bourke, L., Dunbar, T. & Murakami-Gold, L. (2021). Discourses within the roles of remote area nurses in Northern Territory (Australia) government-run health clinics. *Health & Social Care in the Community, 29*(5), 1401–8. https://doi.org/10.1111/hsc.13195

Chiarella, M., Currie, J. & Wand, T. (2020). Liability and collaborative arrangements for nurse practitioner practice in Australia. *Australian Health Review, 44*(2), 172–7. https://doi.org/10.1071/ah19072

Colman, C. (2021). Aged care in rural Australia. *Australian Journal of Rural Health, 29*(3), 483–4. https://doi.org/10.1111/ajr.12770

Cox, T., Hoang, H., Mond, J. & Cross, M. (2022). Closing the gap in Aboriginal health disparities: Is there a place for Elders in the neoliberal agenda? *Australian Health Review, 46*(2), 173–7. https://doi.org/10.1071/AH21098

Department of Health and Aged Care. (2021a). *National Aboriginal and Torres Strait Islander Health Plan 2021–2031*. Commonwealth of Australia.

——— (2021b). *National Preventive Health Strategy 2021–2030*. Commonwealth of Australia.

——— (2023a). *About the Multi-Purpose Services (MPS) Program*. Commonwealth of Australia. www.health.gov.au/our-work/multi-purpose-services-mps-program/about-the-multi-purpose-services-mps-program

——— (2023b). *Nurse and midwives in Australia*: Commonwealth of Australia.

Deravin, L., Anderson, J. & Mahara, N. (2021). Cultural safety for First Nations people in aged care. *Contemporary Nurse: A Journal for the Australian Nursing Profession, 57*(5), 308–11. https://doi.org/10.1080/10376178.2021.1962378

Deravin, L., Francis, K. & Anderson, J. (2018). Closing the gap in Indigenous health inequity – Is it making a difference? *International nursing review, 65*(4), 477–83. https://doi.org/10.1111/inr.12436

Drummond, A. (2021). Working with Aboriginal and Torres Strait Islander health workers and health practitioners. In O. Best & B. Fredericks (eds), *Yatdjuligin: Aboriginal and Torres Strait Islander Nursing and Midwifery Care* (3rd ed., pp. 207–35). Cambridge University Press.

Dwyer, T., Craswell, A. & Browne, M. (2021). Predictive factors of the general public's willingness to be seen and seek treatment from a nurse practitioner in Australia: A cross-sectional national survey. *Human Resources for Health, 19*(1), 21–21. https://doi.org/10.1186/s12960-021-00562-7

Fedele, R. & Dragon, N. (2023). ANMF priorities 2023. *The Australian Nursing Journal, 27*(10), 8–13.

Fitzpatrick, S.J., Handley, T., Powell, N., et al. (2021). Suicide in rural Australia: A retrospective study of mental health problems, health-seeking and service utilisation. *PloS ONE, 16*(7), e0245271–e0245271. https://doi.org/10.1371/journal.pone.0245271

Gilbert, A.S., Owusu-Addo, E., Feldman, P., et al. (2020). *Models of Integrated Care, Health and Housing: Report prepared for the Royal Commission into Aged Care Quality and Safety*. National Ageing Research Institute.

Gott, M., Wiles, J., Mason, K. & Moeke-Maxwell, T. (2023). Creating 'safe spaces': A qualitative study to explore enablers and barriers to culturally safe end-of-life care. *Palliative Medicine, 37*(4), 520–9. https://doi.org/10.1177/02692163221138621

Griffiths, K. & Smith, J. (2020). Measuring health disparities in Australia: Using data to drive health promotion solutions. *Health Promotion Journal of Australia, 31*(2), 166–8. https://doi.org/10.1002/hpja.340

Harding, T., Oetzel, J.G., Foote, J. & Hepi, M. (2021). Perceptions of co-designing health promotion interventions with Indigenous communities in New Zealand. *Health Promotion International, 36*(4), 964–75. https://doi.org/10.1093/heapro/daaa128

Harper, C., Bourke, S.L., Johnson, E., et al. (2021). Health care experiences in rural, remote, and metropolitan areas of Australia. *Online Journal of Rural Nursing and Health Care, 21*(1), 67–84. https://doi.org/10.14574/ojrnhc.v21i1.652

Jacups, S.P. & Kinchin, I. (2021). A rapid review of evidence to inform an ear, nose and throat service delivery model in remote Australia. *Rural and Remote Health, 21*(4), 1–12.

Jennings, N., Lowe, G. & Tori, K. (2021). Nurse practitioner locums: A plausible solution for augmenting health care access for rural communities. *Australian Journal of Primary Health, 27*(1), 1–5. https://doi.org/10.1071/PY20103

Kelly, J., Stevenson, T., Arnold-Chamney, M., et al. (2022). Aboriginal patients driving kidney and healthcare improvements: Recommendations from South Australian community consultations. *Australian and New Zealand Journal of Public Health, 46*(5), 622–9. https://doi.org/10.1111/1753-6405.13279

LaMothe, J., Hendricks, S., Halstead, J., et al. (2021). Developing interprofessional collaborative practice competencies in rural primary health care teams. *Nursing Outlook, 69*(3), 447–57. https://doi.org/10.1016/j.outlook.2020.12.001

Leach, M.J., Gunn, K. & Muyambi, K. (2022). The determinants of healthcare utilisation in regional, rural and remote South Australia: A cross-sectional study. *Health & Social Care in the Community, 30*(6), e4850–e4863. https://doi.org/10.1111/hsc.13894

Matta, G., Longhitano, C., Husodo, C. & McDermott, B. (2021). Mental health service provision in rural Australia: A regional town–city comparison of two continuing care teams. *Australasian Psychiatry: Bulletin of the Royal Australian and New Zealand College of Psychiatrists, 29*(2), 119–23. https://doi.org/10.1177/1039856220928862

McCullough, K., Bayes, S., Whitehead, L., Williams, A. & Cope, V. (2022). Nursing in a different world: Remote area nursing as a specialist–generalist practice area. *The Australian Journal of Rural Health, 30*(5), 570–81. https://doi.org/10.1111/ajr.12899

McPherson, K. & Nahon, I. (2021). Telehealth and the provision of pelvic health physiotherapy in regional, rural and remote Australia. *Australian and New Zealand Continence Journal, 27*(3), 66–70. https://doi.org/10.33235/anzcj.27.3.66-70

Morey, K., Pearson, O., Sivak, L., et al. (2023). An Aboriginal-led consortium approach to chronic disease action for health equity and holistic wellbeing. *Health Promotion Journal of Australia, 34*(3), 634–43. https://doi.org/10.1002/hpja.765

Morgan, J.M. & Calleja, P. (2020). Emergency trauma care in rural and remote settings: Challenges and patient outcomes. *International Emergency Nursing, 51*, 100880–9. https://doi.org/10.1016/j.ienj.2020.100880

Naren, T., Burzacott, J., West, C. & Widdicombe, D. (2021). Role of Aboriginal health practitioners in administering and increasing covid-19 vaccination rates in a Victorian Aboriginal community controlled health organisation. *Rural and Remote Health, 21*(4), 1–4. https://doi.org/10.22605/rrh7043

National Rural Health Alliance. (2021). *Home page.* www.ruralhealth.org.au

New Zealand Flying Doctor Service. (2024). *Home page.* https://www.nzflyingdoctors.co.nz/

New Zealand Health Workforce Advisory Board. (2022). *Annual Report to the New Zealand Minister of Health January 2022.* New Zealand Health Workforce Advisory Board.

New Zealand Minister of Health. (2023a). *New Zealand Health Strategy.* Ministry of Health.

———— (2023b). *Pae Tū: Hauora Māori Strategy*. Ministry of Health.

———— (2023c). *Rural Health Strategy*. Ministry of Health.

Pagone, T. & Briggs, L. (2021). *Royal Commission into Aged Care Quality and Safety, Final Report – Care, Dignity, and Respect*. Commonwealth of Australia.

Royal Flying Doctor Service (RFDS). (2023). *Flying Doctors*. www.flyingdoctor.org.au/

Ryan, E., de Klerk, E. & Green, E. (2024). What are the benefits and opportunities of rural health practice? *The Australian Nursing Journal*, *28*(3), 24–5.

Smith, J.A., Canuto, K., Canuto, K., et al. (2022). Advancing health promotion in rural and remote Australia: Strategies for change. *Health Promotion Journal of Australia*, *33*(1), 3–6. https://doi .org/10.1002/hpja.569

Tipene-Leach, D. (2021). The Choosing Wisely campaign and shared decision-making with Māori. *New Zealand Medical Journal*, *134*(1547), 26–33.

Ung, D.S.K., Goh, Y.S., Poon, R.Y.S., et al. (2024). Global migration and factors influencing retention of Asian internationally educated nurses: A systematic review. *Human Resources for Health*, *22*(1), 17. https://doi.org/10.1186/s12960-024-00900-5

Victorian Auditor-General's Office. (2018). *Community Health Program: Independent Assurance Report to Parliament*. Victorian Government.

Wall, S., Donovan, T., Radford, K., et al. (2022). Reflections on working and walking gently together in collaboration and partnership in Aboriginal ageing research. *The Australian Journal of Rural Health*, *30*(6), 795–800. https://doi.org/10.1111/ajr.12917

Whitehead, J. (2022). Defining rural in Aotearoa New Zealand: A novel geographic classification for health purposes. *New Zealand Medical Journal*, *135*(1559), 24–40.

Whiteing, N., Barr, J. & Rossi, D.M. (2021). The practice of rural and remote nurses in Australia: A case study. *Journal of Clinical Nursing*, *31*(11–12), 1502–18. https://doi.org/10.1111/ jocn.16002

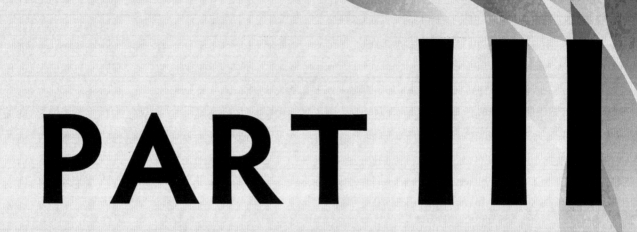

PART III

Skills for practice

9 Interprofessional practice

Kath Peters and Elizabeth Halcomb

LEARNING OBJECTIVES

At the completion of this chapter, you should be able to:

- identify the barriers to and facilitators of multidisciplinary health professionals working well together.
- explain how professional identity and culture influence interprofessional practice.
- describe the behaviours and skills that facilitate effective communication.
- understand the causes of interprofessional conflict and identify conflict resolution strategies.

Introduction

Community and primary health care (PHC) nursing is experiencing a rapid metamorphosis as our population ages and the prevalence of chronic and complex conditions increases. To meet these changing needs, our health workforce has evolved with a range of specialised disciplines now working in diverse health settings. Throughout these changes, nursing continues to be the largest global health workforce providing the most direct client care. Historically, nurses were the original transdisciplinary health care workers, providing basic physiotherapy, occupational therapy, nutritional advice and all other care as required. As more detailed knowledge developed in an area of practice, specialised areas of care evolved, and a variety of allied health professions emerged. In turn, nursing itself became more specialised, due to developments in clinical practice, technological advances and the need for more complex care.

It is widely recognised that PHC nurses are integral to the provision of safe, efficient and high-quality care (Halcomb et al., 2017a; New Zealand Nurses Organisation, 2019) and are seen as key deliverers in the agenda for strengthening PHC services internationally (Karam et al., 2021; World Health Organization (WHO), 2018). While valuable contributions are made by individual groups of health professionals, it has been demonstrated that organised care delivery – where a range of health professionals and support workers provide integrated care to clients – optimises health outcomes, improves patient safety, reduces health costs and improves job satisfaction (Brown et al., 2021; Etz et al., 2019; Saint-Pierre, Herskovic & Sepulveda., 2018).

Characteristics of interprofessional collaboration play a significant role in the effectiveness of the team (Wranik et al., 2019). To be effective, the health team needs to have knowledge and understanding of the various professional roles, an ability to communicate well and, above all else, maintain a person-centred focus (Wranik et al., 2019). Positive workplace relationships between health professionals have benefits for the professionals and the people for whom they are providing care. An enabling workplace culture enhances staff satisfaction, improves retention and reduces stress and burnout (Halcomb, Smyth & McInnes, 2018). A person-centred focus ensures that the needs and preferences of the recipients of care are central to service delivery (Eaton, Roberts & Turner, 2015). In contrast, the failure of multidisciplinary clinicians to work together effectively has been demonstrated to negatively impact the quality of care delivered (Josi, Bianchi & Brandt, 2020) and adversely impact job satisfaction (Halcomb et al., 2018).

The terminology around how health professionals work together is far from consistent, further compounding the complexity and confusion experienced by clinicians. A range of terms including collaboration, interdisciplinary practice, multidisciplinary practice, teamwork, integrated care and variations on these are often used interchangeably to describe the models via which health professionals work together. In this chapter, we use the term **interprofessional practice** to describe the way in which two or more health professionals from different disciplines work in a coordinated way to provide person-centred care. This is achieved through open communication and shared decision making when assessing, planning and evaluating care (Fowler et al., 2020). Health professionals working together in a model, of interprofessional practice facilitate effective teamwork and are vital in alleviating the global health crisis through improved health outcomes (Wagner, 2000; WHO, 2010). In this model practitioners seek to foster team-based activity rather than being defensive of their individual professional boundaries (Flood et al., 2022).

Professional roles, cultures and boundaries

No single health profession is likely to meet all of the health needs of most people (Fiscella & McDaniel, 2018; Rosen et al., 2018). Therefore, different health professionals need to work together to achieve optimal health outcomes (Rosen et al., 2018). While this may seem a simple concept, achieving good working relationships and teamwork between clinicians from different professions can often present significant challenges. One key area which is a potential source of conflict is the mutual understanding of each team member's scope of practice (Szafran et al., 2019).

The scope of practice of each profession is defined in the various regulatory documents within each jurisdiction and refers to the roles, tasks and procedures that the individual is permitted to undertake (Downie et al., 2023). Failure to understand and acknowledge another professional's scope of practice can result in individuals becoming protective of their area of practice and resisting collaboration, particularly if they believe someone else is trying to 'take over' their role (Junod Perron et al., 2019). This is particularly evident, for example, where a GP lacks a clear understanding of the different categories of nurses and their individual scopes of practice (Australian Nursing and Midwifery Federation (ANMF), 2014; New Zealand Nurses Organisation (NZNO), 2019).

Not understanding the scope of each professional's practice may also result in the under-utilisation of expertise and experience (Brown et al., 2021; Junod Perron et al., 2019;

Interprofessional practice – practice that involves two or more health professionals from different disciplines who have common health goals for a client. Working in a coordinated way, health professionals provide client-centred health care, using open communication and shared decision-making when assessing, planning and evaluating care (WHO, 2013).

Szafran et al., 2019). This can result in frustration and reduced job satisfaction for those not practising to the extent of their skills and can negatively impact the retention of skilled staff (Halcomb & Ashley, 2019; Halcomb et al., 2018). Significant gains can be made by having open discussions about the extent of your professional scope and seeking to find out more about the professional scope of others in order to improve the level of shared understanding (Brown et al., 2021;). In their study of Swiss primary care clinics, Josi and colleagues (2020) found that role clarification was the most critical factor in achieving interprofessional collaboration within a team-based model.

REFLECTION

1. How well do you understand the roles and professional scope of your colleagues?
2. How could you improve your understanding of the roles and professional scope of your colleagues?
3. Have a discussion with a health professional from another discipline about their scope of practice. What is their understanding of your scope of practice?

Role blurring may also occur in areas of practice where job descriptions are vague or when health professionals are unsure where their practice responsibilities begin and end (McInnes et al., 2017b). In PHC settings, role blurring may occur where roles and responsibilities are interchangeable, and competencies overlap across professions (Brown et al., 2021). Without clear guidelines, role blurring may be associated with increased conflict and burnout of team members (Conroy, 2019). Improving the understanding of each team member's scope of practice and professional responsibilities as well as open communication can significantly reduce the impact of role-blurring (Halcomb et al., 2017a).

Role and professional identity

Each profession has its own theoretical underpinnings that influence practice, philosophy and approach (Schot, Tummers & Noordegraaf, 2020). Developing a professional identity is an essential aspect of becoming a confident and authoritative health professional and underpins the nurse's values, beliefs and attitudes (Philippa et al., 2021). Experienced professionals who are confident in their individual roles are better able to work across professional boundaries, share knowledge and defer their autonomy to work effectively with professionals from other disciplines (Wranik et al., 2019).

Another feature impacting professional identity within a rapidly evolving primary health care landscape is the rise in corporate structures providing health services. While professional organisations have emerged to regulate and support practitioners through these changes, new nurses must navigate a myriad of challenges as they develop professional roles and identities within this changing landscape. These include demonstrating support for their organisation while at the same time developing a professional identity attuned to nursing.

Additionally, the view of nurses as subordinates continues to pervade contemporary nursing practices in some health care settings, including PHC, and acts as a barrier to integrated care (Taranta & Marcinowicz, 2020). Such perceptions are often exacerbated by the private nature and ownership of many PHC facilities where medical practitioners are often employers of nurses (McInnes et al., 2017a). Given the growth of nursing within private enterprise, there remains a need to evaluate the role and professional identities in this rapidly evolving sector.

While PHC business owners, such as GPs, have a legal and ethical responsibility to monitor the work of their employees, as regulated health professionals, nurses are ultimately responsible for their clinical practice (Nursing and Midwifery Board of Australia (NMBA), 2016; Nursing Council of New Zealand (NCNZ), 2012). Indeed, while administrative and employment-related matters may be overseen by a manager or GP, the clinical care provided by nurses should only be supervised by another nurse (ANMF, 2014; NCNZ, 2012). Nurses, however, need to ensure that they assume a confident and authoritative stance to promote their professional standing and identity.

Professional culture

Professional culture encompasses the values, behaviours and ways of thinking that are passed on to new members as they join the group, and which distinguish one professional group from another (Machen et al., 2019). Professional enculturation commences with discipline-specific education and is facilitated by experiences, values, approaches to problem solving and language (Azzam et al., 2023). In the workplace, incidences of incivility, bullying and horizontal violence can shape an organisation's professional culture. In the pre-industrial period health care was usually provided by women in their community (Nancarrow & Borthwick, 2021). However, during the Industrial Revolution in Britain, several policies regulating health care provision resulted in medical dominance in health care (Nancarrow & Borthwick, 2021). During this time, universities were only accessible to middle- and upper-class men, leading to the delivery of health care being organised around masculine values, needs and desires. Middle-class women were encouraged to enter nursing, creating gender and social class friction that is often still evident today (Snee & Goswami, 2021).

High costs associated with medical education are another aspect driving competition and professional culture in health care. Historically there has been an expectation that medical practitioners take responsibility for decision-making, with an emphasis on action and outcome. An entrenched pattern of hierarchical decision-making, with the medical practitioner at the apex of the hierarchy, is common in most health systems (Macdonald et al., 2023). However, research suggests that hierarchical decision making is largely contrary to good interprofessional practice principles (Al-Worafi, 2024). In PHC settings, these complexities are accentuated by the dual role of the GP as the employer and colleague of nurses (McInnes et al., 2017a; McInnes et al., 2017b). The business model associated with private practice may manifest this hierarchy and the direction of professional culture in this setting.

Nursing practice relies on efficiently exchanging information, collective problem solving and working as part of a team. Professions such as nursing and social work adopt a person-centred approach to care where the client's subjective information and self-determination are valued over the dependence on objective data (Saw et al., 2023). Barriers to communication may be created when differing professional values are unspoken and go unacknowledged between team members (Schot et al., 2020). Focusing on individuals'

Professional culture – the values, behaviours and ways of thinking within each profession, and which distinguish one group from another (Machen et al., 2019).

needs and desires assists professionals to move beyond their professional boundaries, facilitates collaboration and reduces conflict (Flood et al., 2022).

These professional cultural factors can be seen to impact health professionals working together. Successful interprofessional practice is evident when all members are seen as being of equal status, and no single member is considered senior or seeks to dominate decision-making (Wranik et al., 2019).

Working in teams

Team structure and processes, availability of organisational support and a conducive environment are important indicators of successful teamwork (Rosen et al., 2018; Wranik et al., 2019). In the delivery of PHC, the complexity of teamwork is often increased as health professionals, who are working to provide health care to a particular client, are often not a part of a formally constructed team. In reality, they are often employed by a variety of different organisations with competing priorities. This may result in a lack of consistency in the care delivered, as different health professionals will provide care based on factors such as individual needs, preferences for providers, referral patterns and accessibility. This lack of consistency also makes the leadership of the team challenging.

In PHC settings, individual health professionals are often located at different sites or within complex physical layouts. This is problematic as when team members are based at different locations, they tend to be less integrated, and this reduces team functioning and effectiveness. Conversely, co-location enhances information transfer, facilitates communication and increases personal familiarity (Wranik et al., 2019). Team stability and team effectiveness are most apparent when there is a high proportion of full-time staff who have been working together over a long period. PHC settings are often challenged in this regard due to the significant part-time workforce and the regular turnover of staff.

Individual members of a PHC team may be situated in diverse geographical locations and have different communication and medical records systems (Junod Perron et al., 2019). Team processes, including regular formal meetings, are important for effective team functioning and provide important opportunities for members to communicate their perceptions, concerns and understandings (Wranik et al., 2019). Such meetings are often best when they are inclusive of all team members, or at least represent each professional group within the team (McInnes et al., 2017b). As team members gain an understanding of others' competencies, professional barriers begin to break down and interprofessional conflict is resolved promptly. While team meetings provide valuable opportunities to promote positive interprofessional practice, the private business nature of many PHC settings creates a challenge to reconcile the financial cost of staff downtime to attend meetings against the potentially improved performance stemming from a cohesive team (Fiscella & McDaniel, 2018).

Clear team goals promote effective interprofessional practice, help clarify each professional's role and responsibilities and provide the team with a shared vision (Thistlethwaite & McLarnon, 2023; Wranik et al., 2019). Some form of regular critical reflection, evaluation or audit assists in sustaining good performance and improving performance in areas where this is needed. This process facilitates the acknowledgement of a team member's expertise, skills and contribution, and provides the opportunity to discuss problems, provide support and find solutions to improve team functioning. As team members are exposed to the competencies of others, mutual respect and trust are established resulting in more effective teamwork (Szafran et al., 2019).

REFLECTION

1. What factors might challenge teamwork in PHC?
2. What individual attributes might facilitate teamwork in PHC?
3. What are the advantages of teamwork in PHC for clients and for health professionals?

Communication

Miscommunication has been linked to patient safety issues and poor health outcomes (Nora & Beghetto, 2020). The physical environment of PHC may challenge communication between team members and negatively influence interprofessional practice (Seaton et al., 2021). Good formal and informal communication skills enable understanding and differentiation of roles, negotiation and conflict resolution when required, and ensure clarity when sharing information (Rosen et al., 2018). However, each profession tends to report in its individual style and from its own professional perspective (Junod Perron et al., 2019). Effective verbal and written communication between health professionals is a key component of successful interdisciplinary practice and is known to decrease the occurrence of significant errors (Nora & Beghetto, 2020). It is vital, therefore, that workplace guidelines are established to clarify acceptable communication processes, and that all team members have the confidence to approach other members either formally or informally.

Interprofessional communication

Communication between health professionals occurs via various formal and informal means (Donnelly et al., 2019). Common forms of communication include written care notes, referrals, reports and case discussions. Discussions may be held either face-to-face, by email, or via teleconferencing or videoconferencing. How the discussion is framed needs to be considered and non-verbal behaviours, demonstrated during interactions, should be moderated to convey positive messages. Non-verbal communication can convey significant implicit messages that can either enhance or detract from relationships between health professionals.

Communication that supports interprofessional practice is non-hierarchical, acknowledges the skills each professional brings and uses a common language (Szafran et al., 2019). Reaching a consensus between health professionals and presenting a unified opinion to the client is fundamental for the provision of high-quality care (Junod Perron et al., 2019). The use of appropriate assertive negotiation and conflict management skills facilitates the attainment of consensus.

The hierarchical nature of many PHC settings can create a unilateral top-down approach to communication (Fox et al., 2021). Ad hoc communication strategies are frequently used by busy PHC professionals who are working in parallel. Door-stop meetings or electronic messages between professionals may help address immediate client needs. However, regular, structured synchronous communication, utilised in clinical meetings, is vital to achieve deeper communication and mutual understanding between clinicians (McInnes et al., 2017a).

Written communication

One of the key functions of written communication in health care is to share information with other health professionals. This may be through providing a referral, recording history and progress, passing on client information or writing a formal clinical report (Junod Perron et al., 2019). Essentially, written communication should be informative, clear and concise to ensure that the reader receives the message that the sender wanted to deliver. The asynchronous nature of written communication means that there is potential for the reader to misinterpret the message if it is unclear or ambiguous. Health professionals must ensure that their duty of care to their clients is fulfilled by providing sufficient information in a timely manner.

Useful strategies for writing in the health care context include distinguishing between opinion and fact, using positive rather than negative language, avoiding over-generalisations, not being inappropriately critical and using short, familiar words (Junod Perron et al., 2019). Ethical and legal constraints also need to be considered when sharing information, even with other health care providers (Junod Perron et al., 2019). It is therefore important for clinicians to be conversant with policies, guidelines and legal requirements relating to data management within their organisation and local environment.

A key challenge in written communication in PHC is that various health service providers have their own individual medical records systems, and these are rarely transferred or shared between providers. This frequently results in fragmentation of the client's medical history and poor continuity of information. Such fragmentation creates a need for coordination of care and for health professionals to be committed to actively facilitating communication with others to provide integrated care. To enhance such communication and promote coordinated care, the Australian government has initiated the Health Care Homes program. Health Care Homes are general practices or Aboriginal Community Controlled Health Services that provide clients who have multiple and complex health conditions with flexible, tailored and coordinated care (Department of Health and Aged Care, 2022). While co-location is advantageous, the impact of this model on communication is yet to be determined. Aotearoa New Zealand's Ministry of Health (2019a) has set out its standards for published health information to assist the issue of integrated care. The standards are supported and monitored by the Health Information Standards Organisation (Ministry of Health, 2019b).

Electronic communication

Teleconferencing and telehealth, including telemonitoring, are already used in many rural and remote PHC facilities. As a result of COVID-19 telehealth has advanced rapidly and become more mainstream (Halcomb et al., 2023). Such forms of electronic communication remotely monitor and transmit physiological data from the client's residence to the health professional. Telemonitoring has demonstrated a capacity to reduce mortality and length of stay in acute care facilities, improve medication compliance and improve quality of life (Lyth et al., 2021). In Australia, the advent of My Health Record in 2012 provides people with an opportunity to develop an online summary of their health information which they can then share with health providers (Australian Digital Health Agency, 2024; Halcomb et al., 2023). This has significant advantages when multiple providers can contribute to the same record for a single person and share information. From 31 January 2019, all Australians who did not choose to 'opt out' have a My Health Record. My Health Record provides a digital online summary of a person's health record, including up-to-date medical data, test results, referral letters and information about organ donation. My Health Record also seeks to enhance coordinated care for those with chronic and complex health conditions, reduce medication errors and unnecessary duplication of pathology (Healthdirect, 2019). Despite the potential advantages of such electronic records, the uptake and utilisation have been variable among consumers and health providers (Halcomb et al., 2017c). Aotearoa New Zealand's Health Information Standards Organisation has assessed the Patient Summary Standards Set (PSSS) as a source of standards for personal health information and the future national Health Information Platform (nHIP) (Ministry of Health, 2019c). This work is currently ongoing.

Electronic communication within the PHC sector is set to be revolutionised with the increased access of the National Broadband Network in regional and rural areas. Given the speed and video quality associated with these new networks, this high-speed medical-quality internet service will transform the way PHC professionals communicate and deliver care. However, as with all new technologies, there must be a readiness to implement this service and time to participate in professional development opportunities.

The case conference

A **case conference** is a collaborative, interdisciplinary meeting held to discuss and make decisions regarding the health care needs and management of a specific individual (Vest et al., 2021). This kind of meeting is likely to include a range of health care professionals who are involved in the management of the individual and should also include the client and/or family members/carers.

Case conference – a meeting involving consumers (or their representatives) and health professionals at which the needs of the client are presented, and care options are discussed.

Case conferencing has been demonstrated to improve team members understanding of each other and communication between team members (Donnelly et al., 2019; Papermaster, Whitney & Vinas, 2023). Team members report that case conferencing can enhance service delivery, care quality and patient safety, and it has also been shown to enhance health outcomes and reduce health service utilisation (Papermaster et al., 2023; Vest et al., 2021).

Nurses play a key role in the process of case conferencing as a result of their strong advocacy and care coordination responsibilities (Halcomb et al., 2017b). The specific role of the nurse in case conferencing varies between PHC settings but may include tasks such as undertaking baseline client assessments, drawing together various medical records, identifying clinical and client/family problems and priorities, convening the meeting, recording outcomes, distributing records of the conference to participants and other health providers, and monitoring and enacting subsequent care plans. The key to achieving the value of a case conference is ensuring that the care plans and strategies developed from the conference are enacted to enhance the care of clients and optimise their health outcomes.

CASE STUDY 9.1

Harry transitioned into employment within general practice from a busy emergency department three years ago. He is a registered nurse (advanced practice) who identifies and responds to the health and social needs of the local community. Harry works with six GPs, two other general practice nurses (GPNs) and a part-time psychologist. Harry is responsible for running a nurse-led clinic for adolescents two afternoons a week and regularly engages with local community groups to promote the clinic to teenagers. Harry has identified an increase in sexually transmitted infections and discusses his concerns during the weekly team meeting at the general practice.

REFLECTION
1. Who do you think should be present at the team meetings in this general practice?
2. What health promotion activities could the general practice initiate in the local community to address Harry's concerns?
3. What are the professional roles of the various team members in contributing to addressing this issue?

Interprofessional conflict

Due to the diversity in professional backgrounds within PHC, interprofessional conflict is inevitable when collaborative care is required. Sources of interdisciplinary conflict are multiple and complex and include interpersonal and organisational factors (Brown et al., 2021). However, the most common sources of conflict include a lack of understanding and/or confidence in other disciplines, feeling threatened by the blurring of roles, conflicting values and beliefs, poor interpersonal relationships, lack of team goals and poor communication (Brown et al., 2021; Schot et al., 2020). In order to avoid conflict and enhance collaborative care, Brown and colleagues (2021) advocate for greater interdisciplinary dialogue so that health professionals gain a clear understanding of their own and others' roles. Further strategies suggested for avoiding and/or resolving conflict include the development of shared team goals, interprofessional education, open communication and ensuring that all parties respect each other, are willing to listen to varying opinions and assume responsibility for their contribution to the conflict (Brown et al., 2021; Schot et al., 2020). Successful conflict resolution has important implications for interprofessional collaboration (Josi et al., 2020).

Conflict management

Not all conflict is negative. Some conflicts may contribute to the professional development of PHC professionals and the organisation they belong to. However, unresolved interprofessional conflict is detrimental to team functioning and can have a negative impact on job satisfaction and client outcomes (Halcomb et al., 2018).

Ideally, conflict should be resolved using a collaborative and problem-solving approach. This approach is often referred to as 'win-win'. Despite being the most time-consuming approach, the problem-solving process continues until each individual is satisfied with the resolution. Using this approach increases the likelihood of sustainable change.

Barriers to interprofessional conflict resolution include lack of time, power imbalances between health professionals, lack of recognition of conflict or motivation to resolve it and fear of causing emotional discomfort to others (Brown et al., 2021; Wranik et al., 2019). Using a facilitator, who is not invested in the outcome of the conflict, and the development of conflict resolution policies and procedures, may mitigate such barriers. The ability of health professionals to work effectively as a team is a complex process that relies on successful conflict resolution fostered by mutual respect, careful listening, focusing on the issues, and acknowledgement of differences and the emotional aspects of disagreement (Brown et al., 2021).

Negotiation

Negotiation comprises a large part of conflict resolution and is required when there are competing agendas, priorities or perspectives (Ellis, 2021). During all stages of negotiation, verbal and non-verbal communication needs to remain respectful, assertive and non-emotional (Fishman & Slanetz, 2021). The following four strategies may be employed to assist in successful negotiation during the conflict resolution process:

1. Focus on the problem, not the people, and avoid apportioning blame. Focusing on the problem results in the conflict being less emotive and more objective, and blame creates a culture of fear, discourages transparency and decreases collaboration.
2. Identify the cause of the conflict. Conflict is complex and may include personal, professional and organisational issues. Understanding the source of the conflict assists in problem-solving.
3. Ensure all stakeholders are committed and agree to resolve the conflict. It is important to provide the opportunity for all relevant parties to contribute to the solution to maximise collaboration.
4. Focus on common goals (for example, better client outcomes). Interprofessional goals reduce conflict and increase collaboration between co-workers (Brown et al., 2021; Fishman & Slanetz, 2021).

CASE STUDY 9.2

Cindy has been working as a practice nurse alongside a GP for eight years. She has postgraduate qualifications, having completed a graduate certificate in child and family health, and is endorsed as a nurse immuniser. Due to the increased workload at the practice, a second GP has been employed, and today is the first opportunity that Cindy has had to work with him. During a well-baby check on a four-month-old, Cindy was about to administer a scheduled vaccination when the new GP walked into the examination room and insisted on giving the injection. Cindy was embarrassed as this occurred in the presence of the baby's mother. She felt devalued and thought that the GP didn't trust her to carry out the procedure. As she is upset, she decides to confront the GP and let him know how she feels. However, an emergency presentation to the clinic leaves no time for this. After thinking about the scenario, Cindy begins to lack confidence about confronting the GP as she feels intimidated and is doubtful that anything will change.

CASE STUDY 9.2 Continued

REFLECTION

1. What are some possible reasons for the GP's behaviour?
2. What barriers to conflict resolution can be identified in this case study?
3. What possible consequences may there be for Cindy if she continues to avoid conflict in this way?
4. How could the situation be managed differently?
5. What steps can Cindy take to resolve this conflict?

Reflective practice

Critically reflecting on practice is a mechanism that works towards improving the quality of client outcomes. Any health care provider's professional practice can be strengthened by being personally and professionally self-aware. This can be achieved using reflective practice (Linsley & Barker, 2019). The principle underpinning **reflective practice** is that of reflective learning, which has its roots in educational theory. Reflective practice is essentially thoughtful practice. Additionally, critically reflecting on one's personal feelings and responses to situations encountered can assist in facilitating personal growth.

Achieving a standard of professional practice commensurate with safe, client-centred care requires health professionals to individually reflect on their own skills, standards and ethical obligations (Linsley & Barker, 2019). Evidence further suggests that teams that reflect upon their performance and decision-making processes are rewarded with improved efficiency and quality of care (Brown et al., 2021). PHC facilities are able to support the individual insight and reflection of interdisciplinary team members through regular performance reviews and by establishing clinical meetings that are inclusive of all health professionals (Fiscella & McDaniel, 2018).

Reflective practice – 'is a process of thinking clearly, deeply and critically about any aspect of our professional practice' (Clinical Excellence Commission, 2022). 'Reflective practice is purposeful and allows practitioners to critically review, explore, challenge and learn from their practice' (Koh et al., 2022, p. 880).

Conclusion

Interprofessional practice has been demonstrated to enhance health care and provide optimal health outcomes. To ensure the best possible health outcomes for clients, effective teamwork is required between health professionals who have a range of skills and knowledge, and who share common health goals for their clients. Effective teamwork relies on the use of well-developed communication and professional skills by all team members. In a PHC setting – where a range of unique factors impact on interprofessional practice – mastery of communication, conflict management and problem solving skills are paramount to ensure common health goals for clients are met. Further, the use of reflective practice by individuals and the team is essential to ensure optimal team functioning.

CRITICAL THINKING ACTIVITIES

1. Consider Figure 9.1.

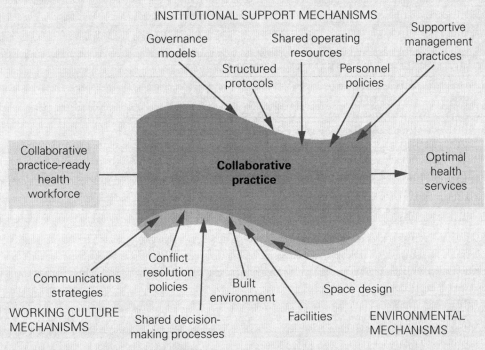

Figure 9.1 Examples of mechanisms that shape collaboration at the practice level
Source: WHO (2010, p. 29).

a. Explain each of the mechanisms that contribute towards collaborative care.
b. Identify and discuss which three mechanisms you consider would have the greatest effect on interprofessional practice. Give your reasons.

2. Consider Figure 9.2.

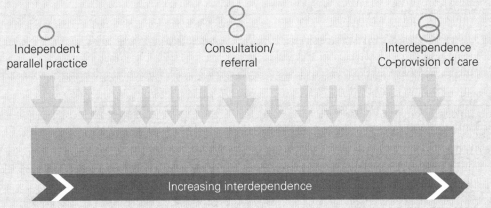

Figure 9.2 The spectrum of collaboration
Source: Oandasan et al. (2006, p. 4).

a. Where would your current practice be positioned within the spectrum of collaboration? What factors impact this?
b. What aspects of the spectrum of collaboration can you identify in terms of multi-morbidity and chronic disease management? Give your reasons.

3. What has your experience been when receiving health care in the community? How have you seen health professionals work together or fail to effectively collaborate? What has the impact been on your care?

4. What skills do you think you might need to develop or improve to optimise your ability to work in an interprofessional manner?

FURTHER READING

Fowler, T., Garr, D., Mager, N.D.P. & Stanley, J. (2020). Enhancing primary care and preventive services through Interprofessional practice and education. *Israel Journal of Health Policy Research*, *9*(1), 1–5. https://doi.org/10.1186/s13584-020-00371-8

Schot, E., Tummers, L. & Noordegraaf, M. (2020). Working on working together. A systematic review on how healthcare professionals contribute to interprofessional collaboration. *Journal of Interprofessional Care*, *34*(3), 332–42. https://doi.org/10.1080/13561820.2019.1636007

Taranta, E. & Marcinowicz, L. (2020). Collaboration between the family nurse and family doctor from the perspective of patients: A qualitative study. *Family Practice*, *37*(1), 118–23. https://doi.org/10.1093/fampra/cmz035

Wranik, W.D., Price, S., Haydt, S.M., et al. (2019). Implications of interprofessional primary care team characteristics for health services and patient health outcomes: A systematic review with narrative synthesis. *Health Policy*, *123*(6), 550–63. https://doi.org/10.1016/j.healthpol.2019.03.015

REFERENCES

Al-Worafi, Y.M. (2024). Interprofessional practice in developing countries. In Y.M. Al-Worafi (ed.), *Handbook of Medical and Health Sciences in Developing Countries* (pp. 1–36). Springer International Publishing. https://doi.org/10.1007/978-3-030-74786-2_300-1

Australian Digital Health Agency. (2024). *My Health Record*. Australian Government. https://myhealthrecord.gov.au/internet/mhr/publishing.nsf/content/home

Australian Nursing and Midwifery Federation (ANMF). (2014). *National Practice Standards for Nurses in General Practice*. www.anmf.org.au/media/ouzgnqft/anmf_national_practice_standards_for_nurses_in_general_practice.pdf

Azzam, M., Drynan, D., Fricke, M., et al. (2023). A case study of organizational and curricular attributes for interprofessional education: A model for sustainable curriculum delivery. *Journal of Research in Interprofessional Practice and Education*, *13*(1). https://doi.org/10.22230/jripe.2023v13n1a351

Brown, J.B., Mulder, C., Clark, R.E., Belsito, L. & Thorpe, C. (2021). It starts with a strong foundation: constructing collaborative interprofessional teams in primary health care. *Journal of Interprofessional Care*, *35*(4), 514–20. https://doi.org/10.1080/13561820.2020.1787360

Clinical Excellence Commission. (2022). *Reflective Practice Workbook*. New South Wales Government.

Conroy, C. (2019). Stereotyping as a major barrier to achievement of interprofession. *Internet Journal of Allied Health Sciences and Practice*, *17*(3), Article 8. https://doi.org/10.46743/1540-580X/2019.1846

Department of Health and Aged Care (2022). *Health Care Homes trial*. Commonwealth of Australia. www.health.gov.au/resources/collections/health-care-homes-trial-evaluation-reports-collection?utm_source=health.gov.au&utm_medium=callout-auto-custom&utm_campaign=digital_transformation

Donnelly, C., Ashcroft, R., Mofina, A., Bobbette, N. & Mulder, C. (2019). Measuring the performance of interprofessional primary health care teams: Understanding the teams perspective. *Primary Health Care Research and Development*, *20*, e125. https://doi.org/10.1017/S1463423619000409

Downie, S., Walsh, J., Kirk-Brown, A. & Haines, T.P. (2023). How can scope of practice be described and conceptualised in medical and health professions? A systematic review for scoping and content analysis. *International Journal of Health Planning and Management, 38*(5), 1184–211. https://doi.org/10.1002/hpm.3678

Eaton, S., Roberts, S. & Turner, B. (2015). Delivering person centred care in long term conditions. *British Medical Journal, 350*, h181. www.bmj.com/content/bmj/350/bmj.h181.full.pdf

Ellis, P. (2021). Conflict management (Part 3). *Wounds UK, 18*(2), 67–9.

Etz, R.S., Zyzanski, S.J., Gonzalez, M.M., et al. (2019). A new comprehensive measure of high-value aspects of primary care. *Annals of Family Medicine, 17*(3), 221–30. https://doi.org/10.1370/afm.2393

Fiscella, K. & McDaniel, S.H. (2018). The complexity, diversity, and science of primary care teams. *American Journal of Psychology, 73*(4), 451–67. https://doi.org/10.1037/amp0000244

Fishman, M.D. & Slanetz, P.J. (2021). Five tips for successful conflict negotiation in the breast imaging workplace. *Journal of Breast Imaging, 3*(3), 381–6. https://doi.org/10.1093/jbi/wbaa094

Flood, B., Smythe, L., Hocking, C. & Jones, M. (2022). Interprofessional practice: The path toward openness. *Journal of Interprofessional Care, 36*(5), 635–42. https://doi.org/10.1080/13561820.2021.1981264

Fowler, T., Garr, D., Mager, N.D.P. & Stanley, J. (2020). Enhancing primary care and preventive services through interprofessional practice and education. *Israel Journal of Health Policy Research, 9*(1). https://doi.org/10.1186/s13584-020-00371-8

Fox, S., Gaboury, I., Chiocchio, F. & Vachon, B. (2021). Communication and interprofessional collaboration in primary care: From ideal to reality in practice. *Health Communication, 36*(2), 125–35. https://doi.org/10.1080/10410236.2019.1666499

Halcomb, E. & Ashley, C. (2019). Are Australian general practice nurses underutilised? An examination of current roles and task satisfaction. *Collegian, 26*(5), 522–7. https://doi.org/10.1016/j.colegn.2019.02.005

Halcomb, E., Ashley, C., Dennis, S., et al. (2023). Telehealth use in Australian primary healthcare during COVID-19: A cross-sectional descriptive survey [Primary care; COVID]. *BMJ Open, 13*(1), e065478. https://doi.org/10.1136/bmjopen-2022-065478

Halcomb, E., Smyth, E. & McInnes, S. (2018). Job satisfaction and career intentions of registered nurses in primary health care: An integrative review. *BMC Family Practice, 19*(136). https://bmcprimcare.biomedcentral.com/articles/10.1186/s12875-12018-10819-12871.

Halcomb, E., Stephens, M., Bryce, J., Foley, E. & Ashley, C. (2017a). The development of professional practice standards for Australian general practice nurses. *Journal of Advanced Nursing, 73*(8), 1958–69. https://doi.org/10.1111/jan.13274

Halcomb, E.J., Stephens, M., Bryce, J., Foley, E. & Ashley, C. (2017b). The development of professional practice standards for nurses working in Australian general practice. *Journal of Advanced Nursing, 73*(8), 1958–69. https://doi.org/10.1111/jan.13274

Halcomb, E., Stephens, M., Smyth, E., Meedya, S. & Tillott, S. (2017c). The health and health preparation of long-term Australian travellers. *Australian Journal of Primary Health, 23*(4), 386–90. www.publish.csiro.au/PY/PY16138

Healthdirect. (2019). *About My Health Record.* www.healthdirect.gov.au/my-health-record

Josi, R., Bianchi, M. & Brandt, S.K. (2020). Advanced practice nurses in primary care in Switzerland: An analysis of interprofessional collaboration. *BMC Nursing, 19*(1). https://doi.org/10.1186/s12912-019-0393-4

Junod Perron, N., Le Breton, J., Perrier-Gros-Claude, O., et al. (2019). Written interprofessional communication in the context of home healthcare: A qualitative exploration of Swiss perceptions and practices. *Home Health Care Services Quarterly, 38*(3), 224–40. https://doi.org/10.1080/01621424.2019.1616025

Karam, M., Chouinard, M.-C., Poitras, M.-E., et al. (2021). Nursing care coordination for patients with complex needs in primary healthcare: A scoping review. *International Journal of Integrated Care, 21*(1), 16. https://doi.org/10.5334/ijic.5518

Koh, D., McNulty, G. & Toh-Heng, H.L. (2022). Reflective practice through clinical supervision: Implications for professional and organisational sustainability. *British Journal of Guidance & Counselling, 50*(6), 879–96. https://doi.org/10.1080/03069885.2021.1978056

Linsley, P. & Barker, J. (2019). Reflection, portfolios and evidence-based practice. In P. Linsley, R. Kane & J.H. Barker (eds), *Evidence-Based Practice for Nurses and Healthcare Professionals* (pp. 157–69). Sage Publications Ltd.

Lyth, J., Lind, L., Persson, H.L. & Wirehn, A.B. (2021). Can a telemonitoring system lead to decreased hospitalization in elderly patients? *Journal of Telemedicine and Telecare, 27*(1), 46–53. https://doi.org/10.1177/1357633X19858178

Macdonald, G., Asgarova, S., Hartford, W., et al. (2023). What do you mean, 'negotiating?': Patient, physician, and healthcare professional experiences of navigating hierarchy in networks of interprofessional care. *Journal of Interprofessional Care*, 1–12. https://doi.org/10.1080/135618 20.2023.2203722

Machen, S., Jani, Y., Turner, S., Marshall, M. & Fulop, N.J. (2019). The role of organizational and professional cultures in medication safety: A scoping review of the literature. *International Journal of Quality Health Care, 31*(10), G146–G157. https://doi.org/10.1093/intqhc/mzz111

McInnes, S., Peters, K., Bonney, A. & Halcomb, E. (2017a). Understanding collaboration in general practice: A qualitative study. *Family Practice, 34*(5), 621–6. https://doi.org/10.1093/fampra/cmx010

———— (2017b). A qualitative study of collaboration in general practice: Understanding the general practice nurse's role. *Journal of Clinical Nursing, 26*(13–14), 1960–8. https://doi.org/10.1111/jocn.13598

Ministry of Health. (2019a). *Health information standards*. New Zealand Government. www.health .govt.nz/our-work/digital-health/digital-health-sector-architecture-standards-andgovernance/ health-information-standards-0

———— (2019b). *Health Information Standards Organisation*. New Zealand Government. www.health .govt.nz/about-ministry/leadership-ministry/expert-groups/healthinformation-standards- organisation

———— (2019c). *Personal health information standards*. New Zealand Government. www.health.govt .nz/our-work/digital-health/digital-health-sector-architecture-standardsand-governance/health- information-standards-0/standards-development/personalhealth-information-standards

Nancarrow, S. & Borthwick, A. (2021). Diversity in the allied health professions. In S. Nancarrow & A. Borthwick, *The Allied Health Professions: A Sociological Perspective* (pp. 57–82). Policy Press.

New Zealand Nurses Organisation (NZNO). (2019). *Aotearoa New Zealand Primary Health Care Nursing Standards of Practice*. www.nzno.org.nz/Portals/0/publications/Primary%20 Health%20Care%20Nursing%20Standards%20of%20Practice%202019.pdf

Nora, C.R.D. & Beghetto, M.G. (2020). Patient safety challenges in primary health care: A scoping review. *Revista Brailiera des Enfermagem, 73*(5), e20190209. https://doi.org/10.1590/0034- 7167-2019-0209

Nursing and Midwifery Board of Australia (NMBA). (2016). *Registered Nurse Standards for Practice*. www.nursingmidwiferyboard.gov.au/Codes-Guidelines-Statements/Professional-standards/ registered-nurse-standards-for-practice.aspx#

Nursing Council of New Zealand (NCNZ). (2012). *Code of Conduct for Nurses*. https://nursingcouncil .org.nz/Public/NCNZ/nursing-section/Code_of_Conduct.aspx

Oandasan, I., Baker, G., Barker, K., et al. (2006). *Teamwork in healthcare: Promoting effective teamwork in healthcare in Canada*. Canadian Health Services Research Foundation.

Papermaster, A.E., Whitney, M. & Vinas, E.K. (2023). Interprofessional case conference enhances group learning and the quality, safety, value, and equity of team-based care. *Journal of Continuing Education in the Health Professions, 43*(1), 4–11. https://doi.org/10.1097/ ceh.0000000000000485

Philippa, R., Ann, H., Jacqueline, M. & Nicola, A. (2021). Professional identity in nursing: A mixed method research study. *Nurse Education in Practice, 52*, 103039. https://doi .org/10.1016/j.nepr.2021.103039

Rosen, M.A., DiazGranados, D., Dietz, A.S., et al. (2018). Teamwork in healthcare: Key discoveries enabling safer, high-quality care. *American Journal of Psychology*, *73*(4), 433–50. https://doi .org/10.1037/amp0000298

Saint-Pierre, C., Herskovic, V. & Sepulveda, M. (2018). Multidisciplinary collaboration in primary care: A systematic review. *Family Practice*, *35*(2), 132–41. https://doi.org/10.1093/fampra/cmx085

Saw, P.S., Balqis-Ali, N.Z., Quek, K.F., et al. (2023). Organizational strategies in promoting person-centered primary care: A participatory concept mapping study. *International Journal of Healthcare Management*, 1–11. https://doi.org/10.1080/20479700.2023.2200604

Schot, E., Tummers, L. & Noordegraaf, M. (2020). Working on working together. A systematic review on how healthcare professionals contribute to interprofessional collaboration. *Journal of Interprofessional Care*, *34*(3), 332–42. https://doi.org/10.1080/13561820.2019.1636007

Seaton, J., Jones, A., Johnston, C. & Francis, K. (2021). Allied health professionals' perceptions of interprofessional collaboration in primary health care: An integrative review. *Journal of Interprofessional Care*, *35*(2), 217–28. https://doi.org/10.1080/13561820.2020.1732311

Snee, H. & Goswami, H. (2021). Who cares? Social mobility and the 'class ceiling' in nursing. *Sociological Research Online*, *26*(3), 562–80. https://doi.org/10.1177/1360780420971657

Szafran, O., Kennett, S.L., Bell, N.R. & Torti, J.M.I. (2019). Interprofessional collaboration in diabetes care: Perceptions of family physicians practicing in or not in a primary health care team. *BMC Family Practice*, *20*(1), 44. https://doi.org/10.1186/s12875-019-0932-9

Taranta, E. & Marcinowicz, L. (2020). Collaboration between the family nurse and family doctor from the perspective of patients: A qualitative study. *Family Practice*, *37*(1), 118–23. https://doi .org/10.1093/fampra/cmz035

Thistlethwaite, J. & McLarnon, N. (2023). Learning in and about interprofessional teams and wider collaborations. In M.Y. Alnaami, D.A. Alqahtani, E.A. Alfaris, et al. (eds), *Novel Health Interprofessional Education and Collaborative Practice Program: Strategy and Implementation* (pp. 67–92). Springer.

Vest, J.R., Blackburn, J., Yeager, V.A., Haut, D.P. & Halverson, P.K. (2021). Primary care-based case conferences and reductions in health care utilization. *Journal of Health Care for the Poor and Underserved*, *32*, 1288–300. https://doi.org/10.1353/hpu.2021.0132

Wagner, E.H. (2000). The role of patient care teams in chronic disease management. *British Medical Journal*, *320*(7234), 569. www.ncbi.nlm.nih.gov/pmc/articles/PMC1117605/pdf/569.pdf

World Health Organization (WHO). (2010). *Framework for Action on Interprofessional Education and Collaborative Practice*. www.who.int/publications/i/item/framework-for-action-on-interprofessional-education-collaborative-practice

——— (2013). *Interprofessional Collaborative Practice in Primary Health Care: Nursing and Midwifery Perspectives*. (Human Resources for Health Observer – Issue No. 13). www.who.int/publications/i/item/9789241505857

——— (2018). *Building the primary health care workforce of the 21st century*. https://apps.who.int/iris/handle/10665/328072

Wranik, W.D., Price, S., Haydt, S.M., et al. (2019). Implications of interprofessional primary care team characteristics for health services and patient health outcomes: A systematic review with narrative synthesis. *Health Policy*, *123*(6), 550–63. https://doi.org/10.1016/j.healthpol.2019.03.015

10 Cultural competence and cultural safety

Diana Guzys and Melanie Eslick
With acknowledgement to Kath Hoare

LEARNING OBJECTIVES

At the completion of this chapter, you should be able to:

- define culture and diversity.
- differentiate between cultural awareness, sensitivity, safety and competence.
- demonstrate an understanding of the impact power, prejudice and discrimination have in health care.
- explain the importance of cultural competence and cultural safety in health practice.
- describe the effect an individual's perceptions of health and health behaviours may have on health outcomes.

Culture – the customs, values, beliefs, material traits, language and behaviours common to a particular group of people.

Diversity – recognition of differences through the dimensions of ethnicity, cultural background, age, generation, socio-economic status, occupation, gender identity, sex, physical abilities, religion, political beliefs and other ideologies.

Person-centred care – a partnership approach to health care focused on elements of care, support and treatment that are most important to the patient and their support people, and that respects and responds to their preferences, needs and values.

Introduction

Cultural competence and cultural safety support health professionals to recognise everyone as unique in order to promote optimal health outcomes (So et al., 2024). This allows for the acknowledgement of diversity that exists within and between individuals and groups in health care. In practice, this represents the broader understanding of **culture** in health care, and encompasses the dynamic influences of culture on attitudes, values and beliefs (McGough et al., 2022). Alongside culture, the understanding of **diversity** is inclusive of – yet not exclusive to – age and generation, sex and gender identity, socio-economic status, occupation, ethnicity or migrant experience, religion or spirituality, and ability or disability (Nursing Council of New Zealand (NCNZ), 2011). Cultural competence and cultural safety align with person-centred approaches in health care as professionals develop a willingness to listen, understand and acknowledge the unique identity of each individual (Ahmed et al., 2018; Stein-Parbury, 2021). Through the integration of cultural competence, cultural safety and **person-centred care** in practice, nurses can actively address social justice in the clinical context.

Health professionals have a responsibility to provide culturally competent and safe care based on mutual respect for all people. A key consideration when working with individuals is to seek an authentic understanding of their cultural context (Curtis et al., 2019; Sharifi, Adib-Hajbaghery & Najafi, 2019).

The concept of cultural competence was introduced in the 1980s based on varying frameworks and with numerous definitions (Curtis et al., 2019). Cultural safety gained prominence in Aotearoa New Zealand around the turn of the century through the work of Māori nurse-scholar Dr Irahepti Ramsden (Chakanyuka et al., 2022; Kaphle et al., 2022). Ramsden described cultural safety as a mechanism that recognises that the power imbalances exist within health care interactions and enables the consumer to say whether health services are safe for them to use (Chakanyuka et al., 2022; Kaphle et al., 2022). The original focus of cultural safety was specifically related to institutional racism; however, this concept has evolved to more broadly acknowledge diversity and may be applied to working with varied marginalised or vulnerable groups. Milligan and colleagues (2021) caution against the conflation of First Nations in Australia with other culturally and linguistically diverse (CALD) groups by health care professionals when considering cultural safety, as this fails to address systemic racism in health care. They argue that recognition of the sovereignty of Indigenous Australians is an essential first step in demonstrating respect for cultural safety in Aboriginal and Torres Strait Islander Health. Please refer to Chapter 5 for a deeper exploration of First Nations health and well-being.

In this chapter, the discussion focuses on understanding culture, cultural diversity and the need for health professionals to integrate cultural competence into everyday care to support culturally safe practice.

Culture, health and health care

Culture influences how people perceive health, illness, disease and their causes. Culture may impact on when people will seek health care and how they behave towards health care providers. Health care providers need to be aware of different values, behaviours and beliefs about health in order to overcome the factors that cause disparities (Curtis et al., 2019; Stubbe, 2020). For example, some cultures may first use complementary and alternative medicine (CAM) or home therapies, including herbal remedies or certain foods, before seeking health care. However, if health professionals convey disapproval of CAM, individuals may not be forthcoming with information about their use of non-biomedical approaches to health care. This also may compromise the care provided by health professionals as there is always the potential for a negative interaction between CAM and biomedical health care. Health professionals who seek to understand CAM are seen to practise in a non-judgemental manner and to convey cultural relativism to optimise health outcomes (Liu et al., 2021).

Understanding the dynamics of different cultural groups, and being conscious of their pre-understandings, supports health professionals to avoid making moral judgements about others (Sharifi et al., 2019). Understanding culture, values and beliefs is an important part of the process of becoming a culturally competent and culturally safe professional. It is inappropriate to think that health professionals know all cultural contexts (Cox & Simpson, 2020). Health professionals must develop the appropriate skills and knowledge required to enable them, in partnership with individuals, to understand how individuals' health behaviour is influenced by culture, as determined by them, to eliminate barriers to health equity (Brottman et al., 2020; Wang et al., 2024).

The premise of cultural competence and cultural safety requires consideration of the diversity that exists in Australia, Aotearoa New Zealand and worldwide. Cultural competence and cultural safety in practice promote positive health outcomes and require health professionals to first develop an understanding of the influence of culture and diversity on individuals, families, groups and populations (NCNZ, 2011; Sharifi et al., 2019).

Culture

Culture can be considered from multiple perspectives and is part of almost every aspect of life. It embraces shared world views among groups and individuals and has been described as learned life patterns and behavioural responses to the world through social interactions (Brottman et al., 2020; Stein-Parbury, 2021). Culture is the understanding that evolves from shared time, ideas and experience that are often intergenerational (Brottman et al., 2020).

For many people, cultural values are reflected in an individual's preferred way of acting or knowing something. A person's ethical approach and/or belief system, whether religious or spiritual, is usually a product of culture or is strongly influenced by it. Culture includes the implicit and explicit beliefs, attitudes, values, customs, norms, taboos, arts, food and recreational activities accepted by individuals and groups (Stein-Parbury, 2021; Wepa, 2015). Interpersonal interactions, family life and kinship are influenced by culture consciously and subconsciously. Culture is primarily learned and transmitted within family and social contexts and has been said to guide decision-making and facilitate feelings of self-worth, self-esteem and resilience (Brottman et al., 2020).

Some cultures value individual decision-making, while others have a collective approach beyond the individual to consider the inclusive family or community (Elbaum, Kinsey & Mariano, 2023). Therefore, it is important to understand the concepts of individualism and collectivism in a population's culture to design and deliver culturally competent and safe approaches to health care. Independence and interdependence are similar terms that may be used to describe individualism and collectivism. These terms are associated with how the 'self' is conceptualised. In cultures where individual goals and self-expression are valued, decisions are made based on individual preferences and values, as people consider themselves autonomous, independent and individualistic in their approach. In collectivistic cultures, the 'self' is considered part of a whole that is enmeshed in the family and/or community. The collective cultural context works towards group goals and draws on social support, whereby behaviours and decisions align with the greater social context and advice sought is more likely to defer to the collective requirements of family or community (Hillman, Fowlie & MacDonald, 2023). Individualism and collectivism are essential concepts for consideration when assessing, planning and implementing health care for individuals, families and communities. Individuals, families and significant others are a potential source of relevant cultural information. When working with different cultures, health professionals must seek guidance and direction from individuals, families and significant others regarding the most appropriate approaches to health care (Brottman et al., 2020). For example, it is relevant to determine who should be present during important meetings as the individual seeking support may also desire a senior person in the family, kinship group or significant other to be involved in decision-making processes.

Culture is not fixed as it occurs in the context of a continuum that moves and changes in response to situations and life experiences. While cultural groups are distinguished by certain characteristics, cultures are dynamic and can change over time. Being open to the potential for change mitigates slipping into cultural stereotypes related to assumed expectations of attitudes and beliefs. Adoption of cultural biases, assumptions or stereotypes by nurses can be incorrect and potentially detrimental to positive health outcomes (Thirsk et al., 2022). As culture is not fixed, it may be necessary to consult with patients and their support networks more than once to discover and respond to changes that may occur over time.

Diversity

In conjunction with the growing recognition for a better understanding of the influence of culture, greater recognition and acknowledgement of diversity is the reality for most countries. Diversity also extends to include ethnicity, age, ability, religion/faith, politics, sex, gender identity, socio-economic status, residence status and language (Brottman et al., 2020; Wang et al., 2024). The need for health care providers and systems to understand and respond appropriately to the impact of the political, socio-economic and geographic factors that led to health disparities is closely linked to the concept of **equity, diversity and inclusion (EDI)**.

Diversity is a result of shifting demographics and contributes to **globalisation**. Diversity requires constructive interactions between all members of different populations with consideration for embracing **multiculturalism**, migration and internationalisation to achieve societal equity (Diamond, 2024). Multiculturalism refers to the conscious consideration of cultural diversity and focuses on the interests of the individual and society as a whole, drawing on human rights and social justice perspectives (Johansson, 2022).

The broadening scope of cultural competency has led to the development of multiple terms, frequently used interchangeably such as culturally appropriate, culturally responsive, culturally sensitive, and culturally informed (Brottman et al., 2020). Transcultural care is another term developed to focus on issues of diversity in health care.

Cultural and linguistic diversity

The term **'culturally and linguistically diverse' (CALD)** is commonly used to describe groups that are different from the English-speaking majority, who were born in non-English speaking countries and/or who do not speak English at home (Pham et al., 2021). When engaging with individuals and families for whom English is a second or subsequent language, health professionals need to remain conscious that people's self-expressions are likely to be different to what they may be if they were using their first language. It is also important to remember that an individual's English proficiency doesn't reflect their educational background or health literacy. If an individual has limited English language skills, it is essential to engage a qualified interpreter to promote effective communication. Professional interpreters improve communication between health professionals, individuals and families, resulting in better health outcomes by reducing errors and increasing satisfaction with care (Kwan et al., 2023).

Interpreters are required to have sophisticated skills in at least two languages and knowledge of how to convey complex concepts. Use of friends, family and other non-professional translators or interpreters may be convenient, or at times inevitable in an emergency situation. However, this is suboptimal for several reasons. This may compromise a person's

Equity, diversity and inclusion (EDI) – a conceptual framework promoting fair treatment, and support of full participation by people from all backgrounds, commonly used in workplaces and educational institutions.

Globalisation – the integration of international world views, products, ideas and other aspects of culture.

Multiculturalism – the promotion of cultural diversity for individuals and society as a whole.

Culturally and linguistically diverse (CALD) – a term describing people born overseas, who speak languages other than the official language of a country and/or have lower proficiency of national language(s) and/ or have parents born overseas.

privacy and confidentiality, the quality of the translation is unknown and there is an increased potential for ineffective or erroneous communication which may hinder the therapeutic process (Habib et al., 2023).

CASE STUDY 10.1

Rahael, a 28-year-old Sudanese woman, presents to the women's health clinic with lower abdominal pain, from which she has been suffering for over a week. She appears pale, anxious and frightened. Her husband and the two children are in the waiting room. She enters the clinical space alone and immediately apologises for her 'poor English'. Rahael expresses that she is fearful that she could die. Apart from her husband and their two children, aged six and two years, she does not have friends or relatives in Australia. She is extremely worried about who would look after her family if anything happened to her.

The female health professional is aware from her previous experience that more than 85 per cent of Sudanese women have undergone female genital mutilation. She vehemently disapproves of this now-outlawed practice. Rahael is visibly frightened by an intimate physical examination and says she is terrified of being sent to the hospital.

REFLECTION
1. What knowledge and skills will the health professional need to best assist Rahael?
2. How could the needs of Rahael's husband and children be met?
3. Is there an opportunity for the health professional to become more culturally sensitive through this encounter?

Language and communication

The provision of health information and education relies on appropriate communication. This has a significant implication for duty of care and consent. A failure of communication due to language barriers can result in inaccurate or incomplete information that leads to sub-standard health care (Al Shamsi et al., 2020). Language is often the key to communication and conveying cultural beliefs, values and norms (Saaida, 2023). Language is an important aspect of delivering health care equitably to all individuals. This includes the acknowledgement of the Australian Aboriginal and Torres Strait Islander Languages and the Aotearoa New Zealand Māori Language within health care services. In Aotearoa New Zealand, the Māori Language, or Te Reo, is one of the three national Languages alongside English and Aotearoa New Zealand sign Language.

Alongside language, non-verbal communication and cultural behaviours can be significant in communication. They can be conveyed through maintaining physical distance, physical touching, facial expressions and gesturing, and vocal cues such as tone, speech rate and intonation.

Power, prejudice and discrimination

Health professionals must recognise their position of power in health care encounters and use this appropriately to enhance health opportunities. Health care professionals need to understand how the history and background of stereotyping and prejudice may influence a person's expectation and perception of care interactions (Byrd & Austin, 2020).

Generalisations and stereotypes

Generalisations and stereotypes can be and are applied to culture and diversity by those who are not part of different groups to make sense of the social world. The difference between these two concepts can be subtle but is important. A stereotype is an oversimplified belief or judgement based on a prior assumption. In contrast, a generalisation is a descriptive statement used in an attempt to portray individual and group similarities (Hall, 2024). However, generalisations can lead to the mistaken assumption that if something suits one person from a particular cultural group, then it will suit the next person with the same background or any other different cultural group.

Applying generalisations and stereotypes to a cultural group or diverse population limits the ability to implement a person-centred approach and creates barriers that may result in judgement and discrimination (Byrd & Austin, 2020). The person may sense this as discrimination through the demonstration of marginalisation and implied prejudice. Stereotyping any individual who is different from the dominant cultural group can result in health professionals engaging in a form of 'othering' (Byrd & Austin, 2020). The process of 'othering' applies to the practice of distancing oneself from those perceived as different. Conveying a sense of 'othering' towards any diverse individual may discourage them from seeking support and endanger health professional-patient relationships (Rosa et al., 2022).

When wielded inappropriately, health professionals can convey a perception of judgement that may result in people not accessing health support due to negative health care experiences (Rivenbark & Ichou, 2020). Prejudice can be described as pre-judgement, which may be enabling or limiting in the health care context. Although some truth may exist in prejudice, as judgements are made in the process of developing knowledge, this becomes problematic when one's perspective remains fixed despite the existence of contradictory knowledge (Wepa, 2015).

Discrimination occurs when a person is treated less favourably than another because of a specific characteristic such as gender, ethnic background or religious belief – the reason for the less favourable treatment is irrelevant. Socially marginalised and vulnerable populations have historically experienced discrimination and exclusion (Byrd & Austin, 2020). According to Drummond (2018), discrimination results from the lack of value placed on cultural understanding. Systemic discrimination may occur across a range of settings. Another form of discrimination occurs when a rule, practice or policy that may appear to be neutral harms a particular group of people. Requiring all staff members to be rostered to work over weekends may indirectly disadvantage employees whose religious observances mean that they may be unable to abide by this policy. This is referred to as 'indirect discrimination', which is unlawful if the rule, practice or policy is not reasonable in the circumstances (Australian Human Rights Commission (AHRC), 2014).

Some individuals, groups and populations report feeling invisible within health care services, resulting in perceptions of marginalisation and discrimination. For example, while health professionals may not assume sexual orientation or gender identity in their interactions, health services predominantly use heteronormative and gender-binary language that can alienate LGBTQIA+ populations (Goldberg et al., 2019). This is seen in health forms, for example, that require individuals to select a category of 'male' or 'female' and use limited terms such as 'Mr' and 'Mrs'. Systemic discrimination continues with the presumption of health needs, information and education. These areas are often directed by the dominant population and thereby presumed for specific cultural groups, such as LGBTQIA+ populations. Previously, it was assumed that LGBTQIA+ health needs were similar to heterosexual, **cisgender** age-matched peers; however, this is not the case.

Cisgender – the term used for people whose self-identity and gender corresponds to their biological sex.

REFLECTION

Imagine a nursing colleague shared this strongly held opinion: 'This transgender thing is a phase, brought about by Hollywood types and social media influencers. We never met so-called trans patients before!'

1. Think about your own gender identity. Do you have in your close circle a family member, friend, colleague or peer who identifies as transgender or non-binary?
2. How might gender identity affect your perceptions of patients or clients?
3. Consider the impact of language and communication in nursing interactions with transgender and non-binary individuals. How can you ensure your language is affirming and respectful?

Cultural conflict

Differences in cultural beliefs, values and practices may cause tension between individuals and professionals, or even within the culture that exists in health care institutions and services. When this occurs, health care professionals must acknowledge and support the individual's cultural identity and sense of autonomy (Clendon & Munns, 2019). Cultural conflict occurs at the boundaries between cultures, as these boundaries define social behaviour. Cultural conflict typically occurs when there is no recognition of cultural differences or no commitment towards similar goals (Clendon & Munns, 2019).

Clendon and Munns (2019) reinforce that when different cultures work together there is no need to relinquish individual values or beliefs. Rather, these encounters are about withholding judgement of others' life views through conscious engagement, open-minded recognition and respect of different practices.

CASE STUDY 10.2

Jack is a 93-year-old Māori war veteran and widower with no children, who lives independently with the support of his extended family and friends in his semi-rural community. Jack recently had a fall at home and following a visit to his doctor, was referred to the district nurse for home visits to dress his lower leg wound. On the first visit, the nurse notices that Jack's house is cold and unkempt and that there is not much food in the cupboard. The nurse suggests that he needs to consider moving into a rest home as she believes that he is having difficulty managing at home. Jack becomes distressed as moving into a rest home would mean moving away from his family, friends and community. The nurse does not know that Jack walks to his local *marae* (Māori community meeting place) daily and has shared meals with his *whānau* (extended family and friends). As the nurse begins to fill in the forms required to begin the aged care assessment process, Jack asks her to leave without doing his dressing.

REFLECTION
1. What is the care priority for Jack?
2. How else could Jack's needs be met?
3. What knowledge and skills do health professionals need to best assist Jack in his situation?
4. How could the nurse have been more culturally supportive in this encounter?

Cultural assumptions, stereotypes and misunderstandings can hinder effective communication increasing the likelihood of poor or adverse health outcomes (Clendon & Munns, 2019). The development of professional communication skills is required to appropriately interact with individuals and families from various backgrounds and to improve participation, satisfaction and health outcomes (Hoare, 2019). Differences in cultural beliefs, values and practices may cause tension with the health professional or the culture of the health system. When this occurs, the health professional's response must be to support and prioritise the individual's cultural identity and autonomy (Stubbe, 2020). This is where cultural competence and cultural safety become imperative in practice.

REFLECTION

Consider your own cultural background.
1. How might this affect how you provide health care to others?
2. What beliefs do you hold about various nationalities, religious or ethnic groups?
3. How or why did you form these beliefs?
4. How easy is it to overcome stereotyping when working with individuals who have different cultural perspectives to your own?

Cultural competence and cultural safety in practice

Developing cultural competence and cultural safety in practice involves recognition of the importance of culture and diversity for individuals, families and populations (Young & Guo, 2020). Cultural competence and cultural safety require health professionals to focus on knowing and understanding themselves, as well as developing knowledge and understanding different cultural contexts or diverse populations via cultural education (Kerrigan et al., 2020). Cultural safety is a process that first requires the integration of cultural awareness and cultural sensitivity (Hoare, 2019).

Culturally safe health professionals engage in a process that enables them to deliver care in a culturally competent manner as determined by its recipients. While it is relevant to everyone who engages with a health professional, cultural safety is especially important for vulnerable or marginalised people, diverse groups and minority populations (Wepa, 2015). Cultural safety is an education process that has three parts (see Figure 10.1):

1. Cultural awareness begins with self-reflection to promote an understanding of differences.
2. Cultural sensitivity uses a process of self-exploration to acknowledge the legitimacy of differences.
3. Cultural safety develops through education and recognising diversity to enable a responsive health care service (NCNZ, 2011; Ramsden, 2002).

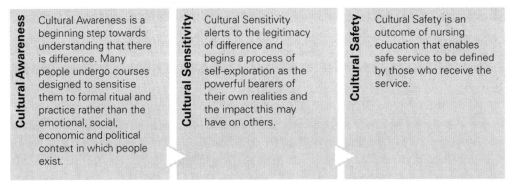

Figure 10.1   The process towards achieving cultural safety in nursing practice
Source: Adapted from NCNZ (2011, p. 8); Ramsden (1992; 2002).

Cultural safety moves beyond awareness and sensitivity to a process that involves health professionals' engagement in self-reflection, self-exploration and education. This enables them to focus on determining their own culture and identity so that they can minimise this potential influence and impact on others from different cultural contexts (Hoare, 2019; NCNZ, 2011). Development of cultural safety skills requires active engagement in critical thinking with attitudinal and behavioural considerations alongside the development of professional and, to some extent, personal skills that engender trust and respect through enhanced open communication in all interpersonal interactions (Hoare, 2019).

Cultural awareness

Differences in the cultural context of individuals, families and groups may present further challenges when assessing an individual's health needs. Some of these differences include variations between language, gender, economic and social groups, and rural/remote and urban groups. It is not expected that health professionals will be able to identify these nuances or intricacies; however, it is important to seek information and actively explore the cultural context through engaging with individuals and their families. Health professionals need to keep in mind that each person's identity is unique, as part of the consideration that people will have different world views, life experiences and approaches to health.

Cultural sensitivity

Cultural sensitivity requires a health professional to have sufficient knowledge about their own thoughts, feelings and reflections to inform how they may react to others from a different cultural background. Self-evaluation as an individual and as a health professional is necessary to understand one's own cultural background and explore the origin of any bias, prejudice and views that may impact on others. Self-aware health professionals are more cognisant of the impact that their own cultural beliefs and values have on their perceptions and understanding of the world. This enables them to be receptive and responsive to different cultural groups and diverse populations. Health professionals use cultural awareness and sensitivity to bracket-off their own beliefs and values in practice and support their progression to becoming culturally competent and culturally safe.

Cultural safety

In practice, cultural safety requires balancing the personal and professional self – a complex process that involves education to support self-reflection and self-exploration alongside personal and professional development (Dawson et al., 2022). Cultural safety complements cultural competence through the acknowledgement of diversity in health care to minimise potential power imbalances (NCNZ, 2011). Any actions that may cause a person to feel that their cultural identity has been demeaned or diminished, or to feel disempowered or alienated, are culturally unsafe (NCNZ, 2011; Ramsden, 2002; Wepa, 2015). While several models for developing culturally competent behaviour exist, all emphasise communication as the key to cultural safety (Hoare, 2019).

Culturally safe care means working from a position that recognises and respects every individual and their differences through the establishment of trust. Cultural safety requires health professionals to engage in practice that acknowledges the unique cultural identity of every person to safely meet their needs, expectations and rights. This means working in a way that respects the cultural perspectives of other people. Health professionals often complete cultural safety education within their undergraduate program requiring authentic reflection on the potential impact of their own cultural values, attitudes and behaviours on others who they will work with in practice (Kurtz et al., 2018; Wepa, 2015). Cultural safety in practice ensures health professionals engage in a partnership approach to make ethical and culturally appropriate decisions with all individuals. In practice, the integration of cultural safety brings social justice and equity to the health professional–consumer relationship through implicit and, at times explicit, acknowledgement of existing power imbalances (Curtis et al., 2019).

REFLECTION

Consider your own health beliefs.

1. What beliefs do you hold about what it means to be healthy?
2. How or why did you form these beliefs?
3. How might these influence your provision of health care to others?
4. How easy is it to accommodate health beliefs that are significantly different to your own?

Health professionals from culturally diverse backgrounds bring a depth of knowledge and skills that may facilitate cultural insights and provide opportunities to enhance other health professionals' cultural safety. Workforce diversity signals to the community that health organisations embrace cultural diversity (Stanford, 2020). However, it can never be assumed that a health professional with a personally diverse background may provide any greater insight into culturally competent care. Every health professional is required to develop their own understanding of cultural awareness, sensitivity and safety.

Conclusion

Health care professionals and health systems have an obligation to facilitate ethical, equitable and appropriate quality services for all. Fundamental to person-centred care is an individualised assessment based on each person's own values, beliefs and practices. This requires cultural competency and culturally safe approaches to practice. Cultural competence and cultural safety acknowledge the benefits and challenges for individuals and health professionals (and health systems) when working with patients from different cultures and diverse populations. This is necessary to achieve equality in health outcomes, providing a social justice response to the inequities frequently experienced by marginalised groups. As a minimum, nurses must reflect on and seek to overcome their own biases, listen carefully, communicate sensitively and demonstrate respect for patients' diverse values, beliefs and practices. Using a person-centred approach to inform cultural competence in health care requires flexibility and a commitment to ongoing learning, allied with well-developed communication skills that evolve over time, to ensure that all people receive culturally safe care.

CRITICAL THINKING ACTIVITIES

Curtis and colleagues (2019) propose an approach to cultural safety which considers focusing on cultural safety activities that go beyond acquiring knowledge about 'other cultures' towards interventions that acknowledge and address biases and stereotypes, and focus on power relationships and inequities in health care interactions that reflect historical and social dynamics.

Consider:

1. Have you observed health professionals engaged in culturally unsafe practice?
2. What occurred to make you conscious of this?
3. How might observing bias or stereotyping of 'others' affect your own nursing practice?
4. When working with Indigenous patients or clients, what historical dynamics could influence interactions?
5. Social dynamics arise from group behaviours that result from interactions of individual group members. Why might this be relevant to community nursing?

FURTHER READING

Baker, K., Adams, J. & Steel, A. (2022). Experiences, perceptions and expectations of health services amongst marginalized populations in urban Australia: A meta-ethnographic review of the literature. *Health Expectations, 25*(5), 2166–87. https://doi.org/10.1111/hex.13386

Hunter, K. & Cook, C. (2020). Indigenous nurses' practice realities of cultural safety and socioethical nursing. *Nursing Ethics, 27*(6), 1472–83. https://doi.org/10.1177/0969733020940376

Peters, L., Bourke, S., Green, J., et al. (2020). Understanding the healthcare needs of Sudanese refugee women settling in Australia. *Clinical Nursing Studies, 8*(2), 40–6. https://doi.org/10.5430/cns.v8n2p40

Ramsey, I., Kennedy, K., Sharplin, G., Eckert, M. & Peters, M.D.J. (2023). Culturally safe, appropriate, and high-quality breast cancer screening for transgender people: A scoping review. *International Journal of Transgender Health, 24*(2), 174–94. https://doi.org/10.1080/26895269.2022.2155289

REFERENCES

Ahmed, S., Siad, F.M., Manalili, K., et al. (2018). How to measure cultural competence when evaluating patient-centred care: A scoping review. *BMJ Open, 8*(7), e021525. https://doi.org/10.1136/bmjopen-2018-021525

Al Shamsi, H., Almutairi, A.G., Al Mashrafi, S. & Al Kalbani, T. (2020). Implications of language barriers for healthcare: A systematic review. *Oman Medical Journal, 35*(2), e122. https://doi.org/10.5001/omj.2020.40

Australian Human Rights Commission (AHRC). (2014). *Racial Discrimination.* https://humanrights.gov.au/sites/default/files/Racial%20Discrimination_2014_Web.pdf

Brottman, M.R., Char, D.M., Hattori, R.A., Heeb, R. & Taff, S.D. (2020). Toward cultural competency in health care: A scoping review of the diversity and inclusion education literature. *Academic Medicine, 95*(5), 803–13.

Byrd, M.Y. & Austin, J.T. (2020). Microaggressions, stereotypes, and social stigmatization in the lived experiences of socially marginalized patients/clients: A social justice perspective. In L.T. Benuto, M.P. Duckworth, A.Masuda & W.O'Donohuename (eds), *Prejudice, Stigma, Privilege, and Oppression: A Behavioral Health Handbook,* (pp. 201–14). Springer.

Chakanyuka, C., Bacsu, J.-D.R., Desroches, A., Walker, J., O'Connell, M.E., Dame, J., Carrier, L., Symenuk, P., Crowshoe, L. & Bourque Bearskin, L. (2022). Appraising Indigenous cultural safety within healthcare: Protocol of a scoping review of reviews. *Journal of Advanced Nursing, 78*(1), 294–9. https://doi.org/10.1111/jan.15096

Clendon, J. & Munns, A. (2019). *Community Health and Wellness: Principles of Primary Health Care* (6th ed.). Elsevier.

Cox, J.L. & Simpson, M.D. (2020). Cultural humility: A proposed model for a continuing professional development program. *Pharmacy, 8*(4), 214. www.mdpi.com/2226-4787/8/4/214

Curtis, E., Jones, R., Tipene-Leach, D., et al. (2019). Why cultural safety rather than cultural competency is required to achieve health equity: A literature review and recommended definition. *International Journal for Equity in Health, 18*(1), 174. https://doi.org/10.1186/s12939-019-1082-3

Dawson, J., Laccos-Barrett, K., Hammond, C. & Rumbold, A. (2022). Reflexive practice as an approach to improve healthcare delivery for Indigenous Peoples: A systematic critical synthesis and exploration of the cultural safety education literature. *International Journal of Environmental Research and Public Health, 19*(11). https://doi.org/10.3390/ijerph19116691

Diamond, A.H. (2024). A globalization diversity ideology. *SN Social Sciences, 4*(2), 35. https://doi.org/10.1007/s43545-024-00847-3

Drummond, M. (2018). *Beyond segmented assimilation: Signaling ethnolinguistic identity with language preference* [Undergraduate honours thesis]. University of North Carolina at Chapel Hill. https://doi.org/10.17615/9402-rs93

Elbaum, A., Kinsey, L. & Mariano, J. (2023). Decision-making across cultures. In C. Banerjee (ed.), *Understanding End of Life Practices: Perspectives on Communication, Religion and Culture* (pp. 85–104). Springer International Publishing. https://doi.org/10.1007/978-3-031-29923-0_7

Goldberg, A.E., Kuvalanka, K.A., Budge, S.L., Benz, M.B. & Smith, J.Z. (2019). Health care experiences of transgender binary and nonbinary university students. *The Counseling Psychologist, 47*(1), 59–97. https://doi.org/10.1177/0011000019827568

Habib, T., Nair, A., Von Pressentin, K., Kaswa, R. & Saeed, H. (2023). Do not lose your patient in translation: Using interpreters effectively in primary care. *South African Family Practice (2004), 65*(1), e1–e5. https://doi.org/10.4102/safp.v65i1.5655

Hall, W.J. (2024). Recognizing stereotypes and their impact on health: A transformative learning activity for undergraduate health science students. *Pedagogy in Health Promotion*, 1. https://doi.org/10.1177/23733799241234069

Hillman, J.G., Fowlie, D.I. & MacDonald, T.K. (2023). Social verification theory: A new way to conceptualize validation, dissonance, and belonging. *Personality and Social Psychology Review, 27*(3), 309–31. https://doi.org/10.1177/10888683221138384

Hoare, K. (2019). *Communicating in a Culturally Safe Manner*. Elsevier.

Johansson, T.R. (2022). In defence of multiculturalism–theoretical challenges. *International Review of Sociology*, 1–15. https://doi.org/10.1080/03906701.2022.2045141

Kaphle, S., Hungerford, C., Blanchard, D., et al. (2022). Cultural safety or cultural competence: How can we address inequities in culturally diverse groups? *Issues in Mental Health Nursing, 43*(7), 698–702. https://doi.org/10.1080/01612840.2021.1998849

Kerrigan, V., Lewis, N., Cass, A., Hefler, M. & Ralph, A.P. (2020). 'How can I do more?' Cultural awareness training for hospital-based healthcare providers working with high Aboriginal caseload. *BMC Medical Education, 20*(1), 173. https://doi.org/10.1186/s12909-020-02086-5

Kurtz, D.L.M., Janke, R., Vinek, J., et al. (2018). Health Sciences cultural safety education in Australia, Canada, New Zealand, and the United States: A literature review. *International Journal of Medical; Education, 9*, 271–85. https://doi.org/10.5116/ijme.5bc7.21e2

Kwan, M., Jeemi, Z., Norman, R. & Dantas, J.A.R. (2023). Professional interpreter services and the impact on hospital care outcomes: An integrative review of literature. *International Journal of Environmental Research and Public Health, 20*(6). https://doi.org/10.3390/ijerph20065165

Liu, L., Tang, Y., Baxter, G.D., Yin, H. & Tumilty, S. (2021). Complementary and alternative medicine – practice, attitudes, and knowledge among healthcare professionals in New Zealand: An integrative review. *BMC Complementary Medicine and Therapies, 21*(1), 63. https://doi.org/10.1186/s12906-021-03235-z

McGough, S., Wynaden, D., Gower, S., Duggan, R. & Wilson, R. (2022). There is no health without Cultural Safety: Why Cultural Safety matters. *Contemporary Nurse: A Journal for the Australian Nursing Profession, 58*(1), 33–42. https://doi.org/10.1080/10376178.2022.2027254

Milligan, E., West, R., Saunders, V., et al. (2021). Achieving cultural safety for Australia's First Peoples: A review of the Australian Health Practitioner Regulation Agency-registered health practitioners' Codes of Conduct and Codes of Ethics. *Australian Health Review, 45*(4), 398–406.

Nursing Council of New Zealand (NCNZ). (2011). *Guidelines for Cultural Safety, the Treaty of Waitangi and Māori Health in Nursing Education and Practice*. NCNZ.

Pham, T.T.L., Berecki-Gisolf, J., Clapperton, A., et al. (2021). Definitions of culturally and linguistically diverse (CALD): A literature review of epidemiological research in Australia. *International Journal of Environmental Research and Public Health, 18*(2). https://doi.org/10.3390/ijerph18020737

Ramsden, I. (1992). *Kawa Whakaruruhau: Guidelines for Nursing and Midwifery Education*. Nursing Council of New Zealand.

——— (2002). *Cultural Safety and Nursing Education in Aotearoa and Te Waipounamu*. Victoria University of Wellington.

Rivenbark, J.G. & Ichou, M. (2020). Discrimination in healthcare as a barrier to care: experiences of socially disadvantaged populations in France from a nationally representative survey. *BMC Public Health, 20*(1), 31. https://doi.org/10.1186/s12889-019-8124-z

Rosa, J., Louise, B., Sandra, Z., Stefan, N. & Kayvan, B. (2022). Conceptualising difference: A qualitative study of physicians' views on healthcare encounters with asylum seekers. *BMJ Open, 12*(11), e063012. https://doi.org/10.1136/bmjopen-2022-063012

Saaida, M. (2023). Language, culture, and power: Exploring the dynamics of communication across differences. *Science for all Publications*, *1*(1), 1–2.

Sharifi, N., Adib-Hajbaghery, M. & Najafi, M. (2019). Cultural competence in nursing: A concept analysis. *International Journal of Nursing Studies*, *99*, 103386. https://doi.org/10.1016/j.ijnurstu.2019.103386

So, N., Price, K., O'Mara, P. & Rodrigues, M.A. (2024). The importance of cultural humility and cultural safety in health care. *Medical Journal of Australia*, *220*(1), 12–13. https://doi.org/10.5694/mja2.52182

Stanford, F.C. (2020). The importance of diversity and inclusion in the healthcare workforce. *Journal of the National Medical Association*, *112*(3), 247–9. https://doi.org/10.1016/j.jnma.2020.03.014

Stein-Parbury, J. (2021). *Patient & Person: Interpersonal Skill in Nursing* (4th ed.). Elsevier.

Stubbe, D.E. (2020). Practicing cultural competence and cultural humility in the care of diverse patients. *Focus (American Psychiatry Publications)*, *18*(1), 49–51. https://doi.org/10.1176/appi.focus.20190041

Thirsk, L.M., Panchuk, J.T., Stahlke, S. & Hagtvedt, R. (2022). Cognitive and implicit biases in nurses' judgment and decision-making: A scoping review. *International Journal of Nursing Studies*, *133*, 104284. https://doi.org/10.1016/j.ijnurstu.2022.104284

Wang, D., Donohue, R., Guo, F., Yang, M. & Luu, T. (2024). A paradox theory lens for developing cross-cultural competence: Mindset, behavior, and work design. *Journal of Business Research*, *177*, 114645. https://doi.org/10.1016/j.jbusres.2024.114645

Wepa, D. (ed.) (2015). *Cultural Safety in Aotearoa New Zealand* (2nd ed.). Cambridge University Press

Young, S. & Guo, K.L. (2020). Cultural diversity training: The necessity of cultural competence for health care providers and in nursing practice. *The Health Care Manager*, *35*(2), 94–102. https://doi.org/10.1097/hcm.0000000000000294

11 Community health needs assessment

Diana Guzys and Melanie Eslick

LEARNING OBJECTIVES

At the completion of this chapter, you should be able to:

- explain the concept of community.
- explain the different types of health needs in a community.
- identify the principles involved in performing a community health needs assessment.
- describe the processes involved in undertaking a community health needs assessment.
- explain how to approach responding to identified needs.

Introduction

Good nursing practice is based on evidence and undertaking a community health needs assessment is a means of providing evidence to guide community nursing practice. A community health needs assessment is a process that examines the health status and social needs of a particular population. It may be conducted at a whole-of-community level, a sub-community level or even a subsystem level. Nursing practice frequently involves gathering data and assessing individuals or families to determine appropriate nursing interventions. This concept is transferable to an identified community when the community itself is viewed as the client.

The primary purpose for undertaking a community health needs assessment is to develop an understanding of a specific community and its health needs. Most often this is done to improve the quality of life and/or health outcomes for those living in that community. The findings from a community health needs assessment contribute to developing informed, relevant and appropriate strategies for health promotion activities and interventions, as well as providing evidence for health service need. This may be through prioritising resource allocation, service redevelopment, and/or workforce development needs, to inform program planning or facilitate community development. The intention of a community health needs assessment is to promote, support and create a healthy community (Pazzaglia et al., 2023; Ravaghi et al., 2023).

A community health needs assessment should be viewed as a tool that focuses thinking on what the client – in this case, the community – requires, rather than focusing on what services are being provided. It provides direction to ensure that nurses (and other health professionals, organisations and governments) are not simply doing what is considered a good idea or what is easy or comfortable to do, but rather are doing what is necessary based on careful analysis of the available data about the specific community context.

The focus of a community health needs assessment is slightly different to that of a health needs assessment, which tends to focus on needs related to specific physical and mental health conditions, rather than considering social factors such as housing, employment and education that influence well-being and health more broadly. Adopting a primary health care (PHC) perspective requires that a community health needs assessment should reflect the social view of health (Ravaghi et al., 2023). It is therefore essential that the process undertaken in determining need incorporates social justice, equity and meaningful **community participation**. Another extremely important consideration when undertaking a community health needs assessment is that the strengths as well as deficits of the community are considered (Kerr et al., 2019; Ravaghi et al., 2023). A community health needs assessment should identify how well the structures, systems and resources already in place are functioning, as well as the issues resulting from the absence of these. Consideration of more intangible aspects of a community, such as **social capital**, **community competency** and **community capacity**, should also be included.

Several models of community health needs assessment have been detailed in the literature, however, the principles that underpin these are the same (Shiomi et al., 2022). This chapter focuses on exploring the principles and processes involved in undertaking a community health needs assessment.

Who or what is a community?

Consistent in most definitions of community is the concept of a group of people who can identify a common interest that links them to the others in the group (Ravaghi et al., 2023). This could be through geography – if they all live in the same neighbourhood, suburb, town or region. Some communities share a common interest or characteristic, such as the farming community, the LGBTQIA+ community, the vegetarian or vegan community, the sporting community, or the homeless community. Culture and religion are other factors that can link a group of people as a community, for example Italian, Indigenous and Islamic communities. Having a shared history can also link members of a community, such as the refugee community, breast cancer survivor community or war veteran community.

What do we mean by 'need'?

Spend enough time in any supermarket or shopping centre, and you are likely to overhear parents telling their children that each item the children so desperately say they need is actually not a 'need' but a 'want'. Ravaghi and colleagues (2023) acknowledge that there is no universally accepted definition of need, as the concept varies in relation to context and resources available to address this. However, we should keep in mind that 'need' is not a value-free concept. Recognition of identified needs frequently depends on the perspective

Community participation – the active, collective involvement of local people in assessing their needs, making decisions, planning and engaging in strategies to meet those needs.

Social capital – the level of trust, social cohesion and connectedness between people, particularly demonstrated through norms and established networks that facilitate cooperation for mutual benefit, resulting in people being prepared to help each other.

Community competency – the demonstration of collective health literacy, as community members have the ability to make informed choices which maintain or result in improvements to their health and the health of the community.

Community capacity – community members who have the appropriate resources, knowledge and skills to ensure that health is prioritised in a community's decision-making.

and values of those identifying them (Diori, 2021; Okura, 2019). The distinction between need and want can be challenging for adults and even health professionals, so it is useful to have a tool to assist in determining this difference. The process involved in undertaking a community health needs assessment simultaneously identifies need and provides evidence to justify responding to these needs.

Bradshaw's typology of need

Bradshaw (1972) identifies four kinds of need, providing a useful way to think about the concept of need and how this may change when considered from different perspectives. This classification is commonly referred to as a typology of need and may be used to help clarify the viewpoint or factors that influence the perception of those identifying the need. Despite the decades that have passed since Bradshaw's work, his typology of needs remains appropriate for the work of health care professionals and is well-established in community assessment practice. These needs are described as felt, expressed, comparative (relative) and normative, and it is important that all are considered when working with a community to plan and implement health intervention strategies.

Felt need

'Felt need' refers to the opinions offered by community members (Bradshaw, 1972; Smart, 2019). This is what people say they need. It reflects what people in the community identify as issues or concerns. However, people may only identify the issues related to what they perceive you are able to do something about or what they believe you wish to be told. Recent events, media attention or vocal minorities could influence the issues identified by a community. On its own, the value of felt need is limited. Public forums, focus groups, interviews and open-question surveys may be used to collect data relating to felt need.

Expressed need

'Expressed need' is measured through the use of services that already exist. Data relating to expressed need is collected by reviewing the demand for health services within the community, such as waiting times or frequency of use (Bradshaw, 1972; Smart, 2019). It is even more limited than felt need, as it does not allow for the identification of new solutions.

Comparative need

'Comparative need', also referred to as 'relative need', is based on comparing the resources or services of one group or area with another similar group or area (Bradshaw, 1972; Smart, 2019). It is assumed that because similarities exist between areas or groups, the response to the need identified in the comparison area or group is also the most appropriate response to the needs of those being assessed. This strategy may be used to quickly identify information to fill in gaps that require attention. Reliance on this type of need assumes that a needs analysis was performed for the original community to determine the appropriate response, although this may not necessarily be a valid assumption.

Normative need

This is determined by the 'experts' on the basis of professional analysis and relies heavily on epidemiological data (Bradshaw, 1972; Smart, 2019). However, experts may have differing opinions depending on their own values and sometimes their political influences. Expert opinion can change over time as new knowledge, evidence and technologies become available. Updated dietary guidelines are an example of shifts in expert advice as a result of adopting a different perspective based on current research and evidence.

The principles of community health needs assessment

A needs assessment should involve a combination of felt, expressed, normative and comparative needs. It should involve formal and informal assessment of needs and resources. The process should create a partnership between the community and health professionals in determining needs and resources (Haldane et al., 2019; Ravaghi et al., 2023). The community should be involved in planning action and evaluating any outcomes. The fundamental principles of undertaking a community health needs assessment are the collection of evidence using primary and secondary data sources. Following analysis and interpretation of the data, the findings must be shared with the community in a way that is understandable and avoids the use of jargon. The community then participates in setting goals for action in response to the findings.

Challenges to undertaking a community health needs assessment

Undertaking a community health needs assessment requires an organisational commitment of time and money, as well as having appropriate research, analysis skills and resources. The scarcity of these resources sometimes leads to organisations and health care professionals relying on informal, anecdotal or perhaps intuitive knowledge to guide activity (Okura, 2019). This tendency potentially results in a lack of innovation, maintaining the status quo and responding inappropriately due to public, media or political pressure. Other challenges to successfully undertaking a community health needs assessment include low participation rates of community members from the most vulnerable groups and the lack of locally relevant good-quality data. Health care professionals are more likely to focus on epidemiological factors and dismiss social and environmental issues, which may result in marginalisation of community members whose priorities may not always be the same (Haldane et al., 2019). Furthermore, a focus on epidemiology and health service provision expenses may be perceived as a means of cost reduction (Ravaghi et al., 2023). Therefore, **community-based participatory research** has been suggested as an alternative to undertaking a community health needs assessment, as it is an empowering process that promotes co-learning thereby building community capacity and competence, as well as facilitating collaborative partnerships that strengthen social capital (Pazzaglia et al., 2023).

Community-based participatory research – a collaborative partnership between community members, organisational representatives and researchers who equally combine knowledge, contribute expertise, share decision-making and ownership of the research process on a topic of importance to the community to achieve social change.

REFLECTION

How can we identify and find ways to include marginalised and difficult-to-reach members of a community who do not respond to mainstream approaches?

The process of undertaking a community health needs assessment

Consideration of the purpose for undertaking a community health needs assessment is an essential first step in the process. A community health needs assessment is a time- and resource-intensive activity. Prior to committing to such an activity, it is important to establish whether the information required could be equally obtained through more focused research activities such as developing a community profile or performing a service evaluation. The next step is to consider whether you or your organisation has sufficient resources to undertake a community health needs assessment. Resources include time, expertise, finances and the capacity to act on the results of the needs assessment (Smart, 2019). There is little point in identifying needs and building community expectations if nothing is going to be achieved from the exercise. It must also be acknowledged that advocacy and lobbying for resources to address identified needs are legitimate activities that may result from a community health needs assessment.

The process involved in undertaking a community health needs assessment is summarised in Figure 11.1.

Developing partnerships

The next step in the process is to determine who is performing the assessment. Most often a team of people is required to do this, although when working with small and well-defined communities it may be possible for an individual to be responsible for the research project. It is important to establish a group of appropriate people who can contribute advice about the processes being used or who might provide insights in relation to the specific community (Ravaghi et al., 2023; Smart, 2019). This group is commonly known as the project advisory or steering committee, or sometimes the reference group. Its expertise contributes to the development of the research plan. This may be through providing advice on the methods best used to obtain the required data or assisting in identifying key informants or 'gatekeepers' who could help in facilitating access to difficult-to-reach subgroups in a community. Developing a realistic time frame to work within is also a fundamental component of health needs assessment planning.

Data collection

Effective planning is an essential foundation for undertaking a genuine community health needs assessment. Planning involves making decisions about the data collection tools and methods, as well as who will be asked to contribute information. Very rarely is it possible to involve every member of a community in data collection. Specific strategies might need to be developed to ensure that under-represented sections of the community are facilitated to engage in the process. Community-based participatory research methodologies provide a theoretical framework for collaborating with community members to collect primary data (Ravaghi et al., 2023).

There is no formula for undertaking a community assessment; it can occur in a variety of ways. What is important is that a range of relevant data is collected, and that the data is analysed in a logical manner to present an understandable picture of what is occurring within the community. You may choose to look at the determinants of health and assess your community against these. Another approach is to use systematic analysis to identify

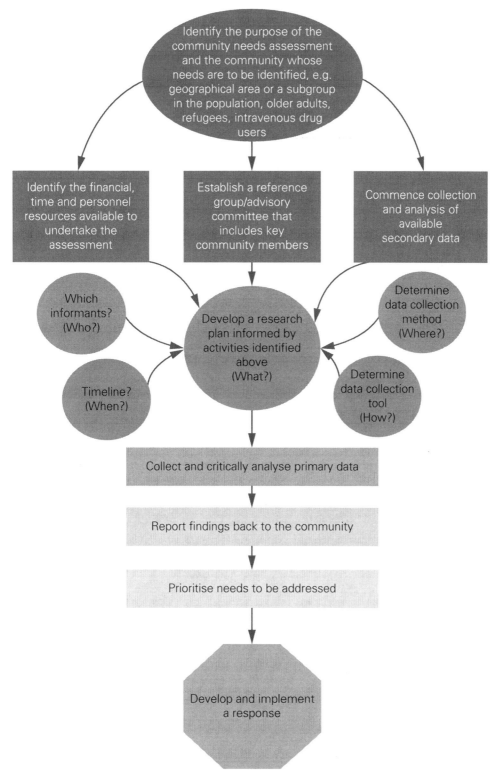

Figure 11.1   The community health needs assessment process

problems, needs, strengths and trends in the community. Using a structured model such as the Community-as-Partner model (Anderson & McFarlane, 2018) may be an appropriate approach to take. This focuses on exploring the community core, which is comprised of its history, social demographics, values and beliefs (Wilbur, 2020). Then a community's subsystems are studied. These include its economy, the physical environment, opportunities to participate in recreation, communication, education facilities, safety and transportation, politics and government, and health and social services (Wilbur, 2020).

Primary and secondary data

There are two types of information or data that are collected when undertaking a community health needs assessment: these are known as primary and secondary data (Shiomi et al., 2022; Smart, 2019). Similar to when undertaking a nursing assessment of an individual, one type of information is subjective data. In this situation, it is known as 'primary data' which comes from the community itself. The other type of data collected equates to the objective data identified in an individual health assessment – this is called 'secondary data'. Secondary data is pre-existing information that comes from statistical and epidemiological reports, as well as information from relevant literature (Smart, 2019). To gain the most accurate understanding of a community and its needs, comprehensive data collection using a variety of primary and secondary sources must occur.

The aim of primary data collection is to gather the opinions and perspectives of community members. This can be achieved via surveys and community forums or public meetings, where members of the community are invited to express their opinions. Community surveys can be conducted by telephone, advertised through local media and made available online, dropped into letterboxes, delivered door-to-door or placed in high-traffic areas frequented by specifically targeted groups (Wilbur, 2020). Focus groups, which gather a small group of people together, are another approach. These provide a good opportunity to explore the responses of community members in detail. Key informants, who are often community leaders holding formal and informal positions within the community, or experts in particular fields, may be interviewed to collect a wide range of information (Smart, 2019). Interviews allow for thorough documentation of an individual perspective and historically have been considered the best method of primary data collection; however, they are time-consuming and therefore usually limited to a small group of participants.

Other primary data collection methods include participant observation – used when informal observations may add depth to understanding of issues – behaviours and values. A windshield survey is another observational technique, involving driving or walking through a community to develop a sense of the available infrastructure as well as its economic and social capital (Kerr et al., 2019). A form of observation that might provide useful data could include recording the number of vacant retail shops, the extent of visible graffiti, home maintenance levels or the number of community members interacting in public places.

A logical starting point for the collection of secondary data is to review the relevant literature. This can assist in identifying potential issues and previously used strategies. Local and national policy documents may contribute information relevant to the community, as may previously conducted community surveys (Department of Health, 2021). One of the most useful sources of demographic and epidemiological information in Australia and Aotearoa New Zealand is the national household census, held every five years and reported by the Australian Bureau of Statistics (ABS) (n.d.) and Statistics New Zealand (Stats NZ)

(2024). In Australia, the census and other data are compiled and presented accessibly by the Australian Institute of Health and Welfare. Primary Health Networks are also increasingly collecting and reporting data related to their local communities and regions. The data available relates to community composition of age, gender and ethnicity. Social and economic indicators as well as mortality and morbidity rates are also presented. Secondary data collection is usually easily obtained and cost-effective in comparison to collecting primary data. However, the value of including data collected from the community outweighs the expense of conducting such research.

Once data are collected, they must be critically analysed. Remember that collecting data does not change anything apart from raising community expectations. Gaps in the data should be included in the analysis as these could be very informative. The results of the analysis should be reported back to the community for comment.

Disseminating results and prioritising actions

Engaging the community in a discussion of the results of a community health needs assessment is another key component of the process. At the most basic level, it shows respect for the community; after all, this is their information. It is also a fundamental part of the research process, confirming the quality of analysis of the data. Finally, it contributes to strengthening community action, as the community becomes involved in prioritising and identifying responses to the identified needs (Haldane et al., 2019). Most commonly, the results of a community health needs assessment are disseminated through the production of a report and/or through community meetings (Ravaghi et al., 2023). A variety of means should be used so as many community members as possible can discuss the findings and take part in setting priorities.

It is essential to explain to community members how the needs identified are drawn from the data collection and analysis. Creating a shared understanding may influence whether the community members recognise the findings as needs, and whether it is possible to address these needs (Haldane et al., 2019). Unless common goals are recognised, it will be difficult to engage with the community and proposed responses are less likely to be successful (Smart, 2019). Sometimes education may be required to enable common goals to be developed with the target community (Smart, 2019). If a community recognises the need, it is more likely to become involved with health-promoting initiatives. Providing information regarding the number of people affected, and the possible consequences of not addressing a need, may assist community members to prioritise action. Understanding the issues from the perspective of the community is invaluable when responding to the needs assessment (Haldane et al., 2019). Ongoing community involvement provides guidance for individual health care workers and organisations in developing the most effective response.

Addressing identified needs

Following prioritisation of needs, the community health nurse (CHN), the employing organisation and other organisations and services that may have been involved in the community health needs assessment process determine how they can best address these needs. A thorough assessment will provide recommendations for action. Responses may involve the expansion or modification of existing services, targeted educational activities, and lobbying or advocating for funds or services to meet the identified gaps.

CASE STUDY 11.1

Cassie is a CHN employed at the Hopefultown Regional Community Service where she runs a number of health education programs and undertakes a range of health promotion activities. She has been nominated by her manager to organise an advisory committee with other interested organisations to undertake a community health needs assessment for the local community to determine where resources should be focused to improve the health of the community. After contacting multiple organisations, agencies and services, a working party was formed consisting of representatives from the local hospital; a GP from the local Primary Health Care Network; a councillor from local government; the President of the Business Association; the principals from the Lutheran primary school and secondary college; as well as the Community Health Service's Community Representative on their board of management.

While negotiating membership of the advisory committee, Cassie commenced collecting secondary data to inform the community health needs assessment. The following information was obtained from national census data, local government information and service directories.

Secondary data

Hopefultown is a regional city located on the Wishes River. It is located about 250 km west of the state capital. The Wishes River and its tributaries provide the main natural feature of the city, which is situated on mostly flat topography. The urban area extends for a 15 km radius around the river. Residential and civic uses of land dominate centrally, and industrial areas are located at the eastern and western edges. However, the larger statistical area is represented by agricultural land surrounding the city. The town's water supply is fully treated drinking water sourced from a nearby lake. When water levels are low this can be supplemented with bore water.

At the last census, Hopefultown had a population of 14 285 and is comprised of approximately 52.1 per cent females and 47.9 per cent males. The municipality has a population of 19 279 and covers an area of 4267 square kilometres. It is the largest city by population in the region, and it is the main administrative centre with a catchment of approximately 95 000 people.

There are two government primary schools, one secondary school, a TAFE and a university campus, plus Catholic and Lutheran primary schools and a Catholic secondary college.

Civic facilities include a regional art gallery, performing arts centre and botanic gardens. There are three privately owned gyms and a martial arts training centre. Sporting facilities include a large indoor stadium with facilities for netball, basketball and other indoor sports. The aquatic centre has one 50-metre heated pool and a toddler pool. There are seven children's playgrounds scattered throughout the residential area, while each primary and secondary school has a football oval and an outdoor netball court. There is one purpose-built stadium, close to the central business district for football and cricket.

The main form of transport is personal vehicles, although rail transport includes both passenger and freight services. Hopefultown has two taxi companies consisting of approximately 18 taxi vehicles. Most are modified station wagons, but also available are two wheelchair-accessible vans. There is a town bus service, consisting of six buses and seven routes. Bus services also run to and from Hopefultown from various outlying areas.

Sixty-one per cent of people living in Hopefultown over the age of 15 identify as being employed. Fifty-seven per cent identify as being employed full time and 34 per cent work part-time. Hopefultown has an unemployment rate of 3.2 per cent.

The main occupations of people living in Hopefultown are:

- 17.7 per cent professionals
- 16.5 per cent managers
- 15.5 per cent technicians and trades workers
- 13.3 per cent community and personal service workers
- 12.9 per cent clerical and administrative workers
- 11.8 per cent labourers
- 9.2 per cent sales workers
- 6.2 per cent machinery operators and drivers, 2.0 per cent have no stated occupation.

The main industries people from Hopefultown work in are:

- 12.4 per cent health care and social assistance
- 10.6 per cent construction
- 9.8 per cent education and training
- 8.2 per cent accommodation and food services
- 7.8 per cent public administration and safety
- 7.3 per cent retail trade
- 6.4 per cent manufacturing.

Forty-eight per cent of people are married, 34 per cent have never married and 9 per cent are divorced. Three per cent are separated and 6 per cent are widowed.

Forty per cent of homes are fully owned and 31 per cent are in the process of being purchased by home loan mortgage. Twenty-six per cent of homes are rented.

The median rent in Hopefultown is $260 per week and the median mortgage repayment is $1500 per month.

The median individual income is $725 per week and the median household income is $1825 per week.

The main long-term health conditions reported in Hopefultown are as follows:

- arthritis: 12 per cent
- asthma: 10 per cent
- mental health condition (including depression or anxiety): 10 per cent
- diabetes (excluding gestational diabetes): 5 per cent
- heart disease (including heart attack or angina): 5 per cent
- cancer (including remission): 4 per cent
- lung condition (including COPD or emphysema): 2.5 per cent
- kidney disease: 1 per cent
- stroke: 1.4 per cent
- dementia (including Alzheimer's): 0.6 per cent
- other long-term health condition(s): 7.5 per cent.

The health services that are available are as follows:

- Wishes Health provides a range of health services including the Wishes Regional Hospital and Medical Centre.

CASE STUDY 11.1 Continued

- Wishes Medical Centre has two permanent independent general practice clinics and several specialists on site.
- Specialist services include an obstetrician/gynaecologist, two physicians and two surgeons.
- Visiting specialists who use the medical centre for consultations include a cardiologist, several dermatologists, an ear, nose and throat surgeon, a neurosurgeon, an ophthalmologist, an orthopaedic surgeon, a renal physician, a respiratory physician, a urologist and a vascular surgeon.

Wishes Regional Hospital is the main hospital for the city of Hopefultown and the surrounding area providing:

- an emergency department
- day procedures, day oncology, dialysis
- an intensive care unit
- general wards
- a sub-acute facility and rehabilitation gym
- a nursing home
- hospice care
- pathology, pharmacy, radiology (X-ray)
- a dietician, audiology, occupational therapy, physiotherapy, podiatry, social work and speech pathology services
- a Hospital Admission Risk Program (HARP)
- a dental clinic
- a continence service
- a day centre
- a district/community nursing service.

Hopefultown Regional Community Service provides an array of programs and services including:

- Aboriginal and Torres Strait Islander health
- alcohol and other drugs support
- carers support and respite
- cardiac and respiratory rehabilitation
- counselling (including youth counselling/psychology)
- diabetes education
- an early childhood intervention service
- exercise groups
- family daycare
- family violence support
- financial counselling
- gamblers' help
- health promotion
- home care packages
- housing support (including youth housing support)

- LGBTQIA+ programs and support (including youth groups)
- men's and women's sheds
- National Disability Insurance Scheme (NDIS) support coordination
- a needle and syringe program
- occupational therapy
- parent support
- physiotherapy
- podiatry
- a school-focused youth service
- social support groups.

REFLECTION

1. Looking at the socio-demographic information provided and health services available, can you identify any service gaps or anticipate what the health needs for the community may be?
2. Can you think of other information that may be useful for Cassie to source to improve the community profile she is developing?

REFLECTION

Visit the ABS or Stats NZ website and look up the community profile information related to a community you know well; perhaps the town or city in which you grew up. Compare your knowledge and perception of that community with the information provided through the data on the website. What are the similarities and differences?

CASE STUDY 11.2

Let us continue exploring Cassie's experience of undertaking a community health needs assessment for the Hopefultown regional community.

Once the members of the community health needs assessment advisory committee reviewed the secondary data that Cassie provided, they met to determine the best approach to undertake the collection of primary data. The committee decided that they did not have the funds to mail out surveys to every household but did want to reach as many people in the catchment region as possible. Following a lengthy discussion, it was decided that primary data would be sought via focus group discussions with several existing groups within the community, such as the Country Women's Association (CWA); men's and women's sheds; Parent and Friends Associations at all the primary schools; Rotary Club and Sporting Association. Two town hall meetings for anyone who wanted to participate would be advertised in the local paper and on local radio. One meeting would be held during the day and one in the evening, to try to make these as accessible as possible to all community members. It was also decided to undertake a less formal survey approach, by giving community members the opportunity to provide written responses to the questions that would be used to stimulate discussion in the focus groups. These surveys would be available to complete

CASE STUDY 11.2 Continued

and submit at a static display in businesses such as pharmacies, supermarkets and general stores, particularly in smaller communities within the catchment area.

The wording of the questions used in the survey document and to stimulate discussion at the focus groups was considered very carefully by the advisory committee. A range of perspectives relating to the purpose of the questions; the model of health informing the advisory committees' understanding of health; and concerns regarding having a deficit-versus-strengths approach, informed the development of the questions to be used. The advisory committee eventually agreed to use the following four questions:

1. How would you know if your community is healthy?
2. What could be done to improve the health of your community?
3. How would you know if your community has the skills and knowledge to be healthy?
4. What could be done to improve the skills and knowledge to be healthy in your community?

Primary data

Primary data were collected over a period of four months. An analysis of the data and the production of a report which incorporated primary and secondary data took place over four months (Table 11.1).

Table 11.1   Themes identified from the primary data

Health expectations	Building health	Contributing to the collective good	The realities of rural life
Sufficient and appropriate services	Accessible trustworthy sources of health knowledge	Thinking beyond self	Social conditions/ social determinants
Behaviour of health care professionals	Skills in assessing the quality of health and health information	Building social connections	Physical environment
Behaviour of various levels of government	Understandable health information	Creating opportunities for participation	Prohibitive costs
Involvement in decision-making	Distributing community information	Supporting each other	Distance and transportation
Health is the norm		Demonstrating community leadership	Access to specialist services
Quality of life			

To better illustrate the dynamic and interdependent relationships of the influences identified as affecting the health of the Hopefultown community, a thematic network (Atrride-Stirling, 2001) was developed that demonstrates the relationship with the basic, organising and global themes, presented as Figure 11.2.

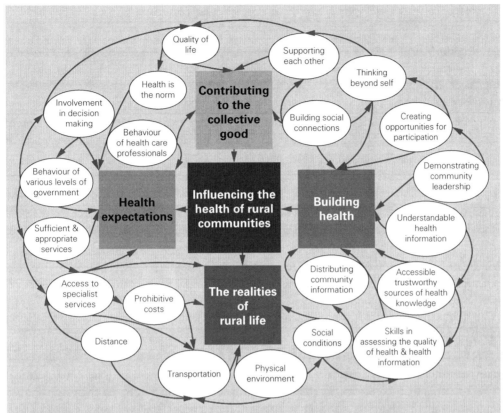

Figure 11.2   Thematic network demonstrating the dynamic interaction of influences on the health of the wider Hopefultown community

Source: Adapted from Attride-Stirling (2001).

Reporting back to the community

To provide community members with the opportunity to provide feedback on the findings of the community health needs assessment, copies of the report were made available from Hopefultown Regional Community Service; Wishes Regional Hospital; Wishes Medical Centre and Hopefultown Regional Council Offices. The availability of the report was advertised on local radio and in the local newspaper. A town hall meeting was held to present the findings, followed by a discussion of what action or responses should then occur. Community members were also invited to send comments and feedback to a dedicated email address that was included in the report.

REFLECTION

1. Looking at the themes derived from the primary data, what do you believe are the main health needs of the community?
2. Can you think of other ways to disseminate the results of the community health needs assessment and prioritise responses?

Responding to identified needs

A community health needs assessment is used to provide evidence to assist with prioritising and informing decisions made in the planning of responses at an organisational and community level. This information is necessary to deploy resources effectively to address the health priorities of local populations (Ravaghi et al., 2023). The results of the needs assessment may indicate that lobbying for extra resources or seeking funding to deliver new or different services are necessary. However, often health promotion activities provide a framework for addressing identified community health needs.

Engaging multiple health promotion strategies, as outlined in the *Ottawa Charter for Health Promotion* (World Health Organization (WHO), 1986), strengthens the likely effectiveness of the response taken to address identified community needs. Organisational responses as well as community-level responses may require intersectoral cooperation to make real and sustained change. The inclusion of representatives from local government and from a wide range of local organisations in planning community-level responses is essential (Department of Health, 2021). Community representation in decision-making committees is also an integral component of this process. Organisational-level responses to needs assessment, which tend to focus on the internal allocation of the organisation's resources, equally benefit from consideration of strategic action based on health promotion principles.

For most nurses working in the community, an educational response of some kind is the most common response. Health education activities may be used in developing personal skills to strengthen community action or as a means of contributing to the creation of a supportive environment (Haldane et al., 2019; Okura, 2019). However, nurses may well be involved in other types of health promotion activities too, such as advocacy via grant writing and lobbying.

Conclusion

A community health needs assessment is a tool that focuses thinking on what a community requires, rather than focusing on what services already exist. It reflects the social view of health in determining the needs and resources of a defined community. When appropriately undertaken, it assists in building strong and meaningful relationships between the community and health professionals. It may provide evidence to guide the allocation of resources and the professional practice of health care professionals, such as CHNs, highlighting areas where the nurse may be able to intervene.

Fundamental to the process of a community health needs assessment is the recognition that the issues identified as needs frequently depend on the perspective and values of those identifying them. Therefore, it is essential to incorporate primary and secondary data drawn from a variety of sources, via various means, in order to achieve a balanced and comprehensive understanding of the community's needs.

We use the evidence provided by a community health needs assessment to ensure that we are not simply doing what we think is a good idea, feel like doing or know we can do (or fund) easily. It should guide our practice and help us to prioritise professional activity, providing a rationale for introducing new programs and activities. The *Ottawa Charter for Health Promotion* (WHO, 1986) provides a useful framework for developing responses to identified need, as is discussed in Chapter 1. The professional activities undertaken by CHNs in response to a community needs assessment, such as writing submissions and grant applications for new programs or services, or planning and delivering health programs, are discussed in greater detail in later chapters.

CRITICAL THINKING ACTIVITIES

1. Develop one potential strategy to address each of the key findings of the community health needs assessment described in the case study.
2. Prioritise the strategies you have developed to address these needs.
3. Identify the criteria you used to prioritise these strategies.
4. Consider the personal values demonstrated in developing your criteria for prioritisation.

FURTHER READING

Collaboration for Evidence, Research, and Impact in Public Health. (2018). *SHBBV Program Planning Toolkit* (2nd ed.). Curtin University. https://siren.org.au/wp-content/uploads/2018/09/SiREN-Toolkit-2nd-Edition.pdf

Community Tool Box (2024). *Section 1. Developing a Plan for Assessing Local Needs and Resources Assessing community needs and resources*. University of Kansas. https://ctb.ku.edu/en/table-of-contents/assessment/assessing-community-needs-and-resources/develop-a-plan/main

Moore de Peralta, A., Davis, L., Brown, K., et al. (2020). Using community-engaged research to explore social determinants of health in a low-resource community in the Dominican Republic: A community health assessment. *Hispanic Health Care International, 18*(3), 127–37. https://doi.org/10.1177/154041531987481

Santana, I.R., Mason, A., Gutacker, N., et al. (2023). Need, demand, supply in health care: working definitions, and their implications for defining access. *Health Economics, Policy and Law, 18*(1), 1–13. https://doi.org/10.1177/1540415319874812

REFERENCES

Anderson, E.T. & McFarlane, J. (2018). *Community as Partner: Theory and Practice in Nursing* (8th ed.). Wolters Kluwer.

Attride-Stirling, J. (2001). Thematic networks: An analytic tool for qualitative research. *Qualitative Research, 1*, 385–405. http:/doi.org/10.1177/146879410100100307

Australian Bureau of Statistics (ABS). (n.d.). *Census*. Australian Government. www.abs.gov.au/websitedbs/D3310114.nsf/Home/Census?OpenDocument&ref=topBar

Bradshaw, J.R. (1972). The taxonomy of social need. In G. McLachlan (ed.), *Problems and Progress in Medical Care* (pp. 69–82). Oxford University Press.

Department of Health. (2021). *PHN Program Needs Assessment Policy Guide 2021*. Commonwealth of Australia.

Diori, H.I. (2021). A critical insight into needs assessment technique and the way social needs are actually assessed. *Advanced Journal of Social Science, 8*(1), 3–9. https://doi.org/10.21467/ajss.8.1.3-9

Haldane, V., Chuah, F.L., Srivastava, A., et al. (2019). Community participation in health services development, implementation, and evaluation: A systematic review of empowerment, health, community, and process outcomes. *PLOS ONE, 14*(5), e0216112. https://doi.org/10.1371/journal.pone.0216112

Kerr, M.J., Gargantua-Aguila, S.D.R., Glavin, K., et al. (2019). Feasibility of describing community strengths relative to Omaha system concepts. *Public Health Nursing, 36*(2), 245–53.

Okura, M. (2019). The process of structuring community health needs by public health nurses through daily practice: A modified grounded theory study. *Asian Nursing Research, 13*(4), 229–35.

Pazzaglia, C., Camedda, C., Ugenti, N.V., et al. (2023). Community Health assessment tools adoptable in nursing practice: a scoping review. *International Journal of Environmental Research and Public Health, 20*(3), 1667.

Ravaghi, H., Guisset, A.L., Elfeky, S., et al. (2023). A scoping review of community health needs and assets assessment: Concepts, rationale, tools and uses. *BMC Health Services Research, 23*(1), 44.

Shiomi, M., Yoshioka-Maeda, K., Kotera, S., Ushio, Y. & Takemura, K. (2022). Factors associated with the utilization of community assessment models among Japanese nurses. *Public Health Nursing, 39*(2), 464–71.

Smart, J. (2019) *Needs Assessment*. Australian Institute of Family Studies, Commonwealth of Australia. https://aifs.gov.au/sites/default/files/publication-documents/1902_expp_needs_assessment_0_0.pdf

Statistics New Zealand (Stats NZ). (2024). *2023 Census*. New Zealand Government. www.stats.govt.nz/2023-census

Wilbur, K.A. (2020). *Community health worker experiences with people who use drugs: A phenomenological study*. University of New Brunswick.

World Health Organization (WHO). (1986). *Ottawa Charter for Health Promotion*. Paper presented to the First International Conference on Health Promotion, Ottawa, Canada.

Health-related program planning and evaluation

Dean Whitehead

12

LEARNING OBJECTIVES

At the completion of this chapter, you should be able to:

- discuss the principles that underpin the planning and evaluation processes for health promotion and health education programs.
- identify commonly used methods and tools for the planning, implementation and evaluation of health promotion and health education programs.
- list related activities that assist and inform the planning and evaluation of health promotion and health education programs.

Introduction

The terms 'health promotion' and 'health education' are often used interchangeably. Often this is a problem as they are distinct and different concepts (see Chapter 2). Whitehead (2004) attempted to overcome this problem by separating and defining the terms. Health education is defined as:

> An activity that seeks to inform the individual on the nature and causes of health/illness and that individual's personal level of risk associated with their lifestyle-related behaviour. [It] seeks to motivate … behavioural change through directly influencing their value, belief, and attitude systems, where it is deemed that the individual is particularly at risk or has been affected by illness/disease or disability already. (Whitehead, 2004, p. 313)

Health promotion is defined as:

> The process by which the ecologically driven sociopolitical-economic determinants of health are addressed as they impact individuals and the communities within which they interact. [It] seeks to radically transform and empower communities through involving them in fundamental activities such as influencing public health. It looks to develop and reform social structures through evolving participation between all representative stakeholders in their different sectors and agencies. (Whitehead, 2004, p. 314)

Health promotion is a broad and complex process that overarches all health strategy related to primary health care (PHC), public health, population health and community health. It is often an overtly political and policy-driven process that includes types of health education activity such as 'radical' health education (Clavier & de Leeuw, 2013; Green et al., 2019). Owing to this, Conrad and colleagues (2019), in their case study findings, stress the importance of earlier and more comprehensive health promotion education to further assist personal knowledge, self-efficacy, and increase the potential for advocacy/public policy involvement and roles.

When it comes to PHC program planning and evaluation, the terms health promotion and health education are also often used interchangeably but this is less of a problem in this specific case than already stated. Health promotion approaches, often by default, include health education interventions. Reflecting this, many 'health' planning and evaluation tools and models incorporate health promotion and health education processes (McKenzie, Neiger & Thackeray, 2023; Raingruber, 2014; Whitehead & Irvine, 2010). For the purposes of detailing **health program planning** and **evaluation**, many of the processes 'overarch' both approaches (Linsley, Kane & Owen, 2011; McKenzie et al., 2023; Watkins & Cousins, 2010). In the case of this chapter, where only the term 'health promotion' is used, it can be assumed that its process will most likely also include health education planning and evaluation.

All health promotion or health education programs ideally require a formal process of planning and evaluation in a systematic manner, especially to secure requested resources and increase the likelihood of meaningful and successful outcomes (Green et al., 2019). Health promotion and health education programs are dynamic and complex processes that cannot be approached in a 'random' manner. It is well established that the more systematic and structured our health promotion and health education activities are, the more likely it is that they will be effective and efficient, assuming that they are also well-resourced and funded (Ervin & Kulbok, 2018; Whitehead & Irvine, 2010). Where health promotion interventions are criticised, it is usually where they are unstructured, opportunistic, ad hoc and fail to follow established and tested processes. PHC nurses should be proficient at incorporating effective and structured processes into their health promotion practice (Clendon & Munns, 2019).

An aspect of successful health promotion programming is adherence to the overall process of health promotion. Therefore, a common criticism is that programs only incorporate elements of the overall process instead of all the identified components. For instance, it is well documented that, while many health professionals are good at planning their activities, they often fail to evaluate their interventions for outcome and effectiveness (Ervin & Kulbok, 2018; Rains et al., 2018; World Health Organization (WHO), 2022). Therefore, this chapter aims to highlight good practice as it applies to essential health promotion and health education programs required to demonstrate effective process. It does so by presenting these in a logical and sequential process and offers an overview of models and frameworks for guiding this process.

Health program planning – a specific phase of the health promotion and health education process that collects available assessment information, makes sense of it, and then identifies the priorities and resources required to 'action' health programs.

Health program evaluation – a specific phase of health promotion and health education process that 'measures' the extent, impact, and effectiveness of health programs.

The theoretical underpinnings of the health promotion process

In trying to understand and help practitioners decide what 'type' of health promotion approach to adopt, it is necessary to identify some of the main seminal and contemporary health promotion theories and models and their related health education concepts. They are useful for helping us to understand the context of our health-related activities and to facilitate an appreciation of the more structured **health promotion process**. They commonly tend to separate out health promotion approaches depending on different degrees of individuals versus population, authority versus empowerment, prevention versus reaction and the amount of political/health policy process involved (Green et al., 2019). Among the most well-known are the Triphasic Map of Health Education (French & Adams, 1986), the Four Paradigms of Health Promotion (Caplan & Holland, 1990), the Strategies of Health Promotion (Beattie, 1991) and Tannahill's Typology of Health Promotion (Downie, Tannahill & Tannahill, 1996).

Often authors, when describing the health promotion process, may also refer to related seminal and contemporary socio-cognitive behavioural models, for example, Becker's (1974) Health Belief Model (incorporating Bandura's elaborations on self-efficacy), Ajzen and Fishbein's (1980) Theory of Reasoned Action/Theory of Planned Behaviour Model, Prochaska and DiClemente's (1984) Transtheoretical Stages of Change (Revolving Door) Model and Tones' Health Action Model (1987). While these models are often useful to consider as part of a health promotion program, they are mostly centred on individualised behavioural change theories and Social Learning Theory (Socio-Cognitive Theory) (Naidoo & Wills, 2016; Raingruber, 2014). These theories are more consistent with health education programs and processes. Health promotion frameworks and models are now more appropriately considered alongside community and population health interventions (Stanhope & Lancaster, 2016; WHO, 2022).

Whatever theoretical frameworks drive our PHC programs, we know that they must be a key feature of what informs the overall process. For instance, Tones (2000, p. 229) states that:

> To critically evaluate the effectiveness and efficiency of any health promotion program which is theoretically and methodologically unsound is either naive or cynical and certainly renders a major disservice to health promotion.

Health promotion process – the systematic approach to health promotion and health education that includes the planning, implementation and evaluation of such programs.

Planning health promotion

From their early stages, the more systematic, structured, and well-planned health promotion activities are, the more likely they are to have effective and successful outcomes (Green et al., 2019; Walsh, Sheridan & Barry, 2023; Wills, 2014). The second 'phase' of health promotion programming is the planning phase. Following on from Chapter 11, it is where the assessment-related 'ideas' that have been formulated and prioritised become more concrete as they begin to take on physical characteristics in preparation for implementation. A community assessment is a comprehensive description of the overall health needs of a population (community) and its existing resources to facilitate this need (Snelling, 2024). Pender, Murdaugh and Parsons (2015) confirm that community assessment is performed as a primary building block for the planning and evaluation of health promotion programs and acknowledge their interrelatedness. For some, it can be difficult to determine where the assessment stage ends and the planning phase begins especially as, with many health programs, the activities can occur at the same time (Stanhope & Lancaster, 2016).

How do we plan health promotion?

Most planning models for health-related programs tend to be 'staged' in their format. They are often 'linear' such as the Flowchart for Planning and Evaluating Health Promotion Model (Ewles & Simnett, 2010). This is an 'easy-to-use' stages model that outlines the broad process in sequence as:

- Identify needs and priorities
- Set aims and objectives
- Decide the best way of achieving the aims
- Identify resources
- Plan 'evaluation' methods (see later in this chapter)
- Set an action plan
- Action! Implement your plan, including your evaluation.

Other authors adopt a similar process in the planning chapters of their texts such as Francis and colleagues (2012) and Naidoo and Wills (2016). Whitehead (2001a) (see Figure 12.1) developed a nursing-related stage-planning model that divides up the activities of health promotion and health education in the same model. Public Health Ontario (2015) has developed the At a Glance: The Six Steps for Planning a Health Promotion Program as:

1. Manage the planning process.
2. Conduct a situational assessment.
3. Identify goals, populations of interest, outcomes and outcome objectives.
4. Identify strategies, activities, outputs, process objectives and resources.
5. Develop indicators.
6. Review the program plan.

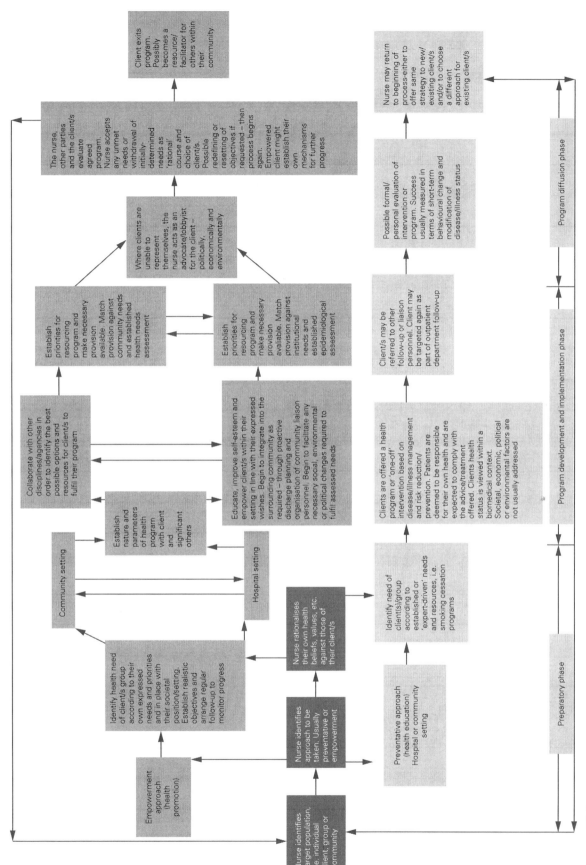

Figure 12.1 Whitehead's Stage-Planning Model

Source: Whitehead (2001a, p. 312).

CASE STUDY 12.1

You are a registered PHC nurse working in a local community clinic. You manage all newly diagnosed diabetes patients of which you have ten or more at any single time. A common 'theme' that emerges from individual health education assessments is that your clients understand their recommended nutritional requirements, but they still struggle with weight loss and exercise. You decide to set up an ongoing support group program to assist the whole group in achieving effective weight loss and exercising.

REFLECTION

1. What type of planning would you make to get this group of clients to initially attend such a support group on a regular basis?
2. What strategies would you consider to ensure that clients regularly attended for the duration of the program?
3. Detail a list of the possible activities that might be most beneficial, considering resources, and in order of priority.

Pender's Health Promotion Model is the most tested nursing-based 'health promotion' planning model (Pender et al., 2015). While acknowledging wider social determinants of health, the model is noted more as a socio-cognitive behavioural (health education) model. Whitehead's (2001b) Socio-Cognitive Model (see Figure 12.2) is similar. Such models are useful, but more suited to individualised health education interventions. On the other hand, Whitehead's (2003a) Effect Planning Model for Health Promotion is representative of a health promotion model that has a socio-ecological community development focus (see Figure 12.3). It is a model that places the nurse in different roles working collaboratively with other disciplines and agencies, especially within a health policy context. As a health promotion planning tool, the Effect Planning Model for Health Promotion allows nurses to see what broad types of activities are involved at the community level, what activities need to be monitored and what outcomes are desirable.

Despite the planning models already mentioned in this chapter, there is one planning model that 'rules them all'. The Precede-Proceed Model is, by far, the most used and tested health promotion program planning model, especially outside of nursing. The fourth edition (2005 version) of the model alone (Green & Kreuter, 2005; see Figure 12.4) has been applied, tested, adapted, and verified in over 960 published studies. Following the third edition, a survey of 253 universities offering graduate or undergraduate degree specialisation in health promotion reported that the Precede-Proceed Model was taught by 88 per cent of respondents, used by 85.7 per cent in teaching and by 74.6 per cent in practice – the most among the top 10 identified health promotion planning models listed (Linnan, Sterba & Lee, 2005). The respondents also ranked Precede-Proceed highest among the 10 planning models on usefulness for research (86%) and usefulness for practice (90.8%). A website exists devoted to the Precede-Proceed Model (www.lgreen.net). It is on this website that the modified and simplified fourth edition revision of the Precede-Proceed Model can also be viewed (www.lgreen.net/precede-proceed). Several nursing-related Australasian studies adopt the Precede-Proceed Model (such as Iannella et al., 2015; Phillips, Rolley & Davidson, 2012; Tramm, McCarthy & Yates, 2011).

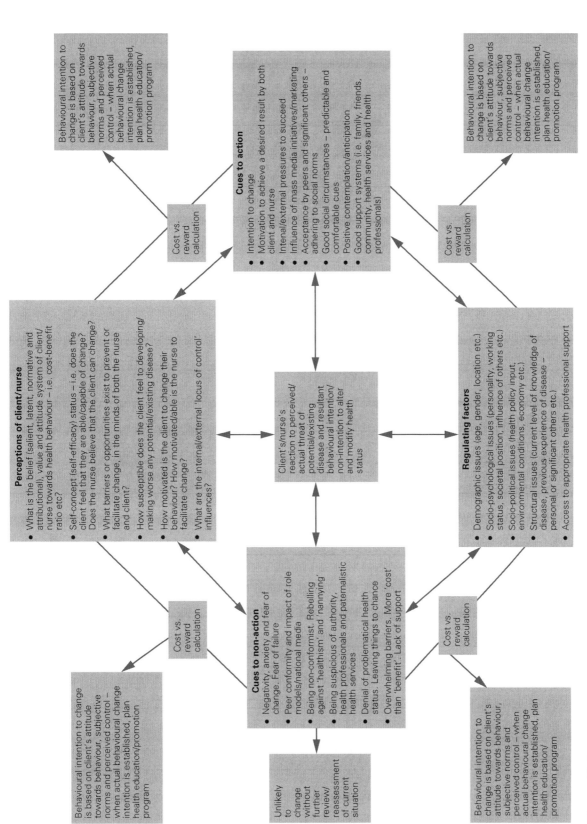

Figure 12.2 Whitehead's Socio-Cognitive Model

Source: Whitehead (2001b, p. 419).

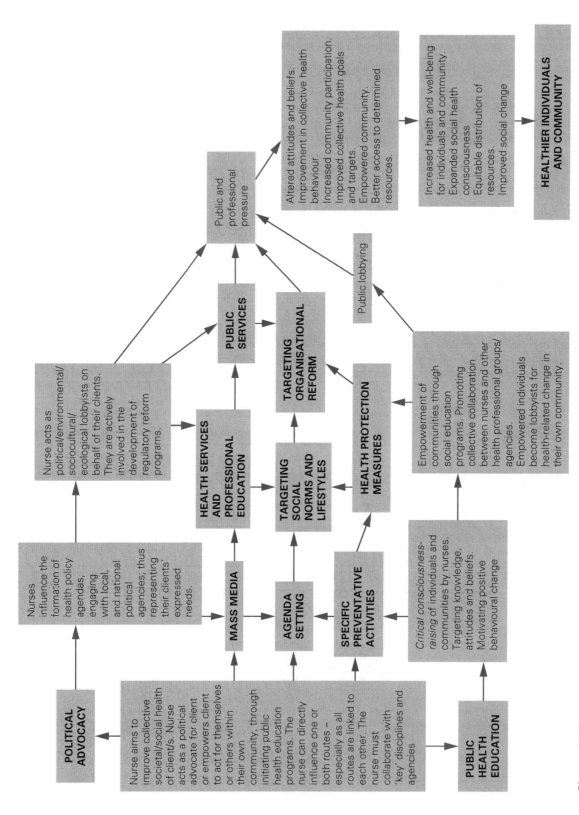

Figure 12.3 Whitehead's Effect Planning Model for Health Promotion

Source: Whitehead (2003a, p. 672).

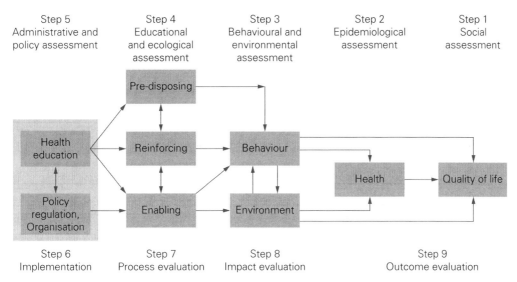

Figure 12.4   Green and Kreuter's Precede-Proceed Model
Source: Green & Kreuter (2005).

The Precede-Proceed Model of Health Program Planning and Evaluation builds on more than 40 years work by Lawrence W. Green and colleagues and was first published in 1980 (Green, 1980). The model was adapted and built upon each time a new edition of *Health Promotion Planning* was published. The original Precede Model was a rather crude four-phase model that drew from the fields of epidemiology, social-cognitive psychology (behavioural diagnosis), and education and management (administrative diagnosis). Its main limitation was that it was a linear, causal planning model that focused on behavioural aspects of health, rather than the wider health promotion social determinants of health that are more common today (Green et al., 2019). In collaboration with Marshall Kreuter, the second and third editions of *Health Promotion Planning* extended the Precede Model to incorporate wider ecological, environmental, policy, organisational and social determinants of health (Green & Kreuter, 1991; 1999). This introduced the 'Proceed' phase of the revised original Precede Model. Green and Kreuter's (2005) subsequent revisions and current thinking on health promotion planning advocate a socio-ecological process with an emphasis on community partnership and a converging systematic, integrative framework for practice. As such, health priorities focus on the structural issues that act as barriers to good health, for example, crime, pollution, lack of health facilities and access to them, poor education, poor standards of housing and so on (Kavanagh et al., 2022; Rains et al., 2018; Walsh et al., 2023).

REFLECTION

There are many frameworks and models that can be adopted with health promotion programs. Many, however, are adaptations of several contemporary models with perhaps the most recognised being the Precede-Proceed Model. Do you know of, or can you readily find, other similar/related models that are not mentioned in this chapter?

Implementing health promotion programs

To describe the implementation stages of a health promotion program process, we might be inclined to believe that the 'doing/action' part deserves the most attention. The paradox, however, is that there is less to write about here than the other part of the health promotion program process. Where comprehensive and sustained assessment and planning have taken place, there is far less likelihood of anything untoward occurring and, hopefully, the health promotion implementation runs relatively smoothly (Green et al., 2019). The main activities to adhere to, in the implementation phase, are that original planned activities and time frames are being adhered to, that due process is being followed, there is effective communication between stakeholders and that any arising issues, barriers and dilemmas are reported and acted on accordingly (Palfrey, 2018). It is by regularly performing these activities that health professionals monitor progress, act on presented issues, and change the nature and course of any intervention where necessary. Programs might deviate along the way from the original plan for several reasons but, where this occurs, the change must be deemed appropriate and be agreed upon between all key stakeholders (Fakoya, et al., 2022; Snelling, 2024). For these activities to take place, once a health promotion program has been implemented, it then needs to be 'monitored' – which brings us to 'evaluation'.

Evaluating health promotion

There are two valid reasons why we need to evaluate. Firstly, there is the need to generate evidence about the health promotion program being delivered and second there is the need to make formal judgements on how effective they are. The sometimes controversial and contested nature of what constitutes health promotion practice means that evidence of best practices and best outcomes must be provided. According to Naidoo and Wills (2016), health promotion can constitute an 'uncertain business' with no guarantees that the outcomes of programs will deliver what is anticipated or required of them. With the evaluation stage of the overall process, health promotion programs can establish whether planned and implemented interventions have been effective, cost-efficient and successful. Programs, such as Goetzel and colleagues' (2019) case study, describes their successful multistage approach applied to the evaluation of an employee wellness program. As an essential activity, health promotion evaluation has a potential role at all stages of health program provision. While effective assessment and planning are essential parts of health promotion programs, on their own they are of limited value (Green et al., 2019). Health promotion programs require that all components of the process are adhered to and this, therefore, must include a concerted evaluation phase (Lederer et al., 2023; Snelling, 2024). Evaluation is therefore conducted for three overarching reasons: knowledge building, accountability and future program development. This way we learn from the strengths and weaknesses of previous programs.

How do we evaluate health promotion?

The WHO (2001) identifies two main types of evaluation for health promotion activity:

1. 'Outcome evaluation' is an evaluation that involves assessing an activity as a measure against specific aims or objectives. Essentially, outcome evaluation refers to the measurement of what has been achieved – usually as the health promotion interventions are

ending – and necessitates that the researcher refers to the original program objectives. Outcome-orientated evaluation is favoured where the objectives are evidence-focused, and effectiveness is an important aspect of the program. Naidoo and Wills (2016) add 'impact evaluation' to the outcome evaluation context in that impact measures immediate effects (increased knowledge) and outcome measures longer-term effects (lifestyle changes) (Simos et al., 2023).

2. 'Process evaluation' aims to measure an activity against a predetermined standard. This approach measures the extent to which the predetermined aims/standards have been achieved as part of the program process as it progresses. For instance, this might involve thinking about how well the different stakeholders collaborated during the health promotion program. Francis and colleagues (2012) broadly characterise it as: 'Is it being done the way that it was said that it would be done?'

Process evaluation might not only consider the success rates of health promotion programs, as outcome evaluation indicators tend to do, but also the processes of how success is achieved, how it is measured and at what cost (Lim et al., 2023; Tchaba et al., 2023). Outcome evaluation is therefore primarily directed at resources and procedure-related indicators (Lederer et al., 2023; WHO, 2022).

Indicator, process and outcome measures need to be known for the effective evaluation of health promotion. It is best practice to incorporate process and outcome techniques in programs when circumstances allow. For instance, a focus on outcome evaluation alone is known to limit the opportunity to learn valuable lessons about the approach itself (Green et al., 2019). When combining a process and outcome approach in the same health promotion program, the evaluation then focuses on the whole process rather than parts of it. In effect, this monitors the overall processes of change that occur as well as the factors that prevent change (Rains et al., 2018).

Process and outcome evaluations are by far the most utilised methods but are by no means the only types of evaluation that can be used in health promotion programs. 'Structural evaluation' – as it relates to the organisational and human resource influences on any health promotion program – and 'developmental, impact and transfer evaluation' processes are also worthy of mention (Kiger, 2004). 'Developmental evaluation' refers to an assessment of the feasibility of a new program and tests the effectiveness of a new approach. 'Impact evaluation' is the assessment of the short-term immediate effect of a program. 'Transfer evaluation' is the assessment of the replicability (repeatability) of program processes and outcomes and their transferability to other settings or populations (Kiger, 2004). Several seminal texts and sources elaborate further on these evaluation methods (for example, Oakley, 2001; Schalock, 2000; Wimbush & Watson, 2000). Later texts elaborate on and expand these earlier texts (Ervin & Kulbok, 2018; Harris, 2016; McKenzie, et al., 2023; Palfrey, 2018). It is worth noting that the earlier-mentioned Precede-Proceed Model (Green & Kreuter, 2005; see Figure 12.4) has several evaluation phases that include process, impact and outcome evaluation.

Difficulties in determining appropriate indicators for measuring success highlight the need for appropriate definitions of anticipated outcomes (Ervin & Kulbok, 2018; Kavanagh, et al., 2022). Perhaps the most used performance indicators in health promotion are the 'three Es': 'effectiveness', 'efficiency' and 'efficacy'. Effectiveness is the extent to which a program has met its intended objectives, and efficiency is a measure of 'relative success' (in other words how successful the program has been overall even if it has not met all its intended objectives and outcomes) and efficacy is a measure used interchangeably between effectiveness and efficiency (Ervin & Kulbok, 2018, Green et al., 2019). As a measurement of the capacity of a program to be accessed by all participants within a targeted community, the term 'equity' can be added to the three Es (Whitehead & Irvine, 2010).

Although some nurses might view health promotion evaluation as a somewhat complex process, modest methods of evaluation can be used routinely in practice (Ewles & Simnett, 2010). Whitehead's (2003b) Evaluation Model (see Figure 12.5) is an example of a simplified stage process model that represents a mostly linear sequence of events to be addressed to ensure that an effective health promotion evaluation process is followed. Evaluation sequences, however, should also be cyclical as this facilitates the redefining and setting of new goals as well as the reformulation of any unmet outcomes. This is highlighted in Whitehead's model. The early stages of this model are aimed at identifying the process and purpose of the evaluation strategy. Following on from these stages are the logistical and resource implications of conducting evaluation research (Ervin & Kulbok, 2018; Harris, 2016; Palfrey, 2018). A comprehensive planning phase is intended to lead to the final evaluation of the program stage. Success is usually measured in terms of the overall outcomes met, although this does not necessarily mean that failing to meet the intended outcomes leads to an unsuccessful program. For example, the program might not meet original objectives but, instead, uncover newer and more appropriate objectives for another project or a continuing project. Therefore, outcomes might change and/or success might be measured in terms of lessons learned and acted upon. Alternatively, the completion of all intended outcomes might lead to the program being 'finished'. Some nursing-specific Australasian examples help to illustrate the health promotion evaluation process, such as Robertson and Neville's (2008) Aotearoa New Zealand-based *Maramataka Korero Hauora* impact evaluation and Banfield, McGorm and Sargent's (2015) multi-method evaluation of an Australian school youth health nurse program. On the theme of school health programs, Santos-Beneit (2022) and colleagues outline the key evaluation lessons learned over 10 years of experience in implementing the SI! Program (Salud Integral–Comprehensive Health) for cardiovascular health promotion in preschool settings in three countries: Colombia (Bogotá), Spain (Madrid), and the United States (Harlem, New York).

CASE STUDY 12.2

You are a registered health professional and part of a team that has performed a community assessment and 'diagnosis'. The assessment and planning 'scoping' exercise mainly drew on objective data – census material – to inform the overall findings.

The community is classed in the lowest socio-economic group with high rates of specific illnesses (such as asthma, diabetes and cancers) against the national average. There are a high proportion of Indigenous and culturally and linguistically diverse (CALD) populations within the community and high levels of unemployment.

Your team presents the results of the assessment to members of the local health board, highlighting the main priority as being the need to resource more health clinics. The board members are enthusiastic about adopting this proposal. The proposal is then promoted among the wider community. However, the wider community is less enthusiastic about opening more health clinics, so the proposal has gone no further.

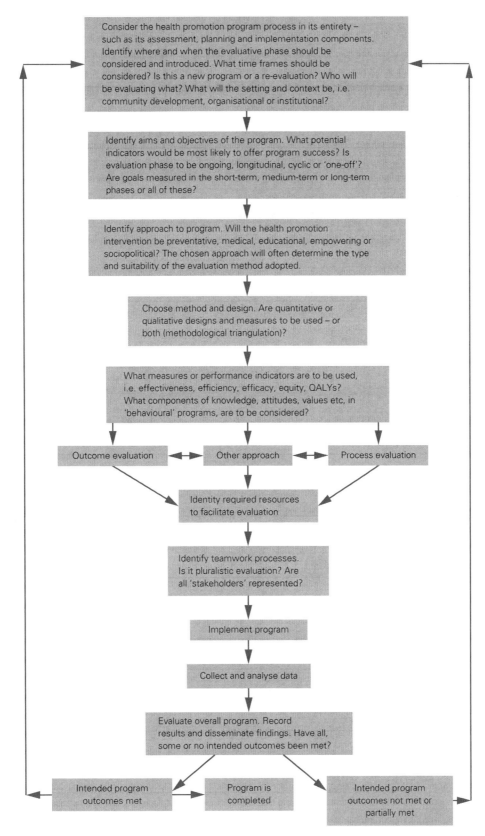

Consider the health promotion program process in its entirety – such as its assessment, planning and implementation components. Identify where and when the evaluative phase should be considered and introduced. What time frames should be considered? Is this a new program or a re-evaluation? Who will be evaluating what? What will the setting and context be, i.e. community development, organisational or institutional?

Identify aims and objectives of the program. What potential indicators would be most likely to offer program success? Is evaluation phase to be ongoing, longitudinal, cyclic or 'one-off'? Are goals measured in the short-term, medium-term or long-term phases or all of these?

Identify approach to program. Will the health promotion intervention be preventative, medical, educational, empowering or sociopolitical? The chosen approach will often determine the type and suitability of the evaluation method adopted.

Choose method and design. Are quantitative or qualitative designs and measures to be used – or both (methodological triangulation)?

What measures or performance indicators are to be used, i.e. effectiveness, efficiency, efficacy, equity, QALYs? What components of knowledge, attitudes, values etc, in 'behavioural' programs, are to be considered?

Outcome evaluation ⟷ Other approach ⟷ Process evaluation

Identity required resources to facilitate evaluation

Identify teamwork processes. Is it pluralistic evaluation? Are all 'stakeholders' represented?

Implement program

Collect and analyse data

Evaluate overall program. Record results and disseminate findings. Have all, some or no intended outcomes been met?

Intended program outcomes met

Program is completed

Intended program outcomes not met or partially met

Figure 12.5 Whitehead's Evaluation Model

Source: Whitehead (2003b, p. 496).

> ## CASE STUDY 12.2 Continued
>
> REFLECTION
>
> 1. The most likely reason for a general lack of enthusiasm from the community would be the lack of consultation with all key stakeholders representing cross-sections of the community. How could you best ensure that all key stakeholders are represented?
> 2. Why do you think that the community might have been particularly opposed to the setting up and resourcing of the program?
> 3. What 'special' requirements could have been put in place to better meet the needs of Indigenous and CALD community members?

Conclusion

Health promotion and health education programs should adhere to a logical, sequential and systematic process. In this chapter, the case has been put forward that – with good, sound and comprehensive attention to the overall process – nursing-related PHC-based programs are far more likely to be successful and result in desirable and effective positive health outcomes. Using frameworks to guide the planning, implementation and evaluation of health promotion and health education programs are major drivers for this process and are complemented by related frameworks such as Whitehead's lifespan/settings-based framework, which was detailed in Chapter 7 (Whitehead, 2011). Health promotion and health education programs are dynamic processes that do not happen by chance or 'run themselves'. Knowing what the overall process is, which parts and stages drive the process, and knowing how and when they can be applied, significantly increases the likelihood of effective health interventions and outcomes within communities and the PHC setting.

CRITICAL THINKING ACTIVITIES

1. You have been tasked with implementing a community-targeted health promotion program. A thorough community assessment has taken place. You must now plan what interventions to use. What do you think are the most common main health-related priorities that generally emerge from community health assessments ready for planning?
2. What do you think might be the most 'difficult' community health priorities to target and tackle?
3. Imagine that you have now implemented the community-targeted health promotion program. In terms of evaluation, identify the factors that would help you determine whether that program has, overall and specifically, been successful or not.

FURTHER READING

Bauman, A. & Nutbeam, D. (2013). *Evaluation in a Nutshell: A Practical Guide to the Evaluation of Health Promotion Programs*. McGraw Hill.

Eldredge, L.K.B., Markham, C.M., Kok, G., Ruiter, R.A. & Parcel, G.S. (2016). *Planning Health Promotion Programs: An Intervention Mapping Approach*. Jossey-Bass.

Hodges, B.C. & Videto, D.M. (2005). *Assessment and Planning in Health Programs*. Jones & Bartlett.

Palfrey C. (2018). *The Future for Health Promotion*. Policy Press.

REFERENCES

Ajzen, I. & Fishbein, M. (1980). *Understanding Attitudes and Predicting Social Behaviour*. Prentice Hall.

Banfield, M., McGorm, K. & Sargent, G. (2015). Health promotion in schools: A multi-method evaluation of an Australian school youth health nurse program. *BMC Nursing, 14,* 21.

Beattie, A. (1991). Knowledge and control in health promotion: A test case for social policy and social theory. In J. Gabe, M. Calnan & M. Bury (eds), *The Sociology of the Health Service* (pp. 162–202). Routledge.

Becker, M.H. (1974). *The Health Belief Model and Personal Health Behaviour*. Slack.

Caplan, R. & Holland, R. (1990). Rethinking health education theory. *Health Education Journal, 49,* 10–12.

Clavier, C. & de Leeuw, E. (2013). *Health Promotion and the Policy Process*. Oxford University Press.

Clendon, J. & Munns, A. (2019). *Community Health and Wellness: Primary Health Care in Practice: Principles of Primary Health Care* (6th ed.). Elsevier.

Conrad, E.J., Becker, M., Brandley, E., Saksvig, E. & Nickelson, J. (2019). Advocacy and public policy perceptions and involvement of college students. *Health Promotion Practice, 20*(5), 730–41. https://doi.org/10.1177/1524839919837619

Downie, R.S., Tannahill, C. & Tannahill, A. (1996). *Health Promotion: Models and Values* (2nd ed.). Oxford University Press.

Ervin, N.E. & Kulbok, P.A. (2018) *Advanced Public and Community Health Nursing Practice: Population Assessment, Program Planning and Evaluation* (2nd ed.). Springer Publishing Company.

Ewles, L. & Simnett, I. (2010). *Promoting Health: A Practical Guide* (6th ed.). Elsevier – Baillière Tindall.

Fakoya, I., Cole, C., Larkin, C., et al. (2022). Enhancing human-centered design with youth-led participatory action research approaches for adolescent sexual and reproductive health programming. *Health Promotion Practice. 23*(1), 25–31. https://doi.org/10.1177/15248399211003544

Francis, K., Chapman, Y., Hoare, K. & Birks, M. (eds) (2012). *Australia and New Zealand Community as Partner: Theory and Practice in Nursing* (2nd ed.). Lippincott Williams & Wilkins.

French, J. & Adams, L. (1986). From analysis to synthesis. *Health Education Journal, 45*(2), 71–4.

Goetzel, R.Z., Berko, J., McCleary, K., et al. (2019). Framework for evaluating workplace health promotion in a health care delivery setting. *Population Health Management, 22*(6), 480–7.

Green, J., Cross, R., Woodall, J. & Tones K. (2019). *Health Promotion: Planning and Strategies* (4th ed.). Sage Publications.

Green, L.W. (1980). *Health Education Planning: A Diagnostic Approach*. Mayfield.

Green, L.W. & Kreuter, M.W. (1991). *Health Promotion Planning: An Educational and Environmental Approach* (2nd ed.). Mayfield.

—— (1999). *Health Promotion Planning: An Educational and Ecological Approach* (3rd ed.). Mayfield.

—— (2005). *Health Program Planning: An Educational and Ecological Approach* (4th ed.). McGraw-Hill Higher Education.

Harris, M.J. (2016) *Evaluating Public and Community Health Programs*. Wiley.

Iannella, S., Smith, A., Post, D.K. & Haren, M.T. (2015). How widespread are the use of frameworks and theories in applied health promotion research in rural and remote places: A review of programs targeted at cardiometabolic risk factors. *Rural and Remote Health, 15,* 3228.

Kavanagh, S., Shiell, A., Hawe, P. & Garvey, K. (2022). Resources, relationships, and systems thinking should inform the way community health promotion is funded. *Critical Public Health, 32*(3), 273–82. https://doi.org/10.1080/09581596.2020.1813255

Kiger, A.M. (2004). *Teaching for Health* (3rd ed.). Churchill Livingstone.

Lederer, A.M., Foster, A.M., Schmidt, N., et al. (2023). A framework for using real-time evaluative interview feedback for health promotion program and evaluation improvement: The Check It case study. *Evaluation and Program Planning, 97*, 102216. https://doi.org/10.1016/j.evalprogplan.2022.102216

Lim, A.S.X., Schweickle, M.J., Liddelow, C., Liddle, S.K. & Vella, S.A. (2023). Process evaluations of health-promotion interventions in sports settings: A systematic review. *Health Promotion International, 38*(5), daad114. https://doi.org/10.1093/heapro/daad114

Linnan, L.A., Sterba, K.R., Lee, A.M., et al. (2005). Planning and the professional preparation of health educators: Implications for teaching, research and practice. *Health Promoting Practice, 6*, 308–19.

Linsley, P., Kane, R. & Owen, S. (2011). *Nursing for Public Health: Promotion, Principles, and Practice.* Oxford University Press.

McKenzie, J., Neiger, B. & Thackeray, R (2023). *Planning, Implementing and Evaluating Health Promotion Programs* (8th ed.). Jones & Bartlett Learning.

Naidoo, J. & Wills, J. (2016). *Foundations for Health Promotion* (4th ed.). Elsevier.

Oakley, A. (2001). Evaluating health promotion: Methodological diversity. In S. Oliver & G. Peersman (eds), *Using Research for Effective Health Promotion* (pp. 16–31). Open University Press.

Palfrey, C. (2018). *The Future for Health Promotion.* Policy Press.

Pender, N.J, Murdaugh, C.L. & Parsons, M.A. (2015). *Health Promotion in Nursing Practice* (7th ed.). Pearson.

Phillips, J.L., Rolley, J.X. & Davidson, P.M. (2012). Developing targeted health service interventions using the Precede-Proceed Model: Two Australian case studies. *Nursing Research and Practice*, 1–8. https://doi.org/10.1155/2012/279431

Prochaska, J.O. & DiClemente, C. (1984). *The Transtheoretical Approach: Crossing Traditional Foundations of Change.* Dow Jones-Irwin.

Public Health Ontario. (2015). *At a Glance: The Six Steps for Planning a Health Promotion Program.* Public Health Ontario.

Raingruber, B. (2014). *Contemporary Health Promotion in Nursing Practice.* Jones & Bartlett Learning.

Rains, C., Todd, G., Kozma, N. & Goodman, M. (2018). Are you making an impact? Evaluating the population health impact of Community Benefit Programs. *Journal of Public Health Management and Practice, 24*(4), 335–9.

Robertson, H.R. & Neville, S. (2008). Health promotion impact evaluation: Healthy messages calendar (The *Maramataka Korero Hauora*). *Nursing Praxis in New Zealand, 24*(1), 24–35.

Santos-Beneit, G., Fernández-Jiménez, R., de Cos-Gandoy, A., et al. (2022). Lessons learned from 10 years of preschool intervention for health promotion. *Journal of the American College of Cardiology, 79*(3), 283–98. https://doi.org/10.1016/j.jacc.2021.10.046

Schalock, R.L. (2000). *Outcome-Based Evaluation.* Kluwer Academic.

Simos, J., Christie, D., Jabot, F., Le Gall, A.R. & Cantoreggi, N. (2023). The ongoing contribution of health impact assessment to health promotion research. In D. Jourdan & L. Potvin (eds), *Global Handbook of Health Promotion Research* (Vol. 3). Springer. https://doi.org/10.1007/978-3-031-20401-2_14

Snelling, A. (2024) *Introduction to Health Promotion* (2nd ed.). John Wiley & Sons.

Stanhope, M. & Lancaster, J. (2016). *Public Health Nursing* (9th ed.). Elsevier.

Tchaba, E., Satur, J., Reid, C. & Burrows, J. (2023). Oral health promotion for rural adolescents: A process evaluation of a co-designed pilot program. *The Australian Journal of Rural Health, 31*(6), 1126–38. https://doi.org/10.1111/ajr.13063

Tones, K. (1987). Devising strategies for preventing drug misuse: The role of the Health Action Model. *Health Education Research, 2*, 305–17.

———— (2000). Evaluating health promotion: A tale of three errors. *Patient Education and Counselling, 39*, 227–36.

Tramm, R., McCarthy, A. & Yates, P. (2011). Using the Precede-Proceed Model of Health Program Planning in breast cancer nursing research. *Journal of Advanced Nursing, 68*, 1870–80.

Walsh, O., Sheridan, A. & Barry, M.M. (2023) The process of developing a mental health promotion plan for the Irish health service. *Advances in Mental Health, 21*(2), 115–28. https://doi.org/10.1080/18387357.2022.2161402

Watkins, D. & Cousins, J. (2010). *Public Health and Community Nursing: Frameworks for Practice* (3rd ed.). Ballière Tindall.

Whitehead, D. (2001a). A stage planning process model for health promotion/health education practice. *Journal of Advanced Nursing, 36*, 311–20.

—— (2001b). A social cognitive model for health promotion/health education practice. *Journal of Advanced Nursing, 36*, 417–25.

—— (2003a). Incorporating socio-political health promotion activities in nursing practice. *Journal of Clinical Nursing, 12*, 668–77.

—— (2003b). Evaluating health promotion: A model for nursing practice. *Journal of Advanced Nursing, 41*, 490–8.

—— (2004). Health promotion and health education: Advancing the concepts. *Journal of Advanced Nursing, 47*, 311–20.

—— (2011). Before the cradle and beyond the grave: A lifespan/settings-based framework for health promotion. *Journal of Clinical Nursing, 20*, 2183–94.

Whitehead, D. & Irvine, F. (2010). *Health Promotion & Health Education in Nursing: A Framework for Practice*. Palgrave Macmillan.

Wills, J. (2014). *Fundamentals of Health Promotion for Nurses* (2nd ed.). Wiley-Blackwell.

Wimbush, E. & Watson, J. (2000). An evaluation framework for health promotion: Theory, quality and effectiveness. *Evaluation, 6*, 310–21.

World Health Organization (WHO). (2001). *Evaluation in Health Promotion: Principles and Practices*. WHO Regional Publications.

—— (2022). *Bending the Trends to Promote Health and Well-Being: A Strategic Foresight on the Future of Health Promotion*. WHO Regional Publications.

13 Digital health

Isabelle Skinner
With acknowledgement to Kerryn Butler-Henderson

LEARNING OBJECTIVES

At the completion of this chapter, you should be able to:

- define digital health and health informatics and outline the role of the health informatician.
- relate the benefits of digital health to community and primary health care (PHC) practice.
- explore developments and uptake of telehealth, mHealth and remote monitoring.
- describe primary care informatics and the impact of consumer health informatics on health care.
- critique the needs of the digital health workforce.
- appraise emerging technologies in health care.

Introduction

Internet of things (IoT) – a network of physical devices (things) sharing data, or connecting with other devices over the internet, e.g. weather stations, animal ear tags, car sensors, vaccine fridges, etc.

The third industrial revolution saw the creation of computers and an increased use of technology in industry and households. We are now in the fourth industrial revolution: cyber, with advances in artificial intelligence (AI), automation and the **internet of things (IoT)**. The third and fourth revolutions have had a large impact on health care, shaping how health and social care are planned, managed and delivered, as well as supporting wellness and the promotion of health. This growth has seen the advent of the discipline of health informatics with several sub-specialty areas emerging over the past two decades. Informatics is used across primary care, allied health, community care and dentistry, with technology supporting the PHC continuum. This chapter explores the development of health informatics as a discipline and how health care innovation, technology, governance and the workforce are supporting digital health transformation.

Digital health and the health informatician

Overview of health informatics

Digital health is integral to health care, with many countries developing digital health strategies to develop and implement legislation, policy and compliance, interoperability and standards, services and applications, investment, infrastructure, leadership and governance and workforce readiness (World Health Organization (WHO), 2021). The WHO has identified that digital health has the potential to close the gap on all five health system challenges: affordability, quality, demand, supply and accountability (WHO, 2019a). The discipline of **health informatics** is one that has emerged because of technological developments. Combining the principles of health, information and computer sciences, this specialised discipline plans, implements, manages and decommissions technology to support health.

The term 'informatics' first emerged in the 1960s, in parallel with developments in organisational computing. In 1974, MedInfo was the first international conference marking the establishment of the discipline. With the increased use of technology in health, there was a transformation in the discipline with several sub-specialty areas emerging. These sub-specialties now include aged-care informatics, biomedical informatics, clinical informatics, consumer informatics, medical informatics, nursing informatics, population/public health informatics and primary care informatics. International and national associations arose to support, promote and advocate for the discipline, and training programs were introduced to provide a theoretical basis for the field. As the body of knowledge in health informatics grew and organisations implemented digital health strategies, dedicated health informatics positions emerged across the health sector.

Digital health – is understood to mean the field of knowledge and practice associated with the development and use of digital technologies to improve health (WHO, 2021).

Health informatics – the interdisciplinary study of the design, development, adoption and application of information technology (IT)-based innovations in health care services delivery, management and planning (Health Information Management Systems Society (HIMSS), 2020, p. 6).

Informatics building blocks

HIMSS (2020) defines health informatics as 'the interdisciplinary study of the design, development, adoption and application of information technology-based innovations in health care services delivery, management, and planning'.

Data integrity

All information communication technology enables the capture of data. For example, an electronic health record captures clinical data during the provision of care, a video teleconference captures audio and visual data, and a wearable device captures digital data such as heart rate. Data can be inputted manually, such as a nurse entering heart rate and blood oxygen level after manually measuring these observations, or automatically, such as a nurse setting up a machine that automatically monitors the heart rate and blood oxygen level over time where the machine automatically updates the electronic health record with these data.

Data integrity ensures that clinical decision making is based on quality data. The first step in digital data integrity is patient identification. Aotearoa New Zealand has the National Health Index (NHI), which is a unique identifier that is assigned to all Aotearoa New Zealand people who receive health care. This number is used to identify patients when admitted to hospital, for medication prescriptions, for pathology tests and discharge, and referrals between sectors of the system. The NHI is also used to identify people in clinical databases such as the

Medical Warnings System, which reports on allergies and other clinical risks, the Aotearoa Immunisation Register, Regional Clinical Data Repositories, which make data available to all registered providers who provide patient care, and the National Enrolment Services, which records a patient's choice of health care provider such as GP. A coded form of the NHI is also used for government reporting, planning and research.

Australia is taking a more networked approach and has recently released the *National Digital Health Strategy 2023–2028* (Australian Digital Health Agency, 2023). This strategy has a priority of transforming the system from siloed document repositories to 'near real-time data exchange' ensuring that there is a single view of an individual regardless of where the data is held and particularly that data is discoverable at the transitions between primary care, aged care and when acute care is needed. Despite this strategy, significant challenges remain in operationalising this in practice.

All technology design must be based on good design principles to ensure the collection of data that is complete, comprehensive, consistent, reliable, relevant and accurate, in a timely, valid and legal manner. Good system design is also informed by national and international standards. Design features may include layout features such as populated drop-down lists, consideration about where to present information on a screen, alerts, such as an alert for missing or contradictory information, or background coding of data. These features ensure data is collected in a uniform, consistent manner which makes it easier to communicate and analyse. Think of all the different ways breast cancer can be written down – breast cancer, cancer of the left breast, BCa, ductal carcinoma of the breast and so on. Providing 'breast cancer' as a term in a drop-down list and capturing location as 'left' ensures that the data is recorded in a clean and easy-to-analyse format. Data integrity needs to be supported with training on how the technology functions, how to use the technology and the importance of data integrity. Organisational governance and international naming standards support data integrity. To date, nursing practice has not been mapped to the SNOMED CT electronic medical record terminology and so nursing practice is not able to be extracted from the electronic medical record (Junglyun et al., 2020).

REFLECTION

Aotearoa New Zealand has the NHI, but Australia does not have an equivalent system for identifying people receiving health care. Consider some of the times when a patient's information may need to be available at the point of care and how this can impact clinical care decisions. What solutions can you come up with to access a discharge summary if the patient reports a recent hospital admission? Perhaps the patient has changes to their regular medications if they report a visit to their GP.

The benefits of digital health

Technology has transformed health care in several ways over the past five decades. The innovations that have had the greatest impact are:

- electronic health records
- digital diagnostics and therapeutics.

Electronic health records

In Australia and Aotearoa New Zealand, most primary care organisations use either an electronic health record or a hybrid paper–electronic health record system. The health record is a legal record of the care planned and provided. The data within an electronic health record can be used for communication between health professionals, for health service planning and management, and for population health. Electronic health records allow forward planning for recalls like the annual cycle of care for people living with diabetes, or immunisation recalls for children. They also help with population-based health promotion planning by identifying the prevalence of conditions in the community.

An electronic health record system will incorporate an alert system that is updated when the patient has an allergic reaction or has a known allergy. In Aotearoa New Zealand these alerts form part of the Medical Warning System (MWS). Currently, the MWS is available in hospitals and work is underway to make this available to primary care clinics. The MWS includes allergies to medications, foods and environmental conditions, anaesthesia, airway and blood product warnings, implanted medical devices, alerts regarding infection control, and organ donor status, as well as child protection alerts and opium substitution alerts and the specific needs of the patients such as the need for an interpreter (Health New Zealand, 2024).

Electronic systems can incorporate clinical decision support to provide prompts to users and map data so clinicians can easily see trends over time. Compared to paper records, electronic health records allow more than one user to view a record simultaneously, are more secure and enable the capture of more and richer data. Electronic health records are reported to improve all aspects of care including clinical decision-making, driving efficiencies and patient safety, and lowering health care costs. In countries where a unique health identifier is available such as Aotearoa New Zealand, a holistic electronic health record allows the capture of information from across organisations and sectors, including health and social services, to support comprehensive health care.

Personal health records are patient portals or electronic health records that are controlled by the individual and include information entered by the individual. In Australia, the 'My Health Record' is a personally controlled electronic health record managed by the Australian Digital Health Agency (2024). All Australians have a My Health Record which contains key health information, such as immunisations; hospital discharge summaries; pathology and radiology results. Individuals can control what information is uploaded to their record, which health professionals can view health summaries and relevant health information, and they can elect to cancel their record. Many health services in Australia also provide patients access to their electronic health records through an online portal or app separate from My Health Record. The Health Hub provides patients access to their records at the Royal Melbourne Hospital, the Royal Women's Hospital, the Royal Children's Hospital and the Peter MacCallum Cancer Centre. This network of agencies in Melbourne, Australia, provides people with information about their care, their pathology and radiology results and upcoming appointments, and provides help desk support (The Royal Melbourne Hospital, 2024). Silver Chain, an Australian in-home aged and community care provider has introduced virtual in-home care for their 115 000 clients. This is supported by a client app giving them access to their own health and care information allowing them to interact with the Silverchain team (www.australianageingagenda.com.au/technology/silverchain-adopts-remote-care-technology/).

In Aotearoa New Zealand, people sign up for a My Health Account where they can then log into a secure online portal, Manage My Health, that allows people and their health care providers to connect seamlessly (Ministry of Health, 2019). There are currently 1.5 million Manage My Health users (Health New Zealand, 2024).

Digital diagnostics and therapeutics

Technology has been used in diagnostics for several decades, particularly in imaging, with more recent developments in point-of-care diagnostics or testing. This has grown from simple urine testing and portable ultrasounds to complex portable test kit technologies. Handheld devices can measure nerve conduction, and benchtop analysers can test blood, saliva or breath for over 100 different tests ranging from blood glucose to human immunodeficiency virus (HIV). Rapid diagnostic tests are being used in many clinics to provide results before the patient leaves, so a treatment plan can be developed immediately, education provided, and prescriptions ordered if necessary.

Similarly, the technology used for digital therapeutics to prevent and manage chronic health conditions has grown more complex over the last two decades. Digital therapeutics can be employed as a standalone or in conjunction with traditional therapy. For example, people living with diabetes can now use equipment such as blood glucose monitors, insulin pumps and wearable devices that provide them with meaningful data about their condition. Many devices are connected to enable the sharing of this data through personally controlled applications, where the person can self-report other information such as diet or exercise or share the data with health professionals such as their diabetes educator, GP or dietician. This information can allow health professionals to detect deviations early and change the treatment regimen instead of waiting until the person presents with symptoms. Digital therapies have expanded to be used to treat people living with psychological and neurological symptoms and conditions. Many mobile phone apps are available to monitor mood and provide activities such as mindfulness exercises and avatars to encourage daily interactions. The use of digital therapies has been shown to change health-related behaviour and increase therapy efficacy and adherence (Kvedar et al., 2016).

The development and uptake of mHealth, wearables and telehealth

mHealth and wearable devices

mHealth – 'the use of mobile wireless technologies for public health' (WHO, 2019a).

Mobile health, or **mHealth**, has become a large commercial market with millions of mobile apps created for the collection of health data accessed through a handheld device or smartwatch. The popularity of smartwatches has increased exponentially with one in three Australians now owning one (Mattison et al., 2023).

The wearable device market is growing exponentially, with a 26 per cent annual increase seen in 2019 and over 225 million units sold (Gartner Press Release, 2018). It is predicted that wearable device vital sign monitoring will grow by 21.7 per cent per year, reaching a US$980 million market by 2024 (Medical Director, 2019). Wearable devices in health range from fitness tracker devices to monitors and wearable therapeutics. Fitness trackers include smartwatches and wristbands, athletic clothing containing sensors, necklaces and rings, clips to hook onto clothing, headphones and bandages. These fitness trackers not only measure how many steps an individual has taken but also the acceleration, elevation and location of any movement, as well as heart rate, blood pressure, blood oxygen, sleep quality and even the electrical activity of the individual's heart, brain or muscles. When used with a mobile or computer app, they can provide users with data about their activity, allow them to track their fitness goals and self-report other data, such as food intake or mood data, set alarms to encourage regular movement, or set daily or weekly goals. Some apps allow individuals to link with friends or join online communities to encourage each other or compete against each other. With very few exceptions (for example, the Apple Watch ECG), fitness trackers have not been approved by the Therapeutic Goods Administration (TGA) for medical use in Australia (Mattison et al., 2023). However, these devices provide individuals with data to allow them to decide what they should do if they detect changes, as well as other functionalities to improve their quality of life.

While fitness trackers have many positives, they come with several challenges. The largest challenge is that they present individuals with recreational grade data which the individuals confuse with medical grade data. Fitness trackers can have variable accuracy with devices reporting 1000 steps varying as much as 700–1200 steps. The second largest area of concern is data security and privacy. Many apps require users to provide the app owner with permission to use their data, with only fine-print information about how they intend to use and share it. The largest opportunity with fitness trackers is the advanced data analytics they can afford users. Such information can be shared through personal health records with health professionals. It is predicted that over time, the use of fitness trackers will eventually form part of a suite of user-friendly, non-invasive, data-rich tools that may lower chronic disease morbidity. They may reduce the need to visit health care professionals, with face-to-face interactions only being required when TGA-approved devices detect any deviation from normal through, for example, advanced machine learning algorithms (Mattison et al., 2023). However, with these data also comes the potential for increased anxiety in response to the information received (Cheung & Saad, 2024). Consideration of these challenges and how best to integrate wearables into usual care is required to optimise their effectiveness.

REFLECTION

1. Do you use wearable technology for health data capture? How do you use the data?
2. How do you think wearable technology can be used to change health behaviours?
3. What do you believe might be the risks of using wearable technology?

Telehealth and remote monitoring

Telehealth is the use of telecommunications and virtual technology to deliver health services (WHO, 2019b). In a country as geographically vast as Australia, telehealth is necessary to provide health care for, and reduce inequities in, rural and remote communities. While not as large, Aotearoa New Zealand has rural and remote areas, such as Fiordland, where telehealth services were also pioneered. While its history started with the delivery of services to people living in geographically remote locations, the COVID-19 pandemic saw its accelerated

Telehealth – the use of telecommunications and virtual technology to deliver health services (WHO, 2019b).

adoption in all settings, particularly primary care (Halcomb et al., 2023). Telehealth can use audio, such as a telephone, video, or email to facilitate clinician contact for care, monitoring, advice or interventions. Telehealth can also be used for reminders, patient education or remote admission. Telehealth enables individuals to seek advice and care sooner, resulting in improved outcomes and a reduction in admissions and time spent away from home.

Telehealth also enables the delivery of health promotion services to communities previously out of reach and for vulnerable or marginalised communities to access a wider range of services in their own language removing or reducing the language barriers to accessing information and care.

Telehealth can be classified as one of three key types:

1. Real-time telehealth allowing a real-time audio or video link between an individual and a health care professional.
2. Asynchronous, or store and forward where digital images, video, audio and text are recorded and stored in the system, then transmitted to the recipient to review, for example, wound images or radiology for a specialist to review and send back advice, or email communication.
3. Remote monitoring, also known as home telehealth, is the continuous transmission of data from the individual to a health care professional, who will remotely review the information and, if an abnormality is detected, implement a management plan.

Vital signs that can be remotely monitored include heart and breathing rate, blood pressure, blood oxygen, blood glucose, temperature and urine. Companies now offer remote monitoring services, where health care professionals are engaged to monitor multiple client vital signs and instigate a predetermined action, such as contacting the individual's GP or health care provider when an abnormality is detected.

There are several innovative uses of telehealth in Australia. Rural emergency departments (ED) are using telehealth to access specialist consultations for stroke care. For example, a stroke specialist on the Victorian Stroke Telemedicine (VST) program roster can be contacted by the partner ED on a toll-free number. The specialist consults with the ED staff, the patient and their family via a telemedicine cart at the bedside that includes video consultation and embedded software for rapid access to a picture archiving system for reviewing brain images. This service allows patients to be thrombolysed close to home without the need for transfer to a specialist centre (Bladin et al., 2020).

Telehealth is facilitating patient discharge and step-down care and supporting multidisciplinary clinical reviews and case conferences across multiple health and social care organisations. Telehealth is also being used for remote skin checks, counselling, rehabilitation and physical therapy services. In Australia, the Medicare Benefits Scheme has changed to make telehealth available more widely than just between patients in geographically remote places and a clinician. This is improving access to services for all people who have difficulties accessing health care services for mobility, transport or financial reasons. Queensland Health recognises the value of telehealth as part of normal business and promotes that all health professionals can provide services via telehealth if they are trained to do so, have access to suitable equipment and their patients are consenting.

Aotearoa New Zealand has the National Telehealth Service which is a fully funded integrated service that brings together a range of support phone lines and other communication channels. This system has been developing over the last 20 years and now consists of more than 35 services supported by 12 clinical teams. Services range from after-hours health care advice from nurses, doctors, paramedics and advisors; quit smoking support and alcohol and other drugs advice; as well as the National Poisons Centre, Diver Emergency Services Hotline and the *puawaitanga*, a service to support people to improve their emotional well-being – their *hauora* for individual counselling. This integrated service uses a scalable clinical and technology platform that allows for economies of scale and ensures that patients can be transitioned from one health advice line to another and link them with appropriate clinical referral pathways to suit their clinical or well-being needs (Health New Zealand, 2024).

CASE STUDY 13.1

Pila is a small community. The town has a population of 300 people, with a significant proportion of people aged over 65 years and retired. The town is located on the coast, with a grocery shop and post office. There is a part-time GP and a full-time registered nurse. The town also has a small pharmacy and a community health centre with rooms for the following visiting health specialists: a physiotherapist (two days a month), an occupational therapist (one day a month), an exercise physiotherapist (one day a week) and a social worker (one day a month). The nearest hospital is located 74 km north of the town.

REFLECTION
1. How can we use technology to support the health needs of this community?
2. How can we use technology to promote wellness in this community?
3. How can technology influence people's decisions to relocate away from major cities?

The impact of primary care, consumer and population health informatics

Primary care informatics

The unique characteristics of primary care have driven the need for the informatics sub-specialty area of 'primary care informatics', which has emerged over the last two decades. As other areas in PHC grow, it is expected that primary care informatics will also expand. The principles of primary care informatics reflect the biopsychosocial model with a focus on holistic, longitudinal care. Primary care informatics reduces fragmented care, improves patient safety and enables evidence-informed care.

In 1997, only 15 per cent of primary care clinicians in Australia used an electronic health record (Kidd & Mazza, 2000). This increased to 71.6 per cent in less than eight years (Britt et al., 2005). By 2014–15, 96.2 per cent of primary care clinicians used a computerised medical record (Britt et al., 2015). The early and rapid adoption of technology was because clinicians were provided financial support for the purchase of the hardware and software, as well as being offered other incentives to integrate electronic functionality into their practices such as billing and prescribing. This has resulted in several innovations emerging from the primary care field. In preparation for electronic health records, the International Classification of Primary Care (ICPC) was developed by the World Organization of Family Doctors' International Classification Committee. This is an extended clinical terminology used in primary care systems to classify morbidity and treatment for reporting purposes. As an international classification, it allows the collection of primary care data for international comparisons.

The impact of technology on clinician-patient interaction was a major turning point in primary care informatics. Computers are now considered part of a triadic relationship. Patients view the computer as a second professional in the relationship. Clinicians also use the computer as an educational tool, showing the patient images or data, such as pathology results recorded in the system. This may in time alter the distribution of power and authority between the clinician and the patient to a mutual partnership.

Technology has enabled several other benefits in primary care. Clinicians can easily print or email health information for the individual to read, using technology as a tool to inform individuals about health literacy. Not only can clinicians electronically prescribe (ePrescribe) but they can also send the prescription directly to the pharmacy so that the order is ready when the individual arrives to collect it or this can facilitate home delivery. Referrals and diagnostic test orders can also be sent electronically. Individuals can book an appointment online and many primary care clinicians offer telehealth appointments for people who are unable or prefer not to attend in person. Technology supports the PHC framework as well as wellness and care focused on health outcomes.

Consumer health informatics

Consumer health informatics – 'the study of consumer information needs and health care technologies, as well as the implementation of methods of making information accessible to consumers' (HIMSS, 2020, p. 6).

The growth in person-centred care has resulted in individuals being more involved in their own health and health care. In turn, the area of **consumer health informatics** has emerged. Individuals are using technology for education, to collect data and to interact with health professionals and organisations, to book appointments and manage recalls. Consumer health informatics enables individuals to use technology and telecommunication to make decisions about their own health.

Health literacy has emerged as an important area in health informatics. As the field of consumer health informatics evolves, the need for health literacy is increasingly highlighted. Health literacy is the capacity to understand and process health information, advice and services to inform decision-making. With an increase in information-seeking behaviour, consumers increasingly need education to ensure that they understand how they are interpreting and understanding information that they find or receive online, how they engage with health and social services through technology, and how they access the internet with the devices they have access to and in the locations they frequent.

Social media platforms have had unprecedented growth in regular monthly users. It was estimated that globally in 2023, there were more than 4.9 billion social media users (Wong, 2023). There are legitimate health organisations providing health information online either as information on a website about various health topics and health podcasts, or in the form of clinicians responding to genuine health questions from the public on social media platforms. Unfortunately, there are just as many untrustworthy websites, social media posts and forums providing inaccurate or misleading health advice. Social media is being employed by health promoters to increase women's awareness of menstrual hygiene, breast and bowel cancer awareness, sexual health promotion, road safety, bushfire and emergency preparedness as well as health behaviours around diet and exercise. Health and social care professionals are constantly looking for better, more effective ways of reaching their target audiences. Social media has provided a way of targeting messages to distinct target groups in discrete geographic locations (Kanchan & Gaidhaine, 2023). Governments are also providing consumers with trusted websites to visit for reliable information and advice.

The growth in consumer health informatics has increased the focus on privacy. Individuals are more aware of privacy, largely due to the media and social media. Health and data literacy education, therefore, needs to include how individuals can keep their information private and safe.

As organisations use technology to interact with individuals, there is also an increased need for digital capabilities. If appointments can only be booked online, users must have the means to access a website and the capabilities to navigate it. The younger generation seeks to interact with health care in an online environment, driving the need for greater technological use, yet the greatest number of health users will be the baby boomer generation (those people born between 1946 and 1964), so organisations need to find a balance. The New Zealand government has developed an innovative scheme to support people to access reliable health information online called Zero Data. The focus of the scheme is to allow people to access a range of digital health services and key information sites through a portal without paying any mobile data fees (Health New Zealand, 2024).

Digital capabilities will be required across all sectors, not just health. Social media has also changed how individuals engage in their own health. Support groups no longer have geographical barriers. For example, parents of a child living with a rare condition are now able to correspond with other parents living in another country for support and advice. Individuals use social media to support their wellness goals, in group competitions or support groups, such as weight loss or smoking cessation. Consumer health informatics will continue to evolve as health care shifts towards a greater PHC framework, placing the person at the centre of the model.

REFLECTION

1. Have you ever searched for health advice on the Internet?
2. How did you decide whether to follow the advice you received?
3. How do you think consumer health informatics will change the future of health?

Population health informatics

Data from different sources can be linked to tell a story. This is known as data linkage. Monitoring large sets of data can inform public health professionals about trends which can indicate when there is a sudden increase in incidence, such as a measles outbreak, or a long-term increase in prevalence, such as an increase in type 2 diabetes. This surveillance informs public health and health promotion strategies. Geographical information systems allow the mapping of trends over time. For example, the linkage of air quality data in certain regions and the dispensing of asthma medication allows public health authorities to gain insight into the correlation between air quality and asthma. So, when the air quality reaches a certain level, public health authorities can implement public health policies such as informing PHC professionals, who can put action plans in place to warn or support those in the community living with asthma or inform pharmacies to allow them to order additional stocks of certain medications.

Data registries exist to collect specific data to evaluate specific health outcomes. In Australia, several data collection registries report to the Australian Institute of Health and Welfare (AIHW) and this includes mental health, acute inpatient, vaccine, cancer and perinatal data. A list of all data collections can be found on the AIHW website (www.aihw.gov.au/about-our-data/our-data-collections). These data collections use metadata items from the AIHW Metadata Online Registry (METeOR), a registry for how data items should be formatted to ensure consistency in data reporting. For example, 'gender' should be captured as a one-character string such as 1 (male), 2 (female), 3 (other) or 9 (not stated/inadequately described). This is to ensure data can be linked against standard criteria to inform health decision-making. In Aotearoa New Zealand, Health and Disability Intelligence produces and maintains population health survey data and Environmental Science and Research manages data on infectious diseases (more information about data collection can be found on the Ministry of Health website (www.health.govt.nz/nz-health-statistics/about-data-collection)).

Developing a digitally ready and enabled health workforce

Information governance

Information governance – managing data and information in an organisation including meeting legal, regulatory, ethics and risk requirements.

Information governance should be a central strategy for any organisation. Information and records management should include policies to support how information is stored, accessed, retained and destroyed. Information management also includes who can access the information and under what circumstances. This is largely governed by privacy laws. Health professionals are required to keep information confidential and private, and organisations are responsible for providing policies, procedures and training to support staff. Information also needs to be kept secure, either physically, including ensuring computer servers are in locked rooms that can only be accessed by authorised personnel, and electronically, such as requiring passwords and two-factor authentication to gain access.

Cybersecurity is an important area for organisations. Health data and information are critical commodities from the personal health information of the individual to the large datasets used to inform health service management. The growth in ransomware over the last two years has resulted in the largest number of reported data breaches in Australia coming from health organisations, with the majority (47%) of breaches being malicious cyberattacks (Office of the Australian Information Commissioner, 2019). The Aotearoa New Zealand health care sector is equally at risk. All organisations should also have a risk and compliance framework including policies, procedures and processes for the detection of risk relating to information governance and fraud, and internal auditing to monitor compliance. An emerging area in information governance is mandatory reporting of data breaches to affected individuals, such as reporting to patients when their health records have been accessed by unauthorised individuals.

Education and training will continue to be an essential tool in keeping information private and secure. All health professionals have a responsibility to treat the information they have collected, curated and used as private and confidential, and to store it safely.

A digital health workforce

The health workforce requires digital capabilities to work in digital services. A digitally capable workforce is one that can use technology to support or enhance the functions of their roles. Furthermore, individuals are required to be adaptable, creative and agile, enabling them to work with new technology with ease (Crawford & Butler-Henderson, 2020). As the use of technology increases, these will become even more important skills in the health workforce.

Several competency frameworks exist for different health professional groups. Competency frameworks for all health professionals include the Health Information Technology Competencies (HITComp) (2016) and the Australian Health Informatics Competency Framework (Australian Institute of Digital Health (AIDH), 2022). The Australian Health Informatics Education Council knowledge and skills domains include informatics knowledge, medicine, health and biosciences, health system organisation, computer science mathematics and biometry. The HITComp domains are administration, informatics, engineering, information systems, information communication and technology, and research.

Specifically, in nursing and midwifery, frameworks are provided by the Australian Nursing and Midwifery Federation (ANMF) (2015) and the Technology Informatics Guiding Education Reform (TIGER) initiative (Hübner et al., 2018), both of which specify that the domains are computer literacy, information literacy and information management. Nursing education providers and all educational providers for health professionals need to ensure that graduates are digitally capable. Health Informatics New Zealand (HiNZ) is a not-for-profit organisation that supports the field of health informatics through the expertise of health sector managers, clinicians, IT experts, industry managers, academics, students and government personnel (HiNZ, n.d.). A workforce with digital capabilities will safely use technology to support and enable the prevention of disease and the management of health.

CASE STUDY 13.2

Rachael is working in a primary care clinic. She is about to provide wound care for Mr Bilal for his leg ulcer.

REFLECTION

1. How will Rachael know if Mr Bilal's ulcer is healing and at what rate?
2. How will she know what care Mr Bilal received for his ulcer during his recent admission to the hospital?
3. There is a wound camera in the clinic how does Rachael ensure she is using it correctly and transferring the data to the electronic medical record?

Emerging technologies in health care

AI

AI is a key advancement in the fourth industrial revolution. It is not a new concept, with one of its founding fathers, John McCarthy, describing AI in the 1950s as 'that of making a machine behave in ways that would be called intelligent if a human were so behaving' (Kaplan, 2016, p. 1). There are four distinct types of AI. Two are currently available:

1. Reactive AI is where a computer is programmed with the millions of moves to play a winning game of chess, or algorithms are built to work out your movie preferences based on your previous choices or what you put into your preference list.
2. Limited Memory AI (LM AI) is where a computer uses learning data to improve and adjust over time. LM AI can complete complex classification tasks and uses historical data to make predictions such as in self-driving cars.

In the future, we may see:

3. Theory of Mind AI is when machines can make decisions the way humans do and react to emotions.
4. Self-aware AI is where the machine is not just aware of the mental and emotional state of others but also their own.

These last two types are very much in the future (Gillis & Petersson, 2023).

Machine Learning (ML), Natural Language Processing (NLP) and Generative AI are forms of Limited Memory AI that are currently widely available. ML is the technology behind chatbots and predictive text and how your social media feed is presented to you. It is also used in machines that can diagnose medical conditions based on a vast number of images. NLP combines computational linguistics with machine learning to enable computers to use voice and text data and understand its meaning. NLP is the technology behind language translation apps, speech-to-text dictation, voice-operated GPS navigation systems and virtual assistants like Alexa. Generative AI is a machine learning model that is trained to create new data. It learns to create more objects like the one it is trained on. The more data it has available, the more new objects it can create. ChatGPT uses all the publicly available text on the Internet. This area of computer science is rapidly evolving to include image-generative AI as well as music and sound generative AI. Working in the community, nurses are often using AI to find their way to the client's home, or to send a text message to their manager. In Australia, the *National Digital Health Strategy 2023–2028* is prioritising health care providers to prepare for and embrace scientific and technological innovations such as AI (Australian Digital Health Agency, 2023).

The New Zealand government has identified that the risks of using Generative AI, which include privacy breaches, inaccurate information, inequities and bias, lack of transparency, data sovereignty and intellectual property rights, have not been adequately assessed and mitigated, and as a consequence are not supporting its adoption (Health New Zealand, 2024).

REFLECTION

1. What beliefs do you hold about AI?
2. Do you currently use Generative AI such as ChatGPT or Google Bard in your everyday life?
3. How do you see AI shaping health care in the future?

Conclusion

The fourth industrial revolution will enable advances in technology to support growth in the delivery of health care in the community. The emergence and growth in new innovations are reducing the gaps across the health sector, supporting interdisciplinary communication and providing the evidence base to inform decision making. The richness of information from the electronic capture of data is not only enabling safer and more effective individual care but also informing community and population health care. Furthermore, it supports the person-centred model, encouraging education to improve health literacy and digital capabilities. The exponential growth of telehealth usage during the COVID-19 pandemic in Australia saw 118.2 million telehealth services provided to 18 million patients and more than 95 000 practitioners using it in the two years between 2020 and 2022 (Australian Digital Health Agency, 2023). We have adapted our models of care in primary care services to incorporate technology into our changing models of care. Being adaptable and continuously learning will be the hallmark of a resilient community-based health system.

CRITICAL THINKING ACTIVITIES

Select one of the issues identified in *Global Top Health Industry Issues: Defining the Healthcare of the Future* (PwC Health Research Institute, 2018: www.pwc.com/gx/en/healthcare/pdf/global-top-health-industry-issues-2018-pwc.pdf).

1. What would be the issue in the context of Australia/Aotearoa New Zealand?
2. How should we address this today?
3. What should we do to plan for the future?
4. What are the health workforce implications?
5. What are the training implications for health professionals?

FURTHER READING

Australian Digital Health Agency. (2023). *Australia's National Digital Health Strategy 2023–2028.* Australian Government. www.digitalhealth.gov.au/national-digital-health-strategy

Australian Institute of Digital Health (AIDH). (2022) *Australian Health Informatics Competency Framework.* https://digitalhealth.org.au/wp-content/uploads/2022/06/AHICFCompetencyFramework.pdf

Australian Institute of Health and Welfare (AIHW). (2024). *Our Data Collections.* Australian Government. www.aihw.gov.au/about-our-data/our-data-collections

Hambleton, S.J. & Aloizos, J. (2019). Australia's digital health journey. *Medical Journal of Australia, 210*(6), S5–S6. https://doi.org/10.5694/mja2.50039

Ministry of Health. (n.d.). *Statistics and research.* New Zealand Government. www.health.govt.nz/nz-health-statistics/about-data-collection

PwC. (2019). *Health Matters. The Future of Health* (1st ed.). www.pwc.com.au/health/health-matters/pwc-australia-health-matters-edition-1-aug19.pdf

World Health Organization (WHO). (2018). *Digital technologies: Shaping the future of primary health care.* https://apps.who.int/iris/handle/10665/326573

REFERENCES

Australian Digital Health Agency. (2023). *Australia's National Digital Health Strategy 2023–2028.* Australian Government. www.digitalhealth.gov.au/national-digital-health-strategy

——— (2024). *My Health Record.* Australian Government. www.digitalhealth.gov.au/initiatives-and-programs/my-health-record/whats-inside

Australian Institute of Digital Health (AIDH). (2022). *Australian Health Informatics Competency Framework.* https://digitalhealth.org.au/wp-content/uploads/2022/06/AHICFCompetencyFramework.pdf

Australian Nursing and Midwifery Federation (ANMF). (2015). *ANMF National Informatics Standards for Nurses and Midwives.* ANMF.

Bladin, C.F., Kim, J., Bagot, K., et al. (2020) Improving acute stroke care in regional hospitals: clinical evaluation of the Victorian Stroke Telemedicine program. *Medical Journal of Australia, 212*(8), 371–7. https://doi.org/10.5694/mja2.50570

Britt, H., Miller, G.C., Henderson, J., et al. (2015). *General Practice Activity in Australia 2014–15.* (General Practice Series No. 38.). Sydney University Press.

Britt, H., Miller, G.C., Knox, S., et al. (2005). *General Practice Activity in Australia 2004–05.* (General Practice Series No. 18. AIHW Cat. No. GEP 18). Australian Institute of Health and Welfare.

Cheung, C.C. & Saad, M. (2024). Wearable devices and psychological wellbeing: Are we overthinking it? *Journal of the American Heart Association, 13*, 15. www.ahajournals.org/doi/10.1161/JAHA.123.033750

Crawford, J. & Butler-Henderson, K. (2020). Digitally empowered workers and authentic leaders: The capabilities required for digital services. In K. Sandhu (ed.), *Leadership, Management, and Adoption Techniques for Digital Service Innovation* (pp. 103–24). IGI-Global Publication.

Gartner Press Release. (2018). *Gartner says worldwide wearable device sales to grow 26 percent in 2019.* www.gartner.com/en/newsroom/press-releases/2018-11-29-gartner-says-worldwide-wearable-device-sales-to-grow-

Gillis, A. & Petersson, D. (2023). *4 main types of AI (artificial intelligence) explained.* Tech Target. www.techtarget.com/searchenterpriseai/tip/4-main-types-of-AI-explained

Halcomb, E., Ashley, C., Dennis, S., et al. (2023). Telehealth use in Australian primary healthcare during COVID-19: a cross-sectional descriptive survey. *BMJ Open, 13*(1), e065478. https://doi.org/10.1136/bmjopen-2022-065478

Health Information Management Systems Society (HIMSS). (2020). *Global Informatics Definitions* (Version 4). HIMSS TIGER Interprofessional Community. www.himss.org/sites/hde/files/media/file/2020/07/29/tiger_informaticsdefinitions-v6.pdf

Health Informatics New Zealand (HiNZ). (n.d.). *About HiNZ.* www.hinz.org.nz/page/AboutHINZ

Health Information Technology Competencies (HITComp). (2016). *Home page.* http://hitcomp.org

Health New Zealand. (2024). *Connected digital health services.* New Zealand Government. www.tewhatuora.govt.nz/our-health-system/digital-health/my-health-account/connected-digital-health-services/

Hübner U, Shaw T, Thye J, et al. (2018). Technology Informatics Guiding Education Reform – TIGER. *Methods of Information in Medicine, 57*(S 01), e30–e42. https://doi.org/10.3414/ME17-01-0155

Jiang, F., Jiang, Y., Zhi, H., et al. (2017). Artificial intelligence in healthcare: Past, present and future. *Stroke and Vascular Neurology, 2*(4), e000101. https://doi.org/10.1136/svn-2017-000101

Junglyun, K., Macierira, T., Mayer, S., et al. (2020). Towards implementing SNOMED CT in nursing practice. A scoping review. *International Journal of Medical Informatics, 134*, 104035. https://doi.org/10.1016/j.ijmedinf.2019.104035

Kanchan, S. & Gaidhaine, A. (2023). Social media role and its impact of public health: A narrative review. *Cureus*, Jan 13, *15*(1), e33737. https://doi.org/10.7759/cureus.33737

Kaplan, J. (2016). *Artificial Intelligence: What Everyone Needs to Know.* Oxford University Press.

Kidd, M.R. & Mazza, D. (2000). Clinical practice guidelines and the computer on your desk. *Medical Journal of Australia, 173*, 373–5.

Kvedar, J.C., Fogel, A.L., Elenko, E., et al. (2016). Digital medicine's march on chronic disease. *Nature Biotechnology, 34*(3), 239–46.

Mattison, G. Canfell, O.J., Forrester, D., et al. (2023). A step in the right direction: The potential of smartwatches in supporting chronic disease prevention in health care. *Medical Journal of Australia, 218*(9), 284–8. https://doi.org/10.5694/mja2.51920

Medical Director. (2019). *The Future of Wearable Devices in Health Care*. Health Communications Network. www.medicaldirector.com/news/future-of-health/new-report-reveals-the-future-of-wearable-devices-in-healthcare/

Ministry of Health. (2019). *Patient portals*. New Zealand Government. www.health.govt.nz/our-work/digital-health/other-digital-health-initiatives/patient-portals

Office of the Australian Information Commissioner. (2019). *Notifiable Data Breaches Statistics Report: 1 April to 30 June 2019*. Commonwealth of Australia. www.oaic.gov.au/privacy/notifiable-data-breaches/notifiable-data-breaches-publications/notifiable-data-breaches-report-1-april-to-30-june-2019?

PwC Health Research Institute. (2018). *Global Top Health Industry Issues: Defining the Healthcare of the Future*. www.pwc.com/gx/en/healthcare/pdf/global-top-health-industry-issues-2018-pwc.pdf

The Royal Melbourne Hospital. (2024). *Health hub portal*. www.thermh.org.au/your-care/hospital-care/your-hospital-stay/your-medical-records/health-hub-portal

Wong, B. (2023). *Top social media statistics and trends of 2024*. Forbes Advisor. www.forbes.com/advisor/business/social-media-statistics/

—— (2019a). *WHO Guideline: Recommendations on Digital Interventions for Health System Strengthening*. WHO.

—— (2019b). *Telehealth*. WHO.

—— (2021). *Global Strategy on Digital Health 2020–2025*. WHO.

14 Managing chronic health conditions

Catherine Stephen, Wa'ed Shiyab and Elizabeth Halcomb
With acknowledgement to Denise Johnston and Eileen Petrie

LEARNING OBJECTIVES

At the completion of this chapter, you should be able to:

- discuss the impact of chronic conditions on individuals, their families and the broader community.
- explain the impact of risk factors on the development of chronic conditions.
- identify the Chronic Care Model and describe its application.
- understand some of the challenges to behaviour change.
- explain how nurses engage in behaviour change communication with clients.
- describe how nurses can contribute to the management of chronic conditions.

Introduction

Chronic conditions –
a broad range of illnesses and diseases that individuals experience over an extended period, usually for longer than six months (Australian Health Ministers' Advisory Council, 2019).

Chronic conditions, or non-communicable diseases, are the leading cause of death worldwide. Chronic conditions are responsible for 41 million deaths and 17 million premature deaths across the world each year (World Health Organization (WHO), 2023). Most of these deaths are due to four major conditions: cardiovascular disease (CVD), cancer, chronic respiratory disease and diabetes (WHO, 2023). However, other chronic conditions, including injuries that result in persistent disability and mental health disorders, also contribute to increased morbidity and mortality. The significant increase in preventable chronic conditions and the need to manage these are major health care concerns of the industrialised world.

Regardless of the specific diagnosis, many chronic conditions are amenable to early identification, risk reduction strategies and facilitating self-management (Australian Health Ministers' Advisory Council, 2019). Interventions focus on the early identification of risk, modification of risky behaviours such as smoking, poor nutrition and low levels of physical activity, optimising evidence-based care and facilitating self-management support (Reynolds et al., 2018). Addressing these factors contributes to reducing the burden of the development and progression of chronic conditions. While this may appear simple, the issues surrounding lifestyle risk and behaviour modification are complex and, therefore, intervention strategies need to be multifaceted and engage multidisciplinary health professionals (James et al., 2019).

Primary health care (PHC) nurses, as part of the multidisciplinary health team, have been demonstrated to have a significant role in health promotion and chronic disease management (Halcomb et al., 2017; Stephen, McInnes & Halcomb, 2018). However, to achieve gains in promoting health and optimising disease management, nurses need to be equipped with the skills and knowledge to intervene effectively (Dobber et al., 2019; James et al., 2019). This chapter presents some of the key considerations and strategies that nurses need to appreciate to assist in reducing lifestyle risk factors and managing chronic conditions.

What is a chronic condition?

A chronic condition is any disability or disease which is long-lasting with persistent effects (Australian Institute of Health and Welfare (AIHW), 2024c). The term 'chronic condition' is used rather than 'chronic disease' as it is inclusive of the broader range of health issues that have ongoing impacts on individuals (Australian Health Ministers' Advisory Council, 2019). In Aotearoa New Zealand, they prefer using the term 'long-term conditions' (LTCs) (Health New Zealand, 2023). Such conditions may occur at any point across a person's lifespan, although they are more prevalent with advancing age. Chronic conditions are usually not immediately life-threatening, although those caused by disease often result in a gradual deterioration of health – punctuated by periods of exacerbation and remission – compromised quality of life and frequently lead to premature death (AIHW, 2024b; Treasury, 2023). There is usually no cure for chronic conditions and priority is placed on initial prevention, self-management, early intervention for exacerbations and quality PHC to optimise well-being and quality of life (Patel, 2022).

In Australia, 89 per cent of all deaths are associated with chronic conditions (AIHW, 2024b). It is estimated that 47 per cent of Australians have at least one chronic condition (AIHW, 2024b). Cancer, musculoskeletal conditions, cardiovascular diseases, mental health conditions and substance use disorders, and neurological conditions account for the most deaths and disability (AIHW, 2022). The impact of chronic conditions is felt beyond the health system with a range of other costs to government, industry and society; these include an increase in reduced productivity, an increase in absenteeism and lost leisure time (Crosland et al., 2019).

Some 20 per cent of Australians and Aotearoa New Zealanders have two or more chronic conditions, termed **multi-morbidity** (AIHW, 2024c; Health New Zealand, 2023). Multi-morbidity increases in prevalence with age (AIHW, 2024b). Those with multi-morbidity have a higher utilisation of health services and are more likely to be receiving polypharmacy (Peters et al., 2019). Multi-morbidity also negatively impacts on quality of life and health outcomes.

Multi-morbidity – the presence of two or more chronic conditions occurring at the same time (AIHW, 2024c).

There is a higher prevalence of chronic conditions in those who are most disadvantaged including the frail, aged, Indigenous Australians and Aotearoa New Zealanders, and those at a socio-economic disadvantage (AIHW, 2024b; Gurney, Stanley & Sarfati, 2020). Additionally, those in the lowest socio-economic groups have significantly lower life expectancy and higher death rates than those who have the highest levels of advantage (AIHW, 2024b).

Risk factors for chronic conditions

Factors such as smoking, hypertension, obesity/overweight, low levels of physical activity and unhealthy alcohol intake are well-recognised antecedents to the development of a range of chronic conditions (Fetherston & Craike, 2020; WHO, 2023). People with a high-risk factor profile are at significant risk of developing chronic conditions. However, reduction in risk improves health outcomes. For example, the successful management of two or more risk factors creates a 50 per cent reduction in the risk of CVD events (Adams et al., 2019; Wong & Sattar, 2023).

Many chronic conditions share common risk factors that can be divided into two broad types: those that are modifiable and those that are non-modifiable (Table 14.1). While non-modifiable factors cannot be changed, modifiable factors can be reduced to improve an individual's overall risk profile. Modifiable risk factors can further be separated into those factors that are amenable to lifestyle change such as smoking, nutrition, alcohol and physical activity and those that require pharmacological management – for example, lipid-modifying drugs and anti-hypertensive drugs (AIHW, 2024e). Early identification of the presence of risk factors can facilitate early intervention and subsequent reduction of risk.

Table 14.1   Risk factors

Modifiable risk factors	Non-modifiable risk factors
Behavioural • smoking • nutrition – including sodium intake, fruit and vegetable consumption • physical inactivity • alcohol intake • stress	• age • sex • family history • social history including ethnicity, culture, socio-economic status
Biological • high blood pressure • high serum lipids • high blood glucose • waist circumference and body mass index (BMI)	
Environmental • air pollution	

Source: Adapted from Prabhakaran, Anand & Reddy (2023).

An estimated 99 per cent of Australians have at least one of the six modifiable risk factors for CVD, with 57 per cent having three or more risk factors at the same time (AIHW, 2024e). Those living in rural and remote areas, First Nations and those in lower socio-economic groups are more likely to exhibit lifestyle behaviours and risk factors that are associated with poor health (AIHW, 2024h; Atkinson-Briggs et al., 2022). The situation is similar in the Aotearoa New Zealand population (Ministry of Health, 2024).

Smoking

Smoking rates in Australia and Aotearoa New Zealand have declined in recent years and are now one of the lowest rates among OECD countries (AIHW, 2024a). However, some 10.7

per cent of Australians and 8.3 per cent of Aotearoa New Zealanders continue to smoke daily (AIHW, 2024a; Ministry of Health, 2023a). Smoking results in the deaths of 19 000 Australians annually (AIHW, 2018) and has been shown to contribute to significant health loss in Aotearoa New Zealand (Ministry of Health, 2023a). Smoking highlights health inequities within Australia, with daily tobacco use more prevalent within Aboriginal and Torres Strait Islander communities and those living in socio-economic disadvantage or with mental health issues (AIHW, 2024a). Similarly, Aotearoa New Zealand Māori are disproportionally affected by higher smoking rates and higher tobacco-related deaths and disabilities than non-Māori (Ministry of Health, 2023a).

Nutrition

The prevalence of overweight and obesity is rising, with two in three Australian adults (67%) and one in three Aotearoa New Zealand adults currently being overweight or obese (AIHW, 2024f; Ministry of Health, 2023a). Between 2011–12 and 2022, the proportion of adults who are overweight or obese weights has increased from 62.8 per cent to 65.8 per cent (Australian Bureau of Statistics, 2023). Additionally, one in four Australian children and 13.5 per cent of Aotearoa New Zealand children are estimated to be above a healthy weight (AIHW, 2024f; Ministry of Health, 2023a). Those living in the lowest socio-economic areas and First Nations are more likely to be overweight (AIHW, 2024f; Ministry of Health, 2023a). The major causes of excessive weight are poor nutrition and inadequate physical activity. Overweight and obesity are the second leading risk factor after tobacco smoking and account for some 8.4 per cent of the total disease burden and 10 per cent of all deaths in Australia (AIHW, 2024f).

It is estimated that 55 per cent of Australian and Aotearoa New Zealand adults do not eat the recommended two serves of fruit daily, while some 91 per cent of Australians and 89 per cent of Aotearoa New Zealanders do not eat the recommended five serves of vegetables per day (AIHW, 2024d; Ministry of Health, 2023a). In addition to the links to increased body weight, diets low in fruit and vegetables have been linked to diabetes, cancer and CVD (AIHW, 2022).

Physical activity

Around 75 per cent of Australian adults aged 18–64 years are not sufficiently active, achieving less than the recommended 150 minutes of moderate- to vigorous-intensity exercise across five sessions each week (AIHW, 2024g). In addition, 83 per cent of those aged 2–14 years and 73 per cent of those aged 15–17 years do not undertake the recommended levels of physical activity (one hour of moderate-to-vigorous activity) every day (AIHW, 2024g). In Aotearoa New Zealand, only 46.5 per cent of adults met physical activity guidelines (Ministry of Health, 2023a), with low activity levels responsible for around 3 per cent of health lost (Ministry of Health, 2019). Inadequate physical activity has been linked to CVD, diabetes, dementia, stroke and some cancers (bowel, breast, uterine), as well as being related to overweight or obesity (AIHW, 2024g). Inactivity contributes to 5.2 per cent of the total deaths and 2.5 per cent of the total disease burden in Australia (AIHW, 2024g). An increase in physical activity by 15 minutes of moderate activity five days each week could reduce the disease burden due to insufficient exercise by 14 per cent (AIHW, 2018). The relationship between physical activity and COVID-19 restrictions is complex. However, the slight reduction in physical activity in recent years is worthy of further monitoring as we return to a new normal.

REFLECTION

Consider what you have learnt about lifestyle risk factors and chronic conditions:

1. Which lifestyle risk factors impact you and/or your family?
2. To what extent do you and/or your family members understand the correlation between lifestyle risk and the development of chronic conditions? How does this influence your/their behaviours?
3. How easy do you think it is to reduce these risk factors?
4. What one or two things could you do immediately to improve your lifestyle risk? What are the barriers and facilitators to doing these things?

The Chronic Care Model

The rising prevalence of chronic conditions and the high incidence of multi-morbidity have highlighted deficiencies within health systems. These include poor application of evidence-based practice, lack of care coordination, limited active follow-up and gaps in self-management support (Australian Health Ministers' Advisory Council, 2019). Much work has gone into investigating how health systems can better support chronic conditions. The Chronic Care Model, developed by Wagner (1998), articulates the fundamental elements required within a health system to facilitate the delivery of high-quality chronic condition management. These essential 'elements are the community, the health system, self-management support, delivery system design, decision support and clinical information systems' (Group Health Research Institute, 2019). Embedding evidence-based practice within each of these elements facilitates productive interactions between informed clients, who are actively involved in their health care, and health professionals with the appropriate resources and expertise to promote health (Group Health Research Institute, 2019). Understanding this sentinel model is important for clinicians and policymakers to ensure that they are promoting access to the best care for those with chronic conditions.

In response to the growing impact of chronic conditions, the Australian Health Ministers' Advisory Council (2019) developed the *National Strategic Framework for Chronic Conditions*. This plan identifies that effective management of chronic conditions must acknowledge the developmental stages of chronic disease from those at-risk to those with varying levels of health impairment and disability, and those requiring palliative care. The framework outlines three key objectives: focusing on preventing chronic conditions; providing efficient, effective and appropriate care to manage them; and targeting priority populations. In a conscious move away from a disease-specific approach, these key objectives are essential considerations when delivering care for those with chronic disease (Australian Health Ministers' Advisory Council, 2019). Aotearoa New Zealand's (Ministry of Health, 2023b) highlights the importance of the use of appropriate and effective health services. These areas include the frequency of health care contact, inclusiveness of health service, availability and affordability, and the continuity of the care provided.

While in this chapter we concentrate on the contribution of the nurse at an individual level, it is important to understand how health system, multidisciplinary team and community-level factors impact the management of chronic conditions, and how lifestyle risk factors in turn impact demand within the health system.

The nurse's role in managing chronic conditions

Nurses play a significant role in providing person-centred, continuous care of individuals with chronic conditions (Hämel et al., 2022). Chronic condition nursing provides person-centred, continuous primary care, with a secondary and tertiary prevention and management focus. Person-centred care places individuals and their families/significant others at the centre of their care (Epperly, Wilson & Kidd, 2023). In this model, the needs, concerns, beliefs and goals of the individual are the main focus rather than the needs of the health system or individual health providers. This focus empowers people to take control of their own health and health care rather than being passive recipients of care so that they feel valued and involved in keeping themselves healthy and managing their chronic condition(s).

While the specific nature of any nursing care will be driven by the individual's diagnosis, comorbidities and health status, there are four key areas in which nurses can work within the multidisciplinary team to improve outcomes. These are:

1. Early identification of risk
2. Support for behaviour modification
3. Optimising evidence-based care
4. Facilitating self-management (Stephen et al., 2022).

Each of these is now discussed in more detail. While these four areas are presented in a linear fashion, they are clearly interwoven and should be considered concurrently when planning care.

Early identification of risk

Regardless of the specific setting in which they work, nurses can contribute to risk identification in several ways. Firstly, during regular consultations, nurses often reveal the presence of risk factors through their assessments and discussions with clients (James et al., 2019; Morris et al., 2022). Opportunistically recording this information in the medical record and offering appropriate advice, support or referral can be the first steps in identifying and managing the risk factor(s). Secondly, nurses can use specific risk-screening tools such as the absolute cardiovascular risk calculator (Australian Chronic Disease Prevention Alliance, 2023) during consultations to actively evaluate individual risk factors and cumulative risk. Finally, nurses can proactively seek out clients with specific risk factors. For example, nurses working in general practice might use the medical records software systems to identify all clients who are recorded as being smokers, or those who are obese, and invite them to attend a dedicated consultation (Stephen et al., 2023). These consultations could then assess risk and offer appropriate advice or referral to other services to support risk factor reduction.

Stages of change

Reduction of modifiable risk factors requires the individual to initiate and sustain behavioural change. Behavioural change is widely understood to be a process that commences with individuals having varying levels of awareness of, or perceptions about, their level of risk

(Pennington, 2021). There is variation in the willingness or intention to change behaviour both between individuals and within a specific individual over time. Therefore, assessing the client's beliefs, behaviour and knowledge is an important first step in understanding where the individual is at in terms of thinking about change (James et al., 2020). Understanding the stage of change that the individual is at during the consultation is vital to the nurse providing appropriate and timely support for behaviour change.

Prochaska and Diclemente (1983) proposed the sentinel Transtheoretical Model of Behavior Change as a way to describe individuals' readiness to modify their behaviour. Although proposed over 40 years ago, this model still informs contemporary behaviour change practice (Del Rio Szupszynski & de Ávila, 2021; Pennington, 2021). By identifying the stage of change that individuals are currently at, the nurses can utilise appropriate types of support to either assist them in recognising the need for change, developing a plan for behaviour modification, or developing and evaluating change strategies. Table 14.2 provides an overview of this model and identifies the task focus that is the most appropriate for the nurse to adopt with a client at each stage.

Table 14.2   Strategies for stages of change

Stage of change	Intervention focus
Pre-contemplation (not yet ready for change)	• Provide information about the need for change. • Raise doubt about the impact of the current behaviours through personalised information about the risks if no change is made.

Contemplation (getting ready – to take action in the next six months)	• Encourage clients to evaluate the benefits and risks of change and help them to choose to change by:
	  – exploring ambivalence and alternatives
	  – identifying the reasons for change and the risks of not changing behaviours
	  – increasing their self-confidence in their capacity to achieve successful change.

Preparation (taking steps towards change but not yet ready for action)	• Work with clients to develop a realistic, achievable plan for making a change and set clear goals. • Use rehearsal and modelling to demonstrate opportunities for success. • Provide support to increase confidence and self-efficacy.
Action (engaging in new behaviour)	• Provide support for change and feedback about performance to sustain motivation. • Address and solve any barriers to implementing the new behaviour and lead to relapse.
Maintenance (sticking to it for > six months)	• Continue to provide support for change as required. • Provide positive feedback and ongoing encouragement that rewards positive behaviour. • Recognise that relapse is normal and plan realistic strategies to prevent relapse. • Use reminder systems to monitor sustained change.
Relapse (learning)	• Work with clients to renew the processes of contemplation and action without becoming stuck or disheartened.

Source: Adapted from Espinosa-Salas and Gonzalez-Arias (2023); Raihan and Cogburn (2020).

REFLECTION

Consider what you have learnt about the stages of change and think about someone you know, such as a family member or friend:

1. Can you identify a person who is in the pre-contemplation stage? What do you notice about the attitudes and behaviours of this individual?

2. Do you know someone who is at the preparation stage? What do you notice about the attitudes and behaviours of this person?

3. Is there anyone who is at the relapse or maintenance stage? What do you notice about their attitudes and behaviours?

4. What are the differences and similarities between the people you have identified at these different stages?

Support for behaviour modification

The identification of the stage of change clearly informs decision-making about the most appropriate focus of intervention for each person. However, there are various ways in which the nurse can facilitate behaviour change. Two key strategies that are used in PHC are the Five As Model and motivational interviewing (MI) (discussed in Chapter 2).

Five As Model

The Five As Model provides a simple summary of the process involved in the development of a personal action plan to enhance behavioural change to reduce modifiable risk factors (Figure 14.1) (Kris-Etherton et al., 2021; Krist et al., 2020; Wharton et al., 2020). This approach was initially developed for smoking cessation but is now considered the

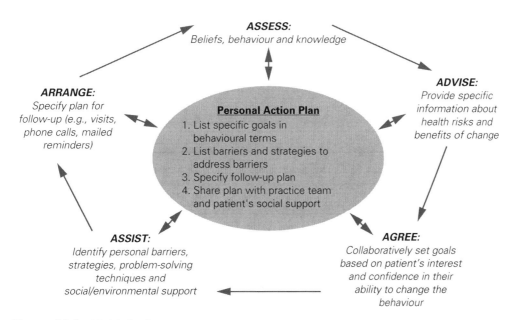

Figure 14.1   Model of self-management
Source: Glasgow et al. (2003, p. 564).

preferred intervention for behaviour change in a range of clinical settings and with various client groups to achieve lifestyle risk reduction (Kris-Etherton et al., 2021; Krist et al., 2020; Stephen et al., 2023).

The Five As Model can be enacted as follows:

1. **A**ssess the client's beliefs, behaviour and knowledge.

   Assessment of current behaviours, knowledge of health and stage of change are important to identify the most appropriate strategies to support health and well-being. Care should be taken to undertake these assessments in a non-judgemental and sensitive manner, building a trusting partnership with the client.

2. **A**dvise the client about health risks and benefits of behavioural change through the provision of specific and relevant information.

   The Health Belief Model describes how the individual's level of perceived personal risk and the potential gains from the new behaviour impact the likelihood of successful behaviour change (Anuar et al., 2020). However, any information provided needs to be easily understood by, and appropriate to, the environmental context of the individual (Dobber et al., 2019; James et al., 2019).

   The level of information provided in this step will be dependent on the stage of change identified in the assessment phase (James et al., 2020). For some clients, broad information about the presence of a risk factor and its potential impact on their health and well-being may be the most appropriate intervention to raise their risk awareness. However, for other clients who are aware of the presence of risk factors, health education may be more about targeting the benefits of lifestyle modification on their health and level of risk.

3. **A**ssist the client to identify personal barriers and use problem-solving techniques to work through these.

   Personal factors and environmental influences make a significant contribution to behaviour change (Green, Murphy & Gryboski, 2020). The process of proactively identifying potential barriers and problem-solving solutions is a positive strategy to optimise the success of behaviour change (Dobber et al., 2019). This can also be important as a way of identifying potential triggers for relapse (for example, stress for those seeking to quit smoking) and planning alternate strategies to promote healthy choices.

   Assisting the client to identify barriers and issues, and facilitating the individual to problem solve is also an important strategy to promote ownership of the process by the client (Kris-Etherton et al., 2021). Such empowerment enhances the individual's level of control in the change process and demonstrates the provision of person-centred care.

4. **A**gree on goals based on the client's interest and on the confidence in the client to change her or his own behaviour.

   Setting realistic, achievable and measurable goals, which the individual feels are achievable, is an important step in the process of behaviour change. Establishing a benchmark for the individual to achieve provides a tangible outcome that progress can be measured against. Writing the goals down and developing an action plan can assist in achieving positive outcomes (Stephen et al., 2018).

While achieving a goal is clearly the desired outcome, not achieving it should not be seen as a failure but rather an opportunity for reframing the objective and reconsidering the strategies to achieve behaviour change (Kris-Etherton et al., 2021).

5. **Arrange** referrals to other services and a specific plan for follow-up, such as visits and phone calls.

The final step of the Five As is for the nurse to facilitate appropriate referrals to relevant allied health or health services and arrange follow-ups to ensure that progress is achieved. The provision of active follow-up by the nurse and the level of accountability between the nurse and the client can be important motivators of change (Kris-Etherton et al., 2021). Planning for follow-up is also a sign of recognition that behaviour change is not easy but rather is an ongoing process and likely to be punctuated by gains and periods of relapse. Additionally, it demonstrates a willingness on the part of the nurse to engage with the client and provide support along the entire process of behaviour change.

Motivational interviewing

Motivational interviewing (MI) is another strategy used to encourage behavioural change to improve health status, particularly to persuade clients to engage with recommended treatments and reduce lifestyle risk factors (Lim et al., 2019). By exploring and addressing individuals' ambivalent attitudes and perceived barriers to behaviour change, MI seeks to enhance their intrinsic motivation (Dobber et al., 2019). Intrinsic motivation exists when the individual is driven by internal rewards, such as enjoyment in the task itself or personal satisfaction. In contrast, extrinsic motivation is external approval/disapproval from peers or health professionals. Change driven by intrinsic motivation has been demonstrated to be more sustainable and enduring than that driven by extrinsic motivation. Motivational interviewing has been discussed in detail in Chapter 2.

CASE STUDY 14.1

Kevin is a 47-year-old male who is 186 cm tall and weighs 119 kg. He works as a self-employed truck driver and lives with his wife Jenny and three children in a comfortable house with a substantial mortgage. While Kevin has never smoked, he does enjoy a bottle of wine with his wife over dinner every evening and has a few social beers at the weekend.

Regular driving jobs have been difficult to secure and lately, Kevin worries about the solvency of his business and his ability to cover the bills. He acknowledges that he has 'gained a bit of weight' over the years but is too busy to go to the gym or think about his diet. While attending his general practice for a flu vaccination, Kevin takes up the nurse's offer of a routine blood pressure check. His blood pressure is measured as 154/90 mmHg. Following a brief consultation with his GP, Kevin accepts the offer of a health assessment with the nurse for the following week.

REFLECTION
Explore the nurse's role in Kevin's health assessment.

1. Identifying the risk factors for CVD relevant in Kevin's case, how would you start a conversation with him about his lifestyle?

CASE STUDY 14.1 Continued

2. Consider where Kevin may be in terms of the Transtheoretical Model of Behavior Change. How might your conversation vary depending on which stage Kevin is at?
3. What motivational interviewing techniques might you use with Kevin?
4. Using the Five As, what person-centred action plan would you develop with Kevin? Consider the factors that may affect his overall mental health, focusing on relevant risk factors, achievable goals (What can I change today?) and potential barriers (Can I overcome them?).

Optimising evidence-based care

There is a strong evidence base for optimal diagnosis, pharmacological treatment and disease management for many chronic conditions. However, despite this plethora of best practice guidelines, a gap remains between these identified gold standards of care and clinical practice (Mazza et al., 2019). The reasons for the evidence-practice gap are multi-factorial and include a complex combination of health system, provider and client issues. While a detailed discussion of these factors is beyond the scope of this discussion, it is important to note that nurses have an important role in bridging this gap and improving the delivery of evidence-based care.

Nurse-led interventions have been demonstrated to improve guideline adherence in a range of client groups and clinical settings (Bulto et al., 2023; Qiu, 2024). Nurses have been able to achieve these gains using several strategies, particularly focused on the identification of:

- those not receiving evidence-based care
- facilitation of the delivery of required care
- empowerment of clients to be aware of the best practice care for their individual circumstances.

Increasingly, nurses are using digital technology to target the delivery of evidence-based care to individuals with the greatest need (Booth et al., 2021). Structured medical records searches enable nurses to identify clients who are either not treated to target (for example, uncontrolled hypertension), have not received indicated diagnostic follow-up (for example, people with diabetes without recorded haemoglobin A1C (HbA1c)) or have specific identified risk factors (for example, smokers with chronic obstructive pulmonary disease (COPD)) (Kademane, Kumar & Chaudhary, 2023; Schwartz et al., 2022). Identified individuals can be recalled to the practice for follow-up. At this visit, the nurse can assess their health and risk factors against relevant guidelines and can either deliver the required treatment for their health and risk factors or refer the client to other health professionals.

REFLECTION

Use the Internet or your library to find best practice guidelines for the management of a chronic condition that you have seen in your clinical practice.

1. What type of evidence exists to support the guidelines?
2. Which aspects of the guidelines have you seen implemented in your clinical experience?
3. What might be some of the barriers to fully implementing the guidelines in clinical practice?

Facilitating self-management

Self-management should be considered along a continuum from prevention and early identification of risk factors to living well with chronic conditions. All individuals should be facilitated to develop good self-care habits from an early age to reduce modifiable risk factors and promote healthy lifestyle habits that reduce the risk of chronic conditions. For those who do progress to develop a chronic condition, self-management includes monitoring and managing the signs and symptoms of the condition, and the effect the condition has on physical, emotional, occupational and social functioning. It also includes the early identification of exacerbations of disease and the implementation of strategies to address this decline in health. Self-management has been shown to be significantly associated with health status and quality of life (Han, Lin & Chen, 2022). Nurses can support self-management by improving **health literacy**, promoting self-care and self-efficacy, and supporting clients to develop care plans which empower them to be active participants in their ongoing health care (Australian Health Ministers' Advisory Council, 2019; Stephen et al., 2022).

Health literacy – the extent to which individuals can access, understand and act upon information relating to their health (Liu et al., 2020).

CASE STUDY 14.2

Karen is a 55-year-old financial accounts manager attending her local general practice, where she is seen by Ben, a registered nurse. The following scenario describes an exchange between Ben and Karen during the appointment.

Ben: Hi Karen, my name is Ben, I'm a registered nurse. What brings you to the practice today?

Karen: Well, I've noticed weight gain over the last few years, and I've started to feel a bit puffed when climbing the stairs, so I thought I'd come and get it checked out by the GP. The receptionist offered a heath check with you first.

Ben: Glad you came in. Is this weight gain something that has been worrying you?

Karen: Since taking on extra hours at work, I've not had time to prepare healthy foods and often rely on takeaways, plus I never have the energy to go to the gym. I'm not too bothered that I've gone up a few dress sizes, but I'm concerned this extra weight could affect my overall health.

Ben: That's a valid concern. What would you like to achieve in terms of health goals?

Karen: I've tried diets in the past but find it really hard to stick to them. Overall, I'd like to eat more fresh fruit and vegetables.

Ben: What could be the barriers to making a change in your diet?

Karen: I have such a busy life schedule and tend to go for the quickest takeaway option on the way home from work. My local grocery offers delivery on fruit and veggie boxes. I've thought of getting that once a week which might help me to prepare healthier food.

Ben: Great strategy! I've also got some pamphlets that outline healthy eating and physical activity guidelines. You're welcome to take those home with you. By visiting the practice today, you've made the first step towards improved health. We can work in partnership with your GP to set goals and an action plan if this is something that you'd be interested in?

Karen: That could be really helpful, thanks.

Ben: Let's work out the best appointment time for you next week and take it from there.

CASE STUDY 14.2 Continued

REFLECTION

1. What stage of the Transtheoretical Model is Karen most likely in? Did this change throughout the discussion?
2. What motivational interviewing techniques are used by Ben to discuss behaviour change?
3. Consider the follow-up appointment for Karen. What key points might the nurse consider for this discussion? What kinds of change might you expect to include in an action plan for Karen?
4. How did Ben address Karen's health literacy? What other aspects of health literacy and self-management should Ben consider?

Conclusion

This chapter has discussed the scope and impact of chronic conditions on the community and the individual. It has highlighted the Chronic Care Model and the importance of person-centred care and multidisciplinary interventions, which provide integrated care to the management of those with chronic conditions. As all nurses will encounter clients who have either lifestyle risk factors and/or chronic conditions, this chapter has outlined the ways in which nurses can contribute to the improvement of health in the community. Through their capacity to build therapeutic relationships and provide ongoing support, PHC nurses can contribute significantly to the identification and reduction of lifestyle risk factors, the optimisation of evidence-based care delivery and can facilitate self-management. Most importantly, PHC nurses can ensure that individuals receive sufficient information and support to make decisions about their own health and health care to promote optimal well-being.

CRITICAL THINKING ACTIVITIES

1. Which lifestyle factors place you at risk of developing chronic disease?
2. How aware are you of the need to change these factors in yourself?
3. What are the barriers and facilitators in changing your behaviour?

FURTHER READING

Australian Institute of Health and Welfare (AIHW). (2024). *Chronic conditions*. Australian Government. www.aihw.gov.au/reports/australias-health/chronic-conditions-and-multimorbidity

Department of Health. (2021). *National Preventive Health Strategy*. Commonwealth of Australia. www.health.gov.au/resources/publications/national-preventive-health-strategy-2021-2030

The Royal Australian College of General Practitioners. (2015). *Smoking, Nutrition, Alcohol, Physical Activity (SNAP): A Population Health Guide to Behavioural Risk Factors in General Practice* (2nd ed.). www.racgp.org.au/clinical-resources/clinical-guidelines/key-racgp-guidelines/view-all-racgp-guidelines/snap

REFERENCES

Adams, M.L., Grandpre, J., Katz, D.L. & Shenson, D. (2019). The impact of key modifiable risk factors on leading chronic conditions. *Preventive Medicine, 120*, 113–18. https://doi.org/10.1016/j.ypmed.2019.01.006

Anuar, H., Shah, S., Gafor, H., Mahmood, M. & Ghazi, H.F. (2020). Usage of Health Belief Model (HBM) in health behavior: A systematic review. *Malaysian Journal of Medicine and Health Sciences, 16*(11), 2636–9346.

Atkinson-Briggs, S., Jenkins, A., Ryan, C. & Brazionis, L. (2022). Prevalence of health-risk behaviours among Indigenous Australians with diabetes: A review. *Journal of the Australian Indigenous HealthInfoNet, 3*(4), Article 6, https://doi.org/10.14221/aihjournal.v3n4.6.

Australian Bureau of Statistics. (2023). *Waist circumference and BMI*. Australian Government. www.abs.gov.au/statistics/health/health-conditions-and-risks/waist-circumference-and-bmi/latest-release

Australian Chronic Disease Prevention Alliance. (2023). *Australian Guideline for Assessing and Managing Cardiovascular Disease Risk*. Commonwealth of Australia. https://d35rj4ptypp2hd.cloudfront.net/pdf/Guideline-for-assessing-and-managing-CVD-risk_20230522.pdf

Australian Health Ministers' Advisory Council. (2019). *National Strategic Framework for Chronic Conditions*. Australian Health Ministers' Advisory Council.

Australian Institute of Health & Welfare (AIHW). (2018). *Australia's Health 2018*. (Australia's Health Series no. 16. AUS 221). Australian Government, https://www.aihw.gov.au/getmedia/7c42913d-295f-4bc9-9c24-4e44eff4a04a/aihw-aus-221.pdf.

—— (2022). *Australian Burden of Disease Study 2022*. (2022). Australian Government. www.aihw.gov.au/reports/burden-of-disease/australian-burden-of-disease-study-2022

—— (2024a). *Alcohol, tobacco & other drugs in Australia*. Australian Government. www.aihw.gov.au/reports/alcohol/alcohol-tobacco-other-drugs-australia/contents/drug-types/tobacco

—— (2024b). *Australia's health*. Australian Government. www.aihw.gov.au/reports-data/australias-health

—— (2024c). *Chronic conditions*. Australian Government. www.aihw.gov.au/reports/australias-health/chronic-conditions-and-multimorbidity

—— (2024d). *Diet*. Australian Government. www.aihw.gov.au/reports/food-nutrition/diet

—— (2024e). *Heart, stroke and vascular disease: Australian facts*. Australian Government. www.aihw.gov.au/reports/heart-stroke-vascular-disease/hsvd-facts

—— (2024f). *Overweight and obesity*. Australian Government. www.aihw.gov.au/reports/overweight-obesity/overweight-and-obesity/contents/overweight-and-obesity

—— (2024g). *Physical activity*. Australian Government. www.aihw.gov.au/reports/physical-activity/physical-activity

—— (2024h). *Rural and remote health*. Australian Government. www.aihw.gov.au/reports/rural-remote-australians/rural-and-remote-health

Booth, R.G., Strudwick, G., McBride, S., O'Connor, S. & López, A.L.S. (2021). How the nursing profession should adapt for a digital future. *British Medical Journal, 373*, n1190. https://doi.org/10.1136/bmj.n1190

Bulto, L.N., Roseleur, J., Noonan, S., et al. (2023). Effectiveness of nurse-led interventions versus usual care to manage hypertension and lifestyle behaviour: A systematic review and meta-analysis. *European Journal of Cardiovascular Nursing, 23*(1), 21–32. https://doi.org/10.1093/eurjcn/zvad040

Crosland, P., Ananthapavan, J., Davison, J., Lambert, M. & Carter, R. (2019). The health burden of preventable disease in Australia: A systematic review. *Australian and New Zealand Journal of Public Health, 43*(2), 163–70. https://doi.org/10.1111/1753-6405.12882

Del Rio Szupszynski, K.P. & de Ávila, A.C. (2021). The Transtheoretical Model of Behavior Change: Prochaska and DiClemente's model. In A.L.M Andrade, D. De Micheli, E.A. da Silva, F.M.

Lopes, B. de Oliveira Pinheiro & R.A. Reichert (eds), *Psychology of Substance Abuse: Psychotherapy, Clinical Management and Social Intervention*, (pp.205–16). Springer. https://doi.org/10.1007/978-3-030-62106-3

Dobber, J., Latour, C., Snaterse, M., et al. (2019). Developing nurses' skills in motivational interviewing to promote a healthy lifestyle in patients with coronary artery disease. *European Journal of Cardiovascular Nursing*, *18*(1), 28–37. https://doi.org/10.1177/1474515118784102

Epperly, T., Wilson, C.R. & Kidd, M. (2023). Person-centered family medicine and general practice. In J.E. Mezzich, W.J. Appleyard, P. Glare, J. Snaedal & C.R. Wilson (eds), *Person Centered Medicine* (pp. 327–40). Springer. https://link.springer.com/chapter/10.1007/978-3-031-17650-0_19

Espinosa-Salas, S. & Gonzalez-Arias, M. (2023). *Behavior Modification for Lifestyle Improvement*. StatPearls Publishing. https://www.ncbi.nlm.nih.gov/books/NBK592418/

Fetherston, H. & Craike, M. (2020). *Australia's Gender Health Tracker Technical Appendix. Australian Health Policy Collaboration*. Mitchell Institute, Victoria University. www.vu.edu.au/sites/default/files/australias-gender-health-tracker-2020.pdf

Glasgow, R.E., Davis, C.L., Funnell, M.M. & Beck, A. (2003). Implementing practical interventions to support chronic illness self-management. *The Joint Commission Journal on Quality and Patient Safety*, *29*(11), 563–74. https://doi.org/10.1016/s1549-3741(03)29067-5

Green, E.C., Murphy, E.M. & Gryboski, K. (2020). The health belief model. *The Wiley Encyclopedia of Health Psychology* (pp. 211–14). Wiley.

Group Health Research Institute. (2019). *The Chronic Care Model*. www.improvingchroniccare.org/index.php?p=Model_Elements&s=18

Gurney, J., Stanley, J. & Sarfati, D. (2020). The inequity of morbidity: Disparities in the prevalence of morbidity between ethnic groups in New Zealand. *Journal of Multimorbidity and Comorbidity*, *10*, 2235042x20971168. https://doi.org/10.1177/2235042x20971168

Halcomb, E.J., Stephens, M., Bryce, J., Foley, E. & Ashley, C. (2017). The development of national professional practice standards for nurses working in Australian general practice. *Journal of Advanced Nursing*, *73*(8), 1958–69. https://doi.org/10.1111/jan.13274

Hämel, K., Röhnsch, G., Heumann, M., et al. (2022). How do nurses support chronically ill clients' participation and self-management in primary care? A cross-country qualitative study. *BMC Family Practice*, *23*(1). https://doi.org/10.1186/s12875-022-01687-x

Han, T.C., Lin, H.S. & Chen, C.M. (2022). Association between chronic disease self-management, health status, and quality of life in older Taiwanese adults with chronic illnesses. *Healthcare (Basel)*, *10*(4). https://doi.org/10.3390/healthcare10040609

Health New Zealand. (2023). *About long term conditions*. New Zealand Government. www.tewhatuora.govt.nz/for-the-health-sector/health-sector-guidance/diseases-and-conditions/long-term-conditions/about-chronic-health-conditions/

James, S., Halcomb, E., McInnes, S. & Desborough, J. (2019). Integrative literature review: lifestyle risk communication by nurses in primary care. *Collegian*, *26*(1), 183–93. https://doi.org/10.1016/j.colegn.2018.03.006

James, S., McInnes, S., Halcomb, E.J. & Desborough, J. (2020). Lifestyle risk factor communication by nurses in Australian general practice: Understanding the interactional elements. *Journal of Advanced Nursing*, *76*(1), 234–42. https://doi.org/10.1111/jan.14221

Kademane, A., Kumar, P., Chaudhary, B. & Castillo-González, W. (2023). The influence of electronic health records on nursing practice within hospital settings. *Salud, Ciencia y Tecnología*, (3), 453.

Kris-Etherton, P.M., Petersen, K.S., Despres, J.P., et al. (2021). Strategies for promotion of a healthy lifestyle in clinical settings: Pillars of ideal cardiovascular health: A science advisory from the American Heart Association. *Circulation*, *144*(24), e495–e514. https://doi.org/10.1161/CIR.0000000000001018

Krist, A.H., Davidson, K.W., Mangione, C.M., et al. (2020). Behavioral counseling interventions to promote a healthy diet and physical activity for cardiovascular disease prevention in adults with cardiovascular risk factors: US Preventive Services Task Force recommendation statement. *Journal of the American Medical Association*, *324*(20), 2069–75. https://doi .org/10.1001/jama.2020.21749

Lim, D., Schoo, A., Lawn, S. & Litt, J. (2019). Embedding and sustaining motivational interviewing in clinical environments: A concurrent iterative mixed methods study. *BMC Medical Education*, *19*(1), 164. https://doi.org/10.1186/s12909-019-1606-y

Liu, C., Wang, D., Liu, C., et al. (2020). What is the meaning of health literacy? A systematic review and qualitative synthesis. *Family Medicine and Community Health*, *8*(2), e000351. https://doi .org/10.1136/fmch-2020-000351

Mazza, D., McCarthy, E., Carey, M., Turner, L. & Harris, M. (2019). "90% of the time, it's not just weight": General practitioner and practice staff perspectives regarding the barriers and enablers to obesity guideline implementation. *Obesity Research and Clinical Practice*, *13*(4), 398–403. https://doi.org/10.1016/j.orcp.2019.04.001

Ministry of Health. (2019). *Annual Update of Key Results 2017/18: New Zealand Health Survey*. New Zealand Government. https://www.health.govt.nz/publications/annual-update-of-key-results-201718-new-zealand-health-survey

——— (2023a). *Annual Data Explorer*. New Zealand Government. https://minhealthnz.shinyapps.io/nz-health-survey-2022-23-annual-data-explorer/

——— (2023b). *Content Guide 2022/23 New Zealand Health Survey*. New Zealand Government.

——— (2024). Health and Independence Report 2023: The Director-General of Health's Annual Report on the State of Public Health. New Zealand Government. www.health.govt.nz/publications/health-and-independence-report-2023

Morris, M., Halcomb, E., Mansourian, Y. & Bernoth, M. (2022). Understanding how general practice nurses support adult lifestyle risk reduction: An integrative review. *Journal of Advanced Nursing*, *78*(11), 3517–30. https://doi.org/10.1111/jan.15344

Patel, A. (2022). Improving chronic disease self-management in high-risk patient populations. *Translational Medicine Communications*, *7*(1), 1–3. https://doi.org/10.1186/s41231-022-00112-w

Pennington, C.G. (2021). Applying the transtheoretical model of behavioral change to establish physical activity habits. *Journal of Education and Recreation Patterns*, *2*(1), 11–20.

Peters, M., Potter, C.M., Kelly, L. & Fitzpatrick, R. (2019). Self-efficacy and health-related quality of life: A cross-sectional study of primary care patients with multi-morbidity. *Health Quality Life Outcomes*, *17*(1), 37. https://doi.org/10.1186/s12955-019-1103-3

Prabhakaran, D., Anand, S. & Reddy, K.S. (2023). *Public Health Approach to Cardiovascular Disease Prevention & Management*. CRC Press. https://doi.org/10.1201/b23266

Prochaska, J.O. & Diclemente, C.C. (1983). Stages and processes of self-change of smoking: Toward an integrative model of change. *Journal of Consulting and Clinical Psychology*, *51*(3), 390–5. https://doi.org/10.1037/0022-006x.51.3.390

Qiu, X. (2024). Nurse-led intervention in the management of patients with cardiovascular diseases: A brief literature review. *BMC Nursing*, *23*(1), 6. https://doi.org/10.1186/s12912-023-01422-6

Raihan, N. & Cogburn, M. (2020). *Stages of change theory*. www.ncbi.nlm.nih.gov/books/NBK556005/.

Reynolds, R., Dennis, S., Hasan, I., et al. (2018). A systematic review of chronic disease management interventions in primary care. *BMC Family Practice*, *19*(1), 11. https://doi.org/10.1186/s12875-017-0692-3

Schwartz, J.L., Duan, D., Maruthur, N.M. & Pitts, S.I. (2022). Utility of an electronic health record report to identify patients with delays in testing for poorly controlled diabetes. *The Joint Commission Journal on Quality and Patient Safety*, *48*(6–7), 335–42. https://doi.org/10.1016/j.jcjq.2022.03.002

Stephen, C., Halcomb, E., Fernandez, R., et al. (2022). Nurse-led interventions to manage hypertension in general practice: A systematic review and meta analysis. *Journal of Advanced Nursing*, *78*(5), 1281–93. https://doi.org/10.1111/jan.15159

Stephen, C., Halcomb, E., Zwar, N. & Batterham, M. (2023). Impact of a general practice nurse intervention to improve blood pressure control: The ImPress study. *Australian Journal of General Practice*, *52*(12), 875–81. https://doi.org/10.31128/AJGP-09-22-6573

Stephen, C., McInnes, S. & Halcomb, E. (2018). The feasibility and acceptability of nurse-led chronic disease management interventions in primary care: An integrative review. *Journal of Advanced Nursing*, *74*(2), 279–88. https://doi.org/10.1111/jan.13450

Treasury. (2023). *Prevalence of Chronic Conditions*. Commonwealth of Australia. https://treasury.gov.au/policy-topics/measuring-what-matters/dashboard/prevalence-chronic-conditions

Wagner, E.H. (1998). Chronic disease management: What will it take to improve care for chronic illness? *Effective Clinical Practice*, *1*(1), 2–4. www.ncbi.nlm.nih.gov/pubmed/10345255

Wharton, S., Lau, D.C., Vallis, M., et al. (2020). Obesity in adults: A clinical practice guideline. *Canadian Medical Association Journal*, *192*(31), E875–E891.

Wong, N.D. & Sattar, N. (2023). Cardiovascular risk in diabetes mellitus: Epidemiology, assessment and prevention. *Nature Reviews Cardiology*, *20*(10), 685–95. https://doi.org/10.1038/s41569-023-00877-z

World Health Organization (WHO). (2023). *Noncommunicable diseases*. www.who.int/news-room/fact-sheets/detail/noncommunicable-diseases

PART IV

Community and primary health care roles

15 Community health nursing

Amanda Moses, Judith Anderson and Melissa Hanson
With acknowledgement to Rhonda Brown, Susan Reid
and Eileen Petrie

LEARNING OBJECTIVES

At the completion of this chapter, you should be able to:

- describe the role and activities of community health nurses (CHNs).
- identify the main focus of the role from a primary health care (PHC) perspective.
- describe the process for identifying and responding to community needs.
- understand the complexity and diversity of the role.
- distinguish this role from other community-based nursing roles.

Introduction

Community health nurses (CHNs) – a specialty role within nursing blending PHC, nursing practice and public health with a community and population focus.

The World Health Organization (WHO) (2017) developed a framework for family and community nursing that identified a role for **community health nurses (CHNs)** identifying the needs of their communities and addressing them. PHC shifted the focus from a disease model treating illness to a preventative model that focused on population and social health, community development, health promotion, illness prevention and early intervention, including community nurses as part of this movement (Gasperini et al., 2023).

CHNs work in community health centres, social service settings, community-controlled health centres, such as those providing health care for Indigenous and Aboriginal populations, schools and a variety of other community settings. They work in partnership with local communities to identify health needs and plan strategies to address health inequities and improve health and well-being (Gasperini et al., 2023; Kiper & Geist, 2020).

This chapter focuses on the practice and role of CHNs. Other chapters focus on other areas of community nursing practice and specialised CHN roles such as working in schools, working with refugee health, maternal, child and family health, sexual health, mental health and working in rural and remote settings.

Community health nursing practice

Community health nursing practice is underpinned by the social model of health and principles of PHC incorporating accessible health care, appropriate technology, health promotion, intersectoral collaboration, community participation and cultural safety (LaMothe et al., 2021). Recognition of the social determinants of health, diversity within and across population groups, empowerment, social justice and advocacy underpin community health nursing practice (Doolan-Noble, et al., 2021). From this perspective, identifying the specific needs of high-risk and diverse populations is essential to ensuring that the needs of the population as a whole are being met in an equitable fashion (Clendon & Munns, 2022).

Community health nursing is defined to a large extent by its interdisciplinary practice that recognises the role of a large variety of organisations in addressing the social determinants of health and focuses on developing supportive links between these organisations and members of the community (LaMothe et al., 2021). The CHNs' unique knowledge, education, experience and skillset prepares them to work with individuals, families and communities across their lifespan. CHN primarily focus on prevention, protection and promotion of health and early intervention (Gasperini et al., 2023). They use principles of **community development** to support capacity-building that is focused on community strengths and community participation (Minkler, 2022).

Community development – strengthening and bringing community members together to identify and take collective action on issues important to them.

CHNs predominantly work in local community health centres, together with other PHC workers, and partner with the local community using a comprehensive PHC approach to address identified community health needs. These broad perspectives on health care are difficult to justify in a political environment where health care often focuses on cures. This has frequently led to community health centres amalgamating to form larger centres. The advantages of larger health centres are that they cover wider geographical areas, they can compete more competitively for funding, and they can increase the diversity and number of multidisciplinary professionals to offer a broader skill set. The focus of these centres is the delivery of **primary care** services, including general medical and nursing care, pharmacy, dental services, dietetics and psychological services (Roussy et al., 2021).

Primary care – the first point of contact an individual has with the health system. In Australia, Aotearoa New Zealand and other similar countries, primary care is delivered mostly through general practice medical clinics and allied health services.

Within this context, the responsibility for PHC and primary care has been given to primary health networks in Australia and primary health organisations in Aotearoa New Zealand. These are predominantly managed by GPs and have resulted in increased funding for programs based in general practice (Hewitt et al., 2021). This, in turn, has resulted in increasing numbers of general practice nurses taking on many of the roles once provided by CHNs, including health education, early intervention, women's health and chronic illness management (see Chapter 24 for more information about the role of general practice nurses). However, examples of comprehensive PHC, in which CHNs have a major role, can still be found particularly in publicly funded community health centres, rural and remote health, child and family health, school health, youth health and Aboriginal and Māori health (Department of Health, 2021; New Zealand Minister of Health, 2023).

REFLECTION

What do you think is to be gained or lost by shifting funding away from community- and population-focused programs to direct care provided by nurses working in general practice mostly to individuals and families?

The role of CHNs

While CHNs work with individuals, families, groups and communities where they live, learn, work and play, much of their work is focused on populations and systems. This includes working closely with government departments, local community groups and services, and specific population groups (particularly high-risk groups and vulnerable communities) to promote, protect and preserve health (Kiper & Geist, 2020). CHNs practice in partnership with community members to encourage their participation and capacity to:

- identify factors affecting their health.
- access health-related resources.
- take action to improve health outcomes (Taylor et al., 2021).

CHNs support the health of the individual, family and community with an emphasis on empowerment and self-determination to enable people to control their own health and ensure they are active partners in decisions that affect health and well-being (Kiper & Geist, 2020). CHNs promote autonomy of the individual and family, while adhering to the public health philosophy of promoting the greatest good for the greatest number of people (Gasperini et al., 2023).

The CHN encourages health-enhancing and health-promoting behaviours and the identification or creation of community structures and networks that support healthy behaviours is fundamental to the role. Another necessary component of CHN practice is to develop and maintain networks with other health and community organisations with whom they work collaboratively to identify needs and develop programs to ensure appropriate health care is provided (LaMothe et al., 2021).

Consistent with PHC, CHNs also adopt an intersectoral approach working closely with a wide range of local, state and federal government and non-government organisations including those involved with housing, education, employment, transport and recreation. CHNs consider the impact of political, cultural and environmental contexts on health and therefore advocate and engage in political action and public health policy development that facilitates healthy living (LaMothe et al., 2021).

While the roles and activities undertaken by CHNs in different communities are fundamentally the same, there may be some differences depending on the specific needs of each community. For example, in some communities, CHNs may provide sexual health and women's health such as Pap smears, while in other communities this may be provided by other health professionals. Many CHNs work with local schools by providing personal development, sexual health and other key health education activities. If these needs can be met by a school nurse or professionals in other services, CHNs will not need to be involved. Therefore, the CHNs' practice roles continually evolve to meet the different and changing health needs of the communities in which they work (Kiper & Geist, 2020).

An understanding of the community that CHNs are working in is integral to their practice. The community can be defined by geographical boundaries, for example, a metropolitan or rural municipality; by cultural or social perspectives, for example, ethnicity, race or sexuality; or by an organisational perspective, such as a school community. Regardless of where CHNs are working, a thorough understanding and knowledge of the community and population group/s ensures that planned and implemented programs are appropriate and address identified needs (Kiper & Geist, 2020).

CASE STUDY 15.1

Toni is a CHN working in a large metropolitan community health program. Toni's role includes a broad range of activities such as coordination of community health promotion events and running a well women's health program that focuses on early intervention and health education. As part of her role, Toni provides cervical screening, health assessment and mental health support. She also runs a women's health discussion group once a month and a walking program for newly arrived migrant women.

Toni has become increasingly aware that several women she is seeing are experiencing intimate partner violence but are reluctant to seek help from family violence-specific services. As a result, Toni arranges several meetings with local service providers and community groups – including representatives from the municipal council's community services, the police, a family counselling service and a community-run emergency housing program – to discuss how to improve support for women and children experiencing violence. After several meetings, it is suggested that women might feel more comfortable initially coming to the community health centre to see a female nurse.

With support from her centre's management, Toni establishes a nurse-led health and well-being program specifically targeting women experiencing family violence. Through the program, Toni is able to give physical and emotional health support, provide information and education, and assist women to develop a safety plan. As women gain confidence, feel more empowered and are ready, Toni is able to link them and their children to other appropriate local medical, health, counselling and community services for ongoing support.

REFLECTION

1. CHNs must be responsive and adapt to a broad range of community needs. What qualities do you think a nurse would need to take on such a complex role in community health?
2. What skills and training would best prepare a nurse to work as a CHN?

Community needs assessment

CHNs gain an understanding of the community they work in through conducting comprehensive **community needs assessments (CNA)**, which provide information about the community's health risks, needs, strengths and resources (Clendon & Munns, 2022). Engaging with the community is vital throughout the process and is key to empowering community members to identify their needs and to plan interventions (Clendon & Munns, 2022). Communities may have specific cultural backgrounds that may require specific models of CNA (Wilson et al., 2021). CHNs also consult with other key stakeholders such as the local community, social and health services, local government and non-government organisations. They obtain information from a range of sources including government documents and statistics, existing community profiles, and reports by other community groups and services. A good starting point is to consider what information would be helpful in determining needs and strengths and how best to collect this information, much of which is now available online (see examples in Table 15.1).

Community needs assessment (CNA) – a systematic process that provides information about the health and social needs, strengths and resources of a community or population group that can be used to prioritise and plan interventions.

Table 15.1   Information collected in a CNA

Guiding questions	Data	Source
1. What are the characteristics of the population?	Population size, age distribution, gender, ethnicity, culture, languages spoken, income, employment, education level	Australian Bureau of Statistics (ABS) Statistics New Zealand (Stats NZ) Local health and municipal reports
2. What is the health of the population? Are some groups more susceptible to some illnesses and conditions?	Common illness and diseases, morbidity and mortality rates, leading cause of death	ABS SNZ Australian Institute of Health and Welfare (AIHW) State and national health department reports
3. What local factors are affecting the health of the community?	Geographic location, sociocultural factors (migration, ethnicity, attitudes, beliefs), education and employment opportunities, local industry, transport, local media such as radio/newspapers, parks and recreational activities, housing, social cohesion, social inclusion, environment (safety, pollution, green spaces)	Local reports ABS SNZ Observation from driving or walking around the local area
4. What does the community say about their health and health needs?	Needs, strengths, priorities, factors impacting on their health, the lived experience of individuals, families and groups	Talking with community members, health and community care providers, teachers, community support workers, the local church and community groups Interviews, focus groups, surveys, local health reports, previous consultations
5. What are the local, state and national health priorities?	Targeted areas, potential funding opportunities	Local, state and national health department reports Health policies Health initiatives
6. What is currently being provided to address the health of the community?	Local health, social and community services and programs; location; accessibility; social support structures; level of community involvement	Local and state government and state reports Local health and community service reviews and reports

An important aspect of assessing community needs is for CHNs to become familiar with the community by walking/driving around, observing activities and health behaviours (Clendon & Munns, 2022), for example, noting if people are out walking, playing sport/other recreational activities and gathering in groups. CHNs also get to know the community by meeting with individuals, families, groups and community leaders. Culturally aware and sensitive CHNs also gain insight into and understanding of the values, attitudes, beliefs, strengths and specific characteristics of a community or group that can promote and protect health (Roden et al., 2016).

The CNA provides the evidence for a planned response (Clendon & Munns, 2022). There are several phases of the assessment process through which CHNs systematically identify needs and develop strategies that address factors impacting health and health outcomes. This cycle is repeated from time-to-time to identify new or changing needs (see Figure 15.1).

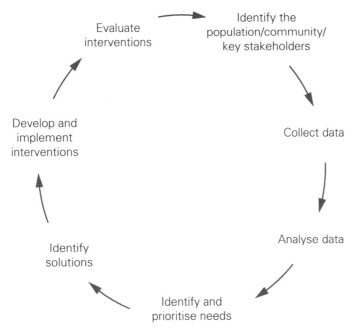

Evaluate interventions

Identify the population/community/ key stakeholders

Develop and implement interventions

Collect data

Identify solutions

Analyse data

Identify and prioritise needs

Figure 15.1   The community needs assessment cycle

Once information and data have been gathered, prioritising health needs can be challenging with competing agendas between different stakeholders. There is likely to be a great range of needs reflecting the diversity of the population. Therefore, it is important that those consulted are aware that it is unlikely that all needs identified can be addressed with limited health funding and resources. For example, a community may demonstrate a need for a heated pool to be used as hydrotherapy for older adults and to provide swimming lessons to improve water safety for local children. Yet insufficient funding or organisational support may be barriers to such a project. Therefore, a process of prioritising needs must follow the needs assessment and decisions made about how to best use available resources. Often, services exist as a historical legacy of earlier identified needs rather than to address newly identified needs. The data collected in a needs assessment helps services respond to changing circumstances and needs, which sometimes leads to the provision of a new activity or service that may displace another. Priorities and subsequent programs will also often align with state or national health priorities where funding is available. Principles of equity and social justice are applied to ensure services and programs are directed towards those with the greatest need and benefit to the community (see Chapter 11 for more detail about community health needs assessment).

REFLECTION

Consider the community where you grew up or are now living.

1. What do you know about the population living in this community and the factors that might impact their health?
2. Can you think of any programs or services that could address health needs and improve the health of this community?

Responding to identified needs

While in the inpatient setting, the focus is on illness and providing care, the community setting has more of a focus on prevention (Taylor et al., 2021). There is increasing awareness of the need to focus on health promotion and disease prevention (Smith, Crawford & Signal, 2016) with the Australian *National Preventive Health Strategy 2021–2030* (Department of Health, 2021) and the *New Zealand Health Strategy 2023* (New Zealand Minister of Health, 2023). These strategies focus on implementing systems that support health promotion and ensuring that interventions are relevant to the community involved, which are often identified by the CNA. With such a diversity of communities in Australia and Aotearoa New Zealand, the information obtained in the CNA is vital to determine relevant and appropriate health promotion and disease prevention activities for each community.

Health promotion and disease prevention occur at primary, secondary and tertiary levels (Clendon & Munns, 2022) and it is clear that CHN plays a pivotal role at each level. At the primary level of prevention, the nurse may be responsible for facilitating immunisation clinics and planning and developing facilities to assist the community in maintaining well-being and reducing risk factors for diseases, such as by supporting smoking cessation programs or educating the community on nutrition. Getting employers involved in health promotion assists in targeting health conditions that may be prevalent in specific industries, whereas community health promotion is beneficial in targeting health conditions related to physical or social environments. Both types of health promotion can involve screening days, where people can get health checks – such as their blood pressure or blood glucose levels – and be referred to their GP if concerns are identified. Education is a large component of tertiary prevention, and nurses play an important role in supporting peoples' understanding of their health and well-being. A nurse may be involved in organising a rehabilitation group, such as a pulmonary or cardiac group for people diagnosed with lung or heart conditions. These programs empower the person in managing their condition and slowing deterioration and also provide opportunities for monitoring and support (Mulligan et al., 2019). CHNs are innovative in seeking opportunities to connect with the community through whatever means are available and accessible in order to promote and improve health, and to promote the development of personal skills and healthy behaviours.

CHNs also provide primary care to the residents of the community, often in the person's home. This supports earlier discharge from acute care, and continuation of the journey to wellness. The CHN might care for wounds, monitor chronic conditions for early identification of change, check medication and blood pressure, and many more activities. This role allows the person to remain at home for care and reduces hospitalisation. It requires close collaboration with the person's health care team and community service providers, and often, being an advocate for the person (Blay et al., 2022). The possibilities of the CHN's role are endless and shaped by the needs of each community. Creativity and flexibility are essential characteristics of the role of CHNs; their practice is as diverse as the communities they work within. Each day is unlikely to be similar.

CASE STUDY 15.2

Katrina is a CHN working in an outer metropolitan suburb with a high proportion of the population under the age of 25. A CNA has identified several health factors affecting the health of the young people in the area including higher-than-average early school leaving age, high levels of unemployment, high rates of underage alcohol consumption and binge drinking, and higher-than-average teenage pregnancy. The young people are reluctant to attend local health services and have limited access to public transport. There are several fast-food businesses operating in the suburb, which have become the meeting place for young people. One of the few recreational activities is the newly built skateboard park.

Katrina is invited to participate in a local committee, which has been set up by the local municipal council to address the growing needs of young people. Other members of the committee include the council community services manager, two council youth workers, a council project officer, a high school welfare officer, a local pharmacist, the coordinator of a local church youth group, a drug and alcohol worker from the city – who provides a local service one day a week – two local teenagers and a GP interested in young people's health.

The committee considers some programs and activities that could improve the health of young people. Katrina suggests that a specific youth health service may improve access to health information and health services.

With support from the local GP and the maternal child and health nurse, Katrina applies for a small start-up grant from the local council to establish a youth health service to run from the community health centre one evening per week. At the service, Katrina provides health information, health screening and assessment, health education and referral. Katrina also agrees to work with the local high school to provide health education sessions on safe sex and the harmful use of alcohol and drugs. She collaborates with the drug and alcohol worker and a mental health worker to provide specialised counselling and support for young people at the youth health service. Katrina and other committee members also apply for an arts and recreation grant to promote health and well-being through young people's participation in circus skills training provided by an experienced circus troupe. The program is designed to provide young people with an opportunity to develop positive connections with each other, to participate in healthy exercise and to build self-esteem. The program is to run for three months at the council-funded recreation hall and be coordinated by the council youth workers.

REFLECTION
1. What are the potential benefits of the CHN being involved in the local committee?
2. Are there any potential challenges for the CHN working within this multidisciplinary team?
3. How would you evaluate the effectiveness of the youth health service?

Community and professional practice

CHNs rely on having strong working relationships with the community and therefore need to build and maintain relationships with key members, specific population groups, community leaders and health and community service providers (Clendon & Munns, 2022). This requires CHNs to establish credibility, which is particularly important for accessing some of the more vulnerable members of the community. Credibility may relate to acceptance, acknowledgement and respect for cultural beliefs and values; knowledge of the local community's social, political and historical context; demonstrated commitment and interest in the community or particular groups within the community; and persistence. Cultivating networks with community members and other service agencies can be time-consuming, may be challenging at times and may show little immediate effect. However, it is often the strength of these 'behind the scene' networks that facilitates successful action and positive health outcomes. Cooperation and coordination between services with a similar community focus usually result in the most effective strategies. This is achieved through well-developed communication, negotiation and interprofessional practice skills (Taylor et al., 2021).

Identifying and addressing diverse community health needs requires a broad range of knowledge, skills and competence. CHNs require a comprehensive understanding of nursing and community practice, health promotion and PHC (Blay et al., 2022). They frequently have additional qualifications in community and public health, health promotion or specialised practice such as women's health, sexual health, youth health, diabetes education or immunisation. Some CHNs also have nurse practitioner qualifications that enable them to provide extended specialised care, such as contraception, or meet other needs as relevant. They are frequently the leaders and coordinators in identifying needs, program development, implementation and evaluation. Therefore, CHNs require strong communication, leadership, research, program planning, financial management and evaluation skills (Roden et al., 2016). CHNs are also frequently involved in seeking additional resources and funding, and therefore must become proficient in grant and report writing. Postgraduate qualifications in primary health nursing are an important factor in successfully meeting the diverse requirements of the CHN role (Taylor et al., 2021).

CHNs also have responsibility and accountability to their employers and funding bodies for the programs and activities that they implement and the resources that they use. Good community nursing practice is guided by evaluation and therefore CHNs should be engaged in a recurring process of assessing, planning, acting, and evaluating, and have a continuous cycle of reflection and action. Evaluation is used to determine the strengths and weaknesses of a program and to determine the effectiveness of the strategies implemented. Findings from the evaluation are used to improve various aspects of a program and to identify inconsistencies between program goals and the implementation process (Taylor et al., 2021). Evaluation findings are reported both to the agency that the CHNs work for and to funding bodies and government departments.

Conclusion

CHNs work in partnership with the community and key stakeholders to identify health needs and service gaps through a CNA. They are involved in developing and implementing a range of activities that address these needs creatively using available means and seeking out additional support and resources. Any response to an identified need requires careful planning and evaluation. CHNs also provide primary care to individuals and families. They frequently identify a need and establish a suitable response, which lays the groundwork for the development of specialist services. Their work incorporates activities representing many of the strategies of broader health promotion, especially health education with groups and the wider community.

CRITICAL THINKING ACTIVITIES

1. How would you define CHN practice?
2. What knowledge, training, skills and experience would best prepare nurses wanting to take on this role?
3. What are some of the challenges CHNs might face in working in such a diverse and autonomous role?
4. How is the role of CHNs similar or different to other community nursing roles?

FURTHER READING

Blay, N., Sousa, M.S., Rowles, M. & Murray-Parahi, P. (2022). The community nurse in Australia. Who are they? A rapid systematic review. *Journal of nursing management, 30*(1), 154–68. https://doi.org/10.1111/jonm.13493

Department of Health. (2021). *National Preventive Health Strategy 2021–2030.* Commonwealth of Australia.

New Zealand Minister of Health. (2023). *New Zealand Health Strategy.* Ministry of Health.

Roden, J., Jarvis, L., Campbell-Crofts, S. & Whitehead, D. (2016). Australian rural, remote and urban community nurses' health promotion role and function. *Health Promotion International, 31*(3), 704–14. https://doi.org/10.1093/heapro/dav018

REFERENCES

Blay, N., Sousa, M.S., Rowles, M. & Murray-Parahi, P. (2022). The community nurse in Australia. Who are they? A rapid systematic review. *Journal of Nursing Management, 30*(1), 154–68. https://doi.org/10.1111/jonm.13493

Clendon, J. & Munns, A. (2022). *Community Health and Wellness: Primary Health Care in Practice* (7th ed.). Elsevier.

Department of Health. (2021). *National Preventive Health Strategy 2021–2030.* Commonwealth of Australia.

Doolan-Noble, F., Tumilty, E., McAuley, K. & Stokes, T. (2021). How rural nurses in southern New Zealand navigate their ethical landscape – A qualitative study. *The Australian Journal of Rural Health, 29*(3), 332–40. https://doi.org/10.1111/ajr.12709

Gasperini, G., Renzi, E., Longobucco, Y., et al. (2023). State of the art on family and community health nursing international theories, models and frameworks: A scoping review. *Healthcare, 11*(18). https://doi.org/10.3390/healthcare11182578

Hewitt, S.L., Sheridan, N.F., Hoare, K. & Mills, J.E. (2021). Understanding the general practice nursing workforce in New Zealand: An overview of characteristics 2015–19. *Australian Journal of Primary Health, 27*(1), 22–9. https://doi.org/10.1071/PY20109

Kiper, V. & Geist, R. (2020). Nurses on the frontline: Improving community health. *Nursing Made Incredibly Easy, 18*(3), 22–6. https://doi.org/10.1097/01.nme.0000658188.17482.9a

LaMothe, J., Hendricks, S., Halstead, J., et al. (2021). Developing interprofessional collaborative practice competencies in rural primary health care teams. *Nursing Outlook, 69*(3), 447–57. https://doi.org/10.1016/j.outlook.2020.12.001

Minkler, M. (2022). *Community Organizing and Community Building for Health and Social Equity* (4th ed.). Rutgers University Press.

Mulligan, H., Wilkinson, A., Chen, D., et al. (2019). Components of community rehabilitation programme for adults with chronic conditions: A systematic review. *International Journal of Nursing Studies, 97*, 114–29. https://doi.org/10.1016/j.ijnurstu.2019.05.013

New Zealand Minister of Health. (2023). *New Zealand Health Strategy 2023*. Ministry of Health.

Roden, J., Jarvis, L., Campbell-Crofts, S. & Whitehead, D. (2016). Australian rural, remote and urban community nurses' health promotion role and function. *Health Promotion International*, *31*(3), 704–14. https://doi.org/10.1093/heapro/dav018

Roussy, V., Russell, G., Livingstone, C. & Riley, T. (2021). Mergers may enhance the legitimacy of community health organisations in neoliberal environments. *Journal of Health Organization and Management*, *35*(6), 717–32. https://doi.org/10.1108/JHOM-04-2020-0160

Smith, J.A., Crawford, G. & Signal, L. (2016). The case of national health promotion policy in Australia: Where to now? *Health Promotion Journal of Australia*, *27*(1), 61–5. https://doi.org/10.1071/he15055

Taylor, J., O'Hara, L., Talbot, L. & Verrinder, G. (2021). *Promoting Health: The Primary Health Care Approach* (7th ed.). Elsevier.

Wilson, D., Moloney, E., Parr, J.M., Aspinall, C. & Slark, J. (2021). Creating an Indigenous Māori-centred model of relational health: A literature review of Māori models of health. *Journal of Clinical Nursing*, *30*(23–24), 3539–55. https://doi.org/10.1111/jocn.15859

World Health Organization (WHO). (2017). *Enhancing the Role of Community Health Nursing for Universal Health Coverage*. WHO.

Home-based care

Amanda Moses, Maryanne Podham and Judith Anderson
With acknowledgement to Jacqueline Allen
and Rhonda Brown

16

LEARNING OBJECTIVES

At the completion of this chapter, you should be able to:

- understand the development of home-based nursing in Australia and Aotearoa New Zealand.
- identify safety issues related to visiting people in their homes from a risk management perspective.
- discuss how nurses work effectively within a multidisciplinary team.
- describe the roles of nurses in palliative and end-of-life care.
- understand case management and the skills nurses require to provide effective case management.

Introduction

Home-based care is common practice in many countries (Gasperini et al., 2023) and has had a long tradition in Australia and Aotearoa New Zealand. Home-based care now takes many forms, including the acute care program Hospital in the Home (HITH), a range of chronic disease programs (Blay et al., 2022) and community aged care. Home-based care provides many benefits to consumers, reducing their need to travel to services and associated costs. It also allows the health care provider to have a holistic picture of the consumers and for the consumers to feel empowered to manage their health care issues in their own homes, while continuing with normal daily activities in a setting that they are comfortable in (Blotenberg, Seeling & Büscher, 2023).

Home-based care is based on a person-centred philosophy that has the potential to deliver individualised and responsive care. The home-based nursing role is not without its challenges. Nurses who undertake home visits go into uncontrolled, and sometimes confronting, environments that may be suboptimal for the delivery of health care (Nix & Altom, 2023). However, the nurse providing care in the home can positively influence health outcomes for individuals and families by delivering tailored assessment, nursing care, case management, care coordination (Dadich et al., 2023; McKinlay, 2021), referral and advocacy.

Home-based care – care provided where people live.

The history of home-based care

Home-based nursing emerged in the late 1800s and was initially associated with charitable and philanthropic organisations that engaged lay personnel and women from religious orders, often without qualifications or professional training, to care for the sick in their homes (Madsen, 2013; Wood & Arcus, 2012). Over time, these organisations attracted government support and funding to enable them to employ professional nurses (Wood & Arcus, 2012). The first Australian district nursing service began in Melbourne in 1885 and, five years later, a similar service began in Aotearoa New Zealand with services spreading ever since (Australian Bureau of Statistics (ABS), 2012).

In the current context, governments and policymakers in Western countries, including Aotearoa New Zealand and Australia, are challenged to ensure health and care services for growing numbers of older people and people living with chronic disease. Many older adults expect to have choice and flexibility about the health and care services they receive and where they receive them (Marsh, Fuller & Anderson, 2021). These issues have resulted in considerable reforms to the funding of home-based care and a split between care models focused on providing personal care (e.g. assistance with activities of daily living) as distinct from clinical health care.

There are now many home-based models of care supporting a diverse range of services including acute care, obstetric and postnatal support and care, palliative care, mental health, home-based alcohol and drug withdrawal support, renal dialysis and **transitional care** with individuals moving between services and care settings (see other chapters for some of these specific roles). Registered and enrolled nurses and registered midwives work alongside other multidisciplinary health professionals within these models of clinical health care. This is distinct from personal carers, who are an unregulated workforce who provide personal care services, particularly in the context of older adults and people living with a disability. The emergence of home-based services has improved access and the financial and logistical barriers of travelling to and receiving care in facilities.

Transitional care –
interventions and approaches that promote the safe and timely transfer of individuals between levels of care including from hospital to the community.

Changing contexts of home-based care

Technological advances have increased the range of services that can be provided in the home. In particular, technology has increased the use of machines and mechanical devices, such as portable intravenous pumps and syringe drivers, and the availability of remote monitoring and telehealth (Halcomb et al., 2023). Nurses require sound practical knowledge regarding a wide variety of devices and technology solutions to ensure that they are used effectively (Ashley et al., 2023). This includes the ability to troubleshoot and educate individuals and/or their families about self-management and the use of equipment.

The high level of autonomy in providing home-based nursing care also brings significant responsibility (Gray, Currey & Considine, 2018; Rusli et al., 2022). Additionally, the environment and facilities may be challenging in home-based settings, and access to resources is limited, requiring an ability to adjust and improvise accordingly to ensure safety (Shahrestanaki et al., 2023). As this population ages, community aged care is also growing.

Community-aged care

In Australia, community-aged care underwent major reforms in 2015, with the implementation of a **consumer-directed care (CDC) model** and the Commonwealth Home Support Program (CHSP) (Moore, 2021). The CHSP is an Australian government initiative that funds domestic assistance, transport, personal care, nursing and allied health care to support independence and improve a person's social connectedness (Department of Health and Aged Care, 2024a). In the CDC model and the CHSP, older adults and their carers can access high-level aged care packages and a range of personal and respite care services through private providers, not-for-profit providers and local councils. The implementation of the CDC means that older adults and their carers have control and choice about how to spend their care package funds. The shift to the CDC has increased the responsibility of older people and their informal carers for the management of their health and care (Department of Health and Aged Care, 2024b). This is because most care within the funded CDC model and the CHSP is directed and planned by the people themselves and focused on personal care needs provided by paid carers such as personal care attendants. Many older adults welcome these changes in home-based care. Health care services and the nursing profession are challenged to rethink what optimal support they can provide to older adults and people living with chronic disease in view of their increased responsibility for their health in the community (Marsh et al., 2021). Older adults living at home with health difficulties can access health care through their GP.

A similar model called self-directed support has also been adopted in Aotearoa New Zealand, although a review has identified the need for sustained investment to improve services, sustainability of the sector and workforce supply.

Consumer-directed care (CDC) model – (also known as 'self-directed care' and 'individualised budgets') developed in the United States in the 1990s, in this model the person manages the care package budget. It is linked to consumer satisfaction, greater choice and responsibility in care-related decision-making and is dependent on the availability of personal care workers, a market economy for personal care and an increased focus on personal care as a transaction.

The HITH program

The HITH program was first piloted in Australia in 1994 to provide acute care to people admitted to a health service in their own home as an alternative to being in a hospital (Hospital in the Home Society Australasia, 2015). In Australia, the state- and territory-based health departments define eligibility criteria to receive care at home through the HITH program. While eligibility criteria vary, they typically include acute conditions that can be safely treated in the home. Examples of HITH services include post-surgical care, complex wound care, intravenous antibiotics and diabetes management. In HITH programs, people are admitted to the relevant health service with access to the same services as inpatients. Care is provided by the HITH team, who are employed by the health service and includes doctors, nurses and allied health professionals (Hecimovic, Matijasevic & Frost, 2020). Health care consumers may also visit the HITH clinic for specified health services as outpatients.

The HITH program has been shown to reduce mortality, inpatient and health care costs in comparison to hospital-based care, as well as increase consumer and carer satisfaction (Montalto et al., 2022). However, it does not reduce the carer burden, as family members have a significant role in supporting the individual to ensure positive outcomes.

In Aotearoa New Zealand, primary and community health services have implemented several programs that support acutely unwell people to be cared for in the community. Some examples of these programs include Primary Options for Acute Care (POAC) and Acute Demand Management Services (ADMS) (Hospital in the Home Society Australasia, 2015).

Chronic disease management

To reduce the demand for inpatient acute care services, Australian state governments have developed, evaluated and implemented a range of chronic disease initiatives. While these vary between states and territories, they are underpinned by the *National Strategic Framework for Chronic Conditions* (Department of Health and Aged Care, 2020). These initiatives are now part of routine health care and focus on improving the management of a range of chronic diseases. Multidisciplinary teams, including nurses and collaborative care arrangements with GPs, support people living with chronic conditions and their families. In Aotearoa New Zealand, as part of the New Zealand Health Strategy, primary and community health services hold contracts with accredited home care providers to provide designated publicly funded services (Ministry of Health, 2023).

Palliative and end-of-life care

Palliative care involves the delivery of person- and family-centred care aimed at improving the quality of life for individuals who have been diagnosed with an incurable, active, progressive and/or advanced disease (Department of Health and Aged Care, 2023). Palliative care that is provided in the community allows the individual to maintain some aspects of normality in their lives alongside the management of their conditions (Dadich et al., 2023). The provision of palliative care in the community should focus on establishing a rapport with the individual, rather than the disease causing the symptoms, in order to support more personal interactions (Dadich et al., 2023). Nurses are involved in providing these individuals with physical (e.g. pain), emotional (e.g. fear), spiritual and cultural (e.g. loss of meaning) and social (e.g. stigma) care options to enhance their quality of life through the management of symptoms (Palliative Care Australia, 2018; Saurman, Wenham & Cumming, 2021).

An assessment of a person's needs and preferences for care should be identified at diagnosis and reassessed regularly (e.g. yearly) and when there is a change in condition or needs. Family members' needs and wishes should also be considered at these times as they are pivotal to the support of the person receiving palliative care (Palliative Care Australia, 2018).

An advanced care plan enables people to discuss their values and future wishes regarding their health care and interventions. Nurses can use the plan to be informed of their care at a later point in time when they are unable to articulate their preferences (Landefeld & Incze, 2020). While there are variations across jurisdictions regarding the specifics of documenting these wishes, creating an advanced care directive (or living will) is a legally binding document that helps both health professionals and family members make decisions.

End-of-life care occurs when an individual with an incurable condition, an acute exacerbation of a pre-existing condition that they are unlikely to recover from or a life-threatening condition due to a catastrophic event, such as a motor vehicle accident or self-harm, is expected to die within a few hours or days (Australian Commission on Safety and Quality in Health Care (ACSQHC), 2023). There has been an increase in people wishing to die in their homes. To support this demand, various services have been established or expanded. In Aotearoa New Zealand an End of Life Choice Act has been legislated since 2019 and there is a centralised Assisted Dying Service (Health New Zealand, 2024). Most Australian states and territories have a last days of life home support service, which assists community nurses in providing care and support for individuals to die in their own homes supported by their family and friends (New South Wales (NSW) Health, 2018).

In addition to unassisted death, nurses working within home-based care organisations may be involved in the delivery of voluntary assisted dying (VAD), which has been introduced in recent years in both Australia and Aotearoa New Zealand. This right allows a person with a terminal illness to request medication to end their life. The specific criteria a person must meet to be eligible for VAD varies across Australian states and territories and in Aotearoa New Zealand. While this kind of program is in its infancy in Australia and Aotearoa New Zealand, it raises numerous ethical and professional issues for nurses delivering care in the home and requires specific training to perform (Ministry of Health, 2024; NSW Health, 2023).

Home visiting and risk management

Risk assessment should be undertaken before a first visit to a client's home. Nurses should become familiar with their organisation's policies, procedures and reporting arrangements about risk assessment, any risks identified or any **adverse event** that may occur. Risk assessment should be undertaken proactively as standard practice on a first visit and as soon as a potential hazard has been identified. Once a risk has been identified, action is required. The seriousness of the situation is considered, followed by consideration of actions that may reduce or eliminate the risk (ACSQHC, 2021). In many organisations, if a visit is considered to be high-risk, nurses may be required to visit in pairs (Small, 2020).

Adverse event – an event that has resulted or may have resulted in harm to a health care consumer or staff member (ACSQHC, 2021).

Common risks to nurses practising in client homes are trip hazards, poor air quality, pests and rodents (Polivka et al., 2015). However, concerns about workplace violence, particularly when working alone, in unsafe neighbourhoods or when seeing clients with a history of violence, are important to consider (Nix & Altom, 2023).

Preparing for a home visit

A comprehensive referral document can detail information to the health care provider about the cultural background, safety of access; history of mental illness, violence, or drug abuse in the home, and the presence of animals and/or other people who may reside there. A pre-visit phone call is often part of an organisation's intake protocol. This usually involves a checklist that covers aspects of safety and security (Small et al., 2020).

REFLECTION

Consider what information the nurse needs to know about a person's home environment before a visit. How would you structure questions to obtain this information?

When risks have been identified, strategies to control those risks should be determined. Table 16.1 provides an example of possible risk control strategies.

Once the plan for risk management has been decided, it is important that this information is communicated to all relevant health care workers who could be exposed to the hazards identified. It is important to revisit the document regularly to review and revise the assessment as necessary (Small et al., 2020).

Table 16.1   Examples of risk control strategies

Risk control	Explanation	Examples
Elimination	Can the risk be eliminated?	Can a smoker agree not to smoke during the time of the visit?
Substitution	Can the risk be reduced by using something else?	Can health care workers use an alternate entry to the location due to environmental risks?
Isolation	Can the risk be reduced by isolating the hazard from the people?	Can a pet be put outside and on a leash during the visit?
Engineering	Can the risks be reduced using mechanical/electrical devices?	Use a mechanical aid to help a client with manual handling
Administrative means	What procedures are required to ensure the controls are followed?	Ensure safe work procedures for taking blood.
Personal protective equipment (PPE)	Having considered all other options, what items of PPE will be required to minimise the risk?	Wear gloves while taking bloods.

Source: Adapted from Safe Work Australia (2024).

Telephoning the client before visiting alerts them to the impending visit, enabling them to confirm they are at home and restrain any pets before the nurse's arrival. Managers or other staff should be aware of the nurse's planned movements with a list of client names, addresses and phone numbers, the anticipated time of return or the expected time to call in, following the visit.

During the visit

Most home visits are welcoming, but professionals must consider that this workspace is someone's home. On arrival, nurses should state who they are and why they have come and show their identity badge. Encouraging clients to ask to see identification protects the client as well as the professional. Nurses should be sensitive to the cultural background, asking about cultural practices and seeking guidance regarding these. It is not always obvious if someone is from a different cultural background and many people will adapt their cultural practices as they see fit, so it is important not to label people or expect them to behave in specific ways (Kelly et al., 2022). Nurses should identify if there are any other people in the home, understand the layout of the house and note exit points. Nurses should ensure that they have a charged mobile phone with pre-programmed emergency contacts to enable easy access. Personal alarms are also useful in some situations and can call attention to a difficult situation (Small et al., 2020).

Nurses should not react to conditions that may seem unacceptable to them such as a dirty or smelly environment. Establishing trust can be assisted by the health care professional focusing on addressing the reason the client requires professional care and not appearing judgemental. An altered mental state caused by pain, feeling scared, substance use, cognitive impairment, mental illness and previous trauma can increase the risk of aggression and violence. Nurses must remain alert for cues of increasing agitation that could escalate into aggression. Threats should be taken seriously. It may be necessary to decide if the situation can be de-escalated or if it is safer to shorten the visit and leave the premises. Nurses should trust their instincts and not wait until there is an incident if uncomfortable feelings are building up (Small et al., 2020).

If de-escalation is to be attempted, it may involve various actions depending on the specific situation. Sensory overload can result in confusion and agitation, particularly in older adults or those with sensory issues. Turning the television off or minimising other sources, such as noise or people talking to the client, may de-escalate the situation (Somes, 2023). When the situation involves an agitated person, only one person should talk to them in a slow, calm, gentle and direct manner, giving one clear instruction at a time with an emphasis on reassurance. Distraction is another useful technique. This might be achieved by asking if the person is in pain or uncomfortable, as pain relief, food, hydration or toileting may be needed (Somes, 2023).

When clients are at-risk

Nurses need to be aware of the relevant policies for the protection of their clients; for example, mandatory reporting of child or elder abuse, bearing in mind that these requirements vary across jurisdictions (Australian Law Reform Commission, 2024). However, some client risks may be less well-defined. A frail, elderly client may live in suboptimal circumstances and be unable to adequately look after themselves. If the client has the cognitive capacity to make informed decisions, their autonomy must be respected. When a client refuses care or the help of services, it can be ethically challenging for nurses to support this right to choose and place themselves at-risk.

Medication management, including polypharmacy, is another potential risk for clients, particularly those transitioning home following hospitalisation. Periods of transition increase the risk of medication errors (Mohammad, DiTommaso & Jacobsen, 2020). Nurses can provide education, resources and referrals for safe medication self-management, ensuring that clients understand how to take their medication correctly (Shang et al., 2021).

CASE STUDY 16.1

Jeremy, a nurse who provides community-based clinical care, has been visiting Mary twice a week to manage a slow-healing leg ulcer. Mary lives in a small, well-maintained house on a large block of land on the outskirts of town. When Jeremy arrives, he notices several cars that he has never seen before. Jeremy recalls Mary mentioning that her grandson was coming to visit her. Mary had been quite excited about this, as she had not seen her grandson for over five years due to family conflict.

When Jeremy knocks on the door, it is violently yanked open by a shirtless and dishevelled young man. In an angry tone, the man asks Jeremy what he wants and what he is doing there. Jeremy explains that he has come to attend to Mary's leg and asks if he is Mary's grandson. The young man says that he is not Mary's grandson, but a friend of his, and opens the door to let him in. He then tells Jeremy that 'the old lady is in her bedroom' and walks back into the lounge room, where almost a dozen young men are sleeping. As Jeremy surveys the usually spotless room, he notices drug paraphernalia, empty beer bottles and fast-food wrappers strewn across the floor. As he is about to enter Mary's bedroom, he meets the eye of a young man, which makes him feel uncomfortable.

CASE STUDY 16.1 Continued

When Jeremy enters Mary's bedroom, he observes that she is pale and appears teary. Mary apologises to Jeremy for the state of her house and says that she hopes the boys were not rude to him. Jeremy expresses his concern for Mary and comments that she does not appear to be her usual self. Mary explains that her grandson has brought several friends with him on his visit, and the boys have been partying late into the night so she has not had much sleep. Mary also informs Jeremy that the boys have broken a few of her things. She concludes this with the comment that 'boys will be boys'. Jeremy asks Mary if she would like him to ask the young men to leave. Mary appears a little frightened and tells Jeremy that he should just attend to the dressing and go.

REFLECTION

1. What are the potential risks in this situation?
2. Who do you think is at-risk?
3. How should this situation be best managed?

Multidisciplinary practice

Nurses conducting home visits often work as part of a multidisciplinary team or alongside multidisciplinary health care professionals. Nurses must collaborate with and make referrals to various providers including those within their multidisciplinary team and health service, such as allied health professionals, and those outside their health service such as dentists or optometrists. Nurses may also refer to other community health and social care agencies. They may also take on the role of **care coordination** and **case management** (Putra & Sandhi, 2021).

Care coordination – the organisation of care and the sharing of information between services to ensure safer and more effective care.

Case management – assessment, planning, facilitation and advocacy for services to meet the needs of the individual. Often extending beyond health care needs to include social needs.

REFLECTION

1. Consider how you work with other health care professionals during your day. How do you adapt to meet somebody's health needs?
2. Consider how technology supports your work. How could you use it more effectively to improve the health care that you provide?

In the home setting, nurses may be required to make care decisions, acting decisively and proficiently while remaining within their scope of practice and practice guidelines (Nursing and Midwifery Board of Australia (NMBA), 2016; Nursing Council of New Zealand (NCNZ), 2007). This requires the nurse to have the essential clinical expertise and confidence to manage a range of issues in sometimes ambiguous circumstances. In these situations, quality communication of assessment information with members of the multidisciplinary team and network is crucial. Nurses in the home are often required to contact other health practitioners in public and private health networks and hospitals, in community health and general practice, and in emergency services. In remote areas where nurses may have difficulty accessing the multidisciplinary team, for example, due to limited telephone coverage, their scope of practice is also driven by defined protocols to enable timely care and first aid (NMBA, 2016; NCNZ, 2007).

CASE STUDY 16.2

Jen is a registered nurse who works for the HITH program at a rurally-based health service. She is called on Saturday evening to go to visit a farmer out of town. James Bird is 60 years old and lives on a large 5000 ha property with his wife Sue, who is a teacher. Jen first visited James two days ago after he was transferred to the HITH program from the acute medical ward in the hospital for treatment of cellulitis in his lower left leg following a superficial laceration that he sustained after falling from his quad bike while checking cattle.

This was James' first experience of being in the hospital. He was anxious about being away from his farm and preoccupied with the risk of fire to his property. James had insisted on returning home and the doctors agreed to transfer him to the HITH program as he was well supported at home by his family. With this in place, he returned home on oral antibiotics and required a daily wound dressing to his leg.

Sue calls Jen, worried that James is unwell and has developed a fever again. The visit to the property involves a 45 km drive on an unsealed road, taking an hour due to poor road conditions. Jen arrives at the house at 9.30 p.m. to find James in bed. He has not eaten since breakfast and appears dehydrated. He is shivering and has a temperature of 39.5°C. James also appears to be in a low mood, stating: 'I'm useless. I can't even get to the toilet, let alone take care of the farm.' He is also experiencing significant leg pain.

On discussing James' return home, Jen learns that Sue is working full-time as a teacher, which is taking her away from the farm for long periods of time. This leaves James alone during the day. James and Sue have three sons who live and work in neighbouring properties, with the closest being 30 km away. The farmhouse, built on stilts, is very old and has six steps up to the entrance. The toilet is external to the house and is about 50 m away.

REFLECTION

1. What assessment and interventions should Jen implement to ensure appropriate care for James?
2. What are some of the challenges in delivering care for James?
3. What additional support is needed for both James and Sue to enable an effective outcome for James?

Case management

Case management involves a multidisciplinary team, including a nurse, that assists the individual, their family and support networks to attain identified health and health care goals. The phases of case management are described in Table 16.2. During the case management process, a case manager is involved to assist in the navigation of resources (Putra & Sandhi, 2021).

Table 16.2   Phases of case management

Phase	Description
Identification	Individual identified as meeting criteria for case management Consent obtained to begin process
Assessment	Comprehensive personal and medical data gathered from the individual regarding their needs Family and support people also interviewed to determine their needs
Planning	Goals of care/needs identified and prioritised Identification of appropriate services and resources that address the needs
Implementation	Case management activities and plans implemented Outcomes monitored
Evaluation and follow-up. Transition to self-care	Review, evaluation, monitoring and reassessment of individual's health status and goals
Termination of case management	Following reassessment, if individual has met goals and their functional abilities increased, case management can cease
Post transition	Further follow-up to ensure goals are still being met and to identify any new considerations for review/assessment

Source: Adapted from Case Management Body of Knowledge (n.d.).

A nurse's role in case management

The specific skills required for effective case management will be dependent on the health needs of the individual, the nature of the organisation and the scope of the case management being undertaken. However, key skills for effective case management include highly developed clinical knowledge and practice skills, excellent communication and interpersonal skills, and well-developed skills in client advocacy and negotiation (Joo & Liu, 2019). Case management depends on effective communication, interprofessional practice and skills in health education. Case managers need to develop and sustain relationships with individuals and their carers/families to build trust, facilitate open communication and develop therapeutic relationships. Facilitating client self-determination and supporting the development and maintenance of self-management strategies are also key aspects of the role. Additionally, case managers need to work collaboratively within the broad multidisciplinary care team to facilitate optimal access to appropriate services (Putra & Sandhi, 2021). While all nurses advocate for their clients, the case management role requires a high level of advocacy to connect individuals to relevant services (Baker, 2020). Advocacy involves representing the needs and interests of the individual to obtain the services required, which may include persuading those in positions that facilitate action and resources to provide assistance. It may also involve ensuring that reasonable adjustments or alternatives are made to meet any special needs of the individual and promoting opportunities for independence in the community. Case managers need to be knowledgeable about local providers, resources and support groups from whom the individual could benefit. They need to know any specific participation criteria for various programs, services and resources the individual might be able to access, as well as any rules or regulations that may influence eligibility for particular services. When a case manager is unable to broker care that completely meets the specific needs of the individual, the manager may need to advocate for the removal of barriers that impede service access, or for new resources to help meet individual needs.

Conclusion

The availability of a range of programs enables care to be provided to individuals and families in their own homes. Care in the home aims to promote individuals' autonomy and control over their own health. Chronic disease management and palliative care are particularly suitable for home-based management. Within a home-based care program, nurses may provide a range of interventions, care coordination and case management for individuals and their families, working in collaboration with other health care practitioners and support workers from a range of disciplines in community- and hospital-based settings.

Working in people's homes requires nurses to be adaptable and flexible. At times, they may also need to manage potential risks to both themselves and the people in their care. Providing care in the home can be challenging because the environment is constantly changing. Despite this, nurses can positively influence health outcomes for individuals and support greater choices for individuals and families in terms of where health care is provided.

CRITICAL THINKING ACTIVITIES

1. What are the advantages and challenges of providing care in people's homes?
2. What does the future of home-based nursing look like with current technological developments?
3. How would you prepare yourself for being a case manager?

FURTHER READING

Dadich, A., Hodgins, M., Womsley, K. & Collier, A. (2023). 'When a patient chooses to die at home, that's what they want... comfort, home': Brilliance in community-based palliative care nursing. *Health Expectations: An International Journal of Public Participation in Health Care and Health Policy, 26*(4), 1716–25. https://doi.org/10.1111/hex.13780

James, S., Ashley, C., Williams, A., et al. (2021). Experiences of Australian primary healthcare nurses in using telehealth during COVID-19: A qualitative study. *British Medical Journal Open, 11*(8), e049095–e049095. https://doi.org/10.1136/bmjopen-2021-049095

Rusli, K.D.B., Ong, S.F., Speed, S., et al. (2022). Home-based care nurses' lived experiences and perceived competency needs: A phenomenological study. *Journal of Nursing Management, 30*(7), 2992–3004. https://doi.org/10.1111/jonm.13694

REFERENCES

Ashley, C., Williams, A., Dennis, S., et al. (2023). Telehealth's future in Australian primary health care: A qualitative study exploring lessons learnt from the COVID-19 pandemic. *British Journal of General Practice Open, 7*(2), BJGPO.2022.0117. https://doi.org/10.3399/BJGPO.2022.0117

Australian Bureau of Statistics (ABS). (2012). *History of home nursing in Australia*. Australian Government. www.abs.gov.au/ausstats/abs@.nsf/0/911b5af72f818795ca2569de0024ed5a?OpenDocument#:~:text=Home%20nursing%20began%20in%20Australia,disadvantaged%20sick%20people%20at%20home

Australian Commission on Safety and Quality in Health Care (ACSQHC). (2021). *Incident Management Guide*. ACSQHC.

——— (2023). *Essential elements for safe and high-quality end-of-life care: National Consensus Statement*. ACSQHC. https://www.safetyandquality.gov.au/sites/default/files/2023-12/national_consensus_statement_-_essential_elements_for_safe_and_high-quality_end-of-life_care.pdf

Australian Law Reform Commission. (2024). *Mandatory reporting*. Australian Government. www.alrc.gov.au/publication/family-violence-a-national-legal-response-alrc-report-114/8-family-violence-and-the-criminal-law-an-introduction-2/mandatory-reporting/

Baker, M. (2020). "Boots-on-the-Ground" advocacy: Field case management and transitions of care. *Professional Case Management, 25*(1), 46–7. https://doi.org/10.1097/ncm.0000000000000411

Blay, N., Sousa, M.S., Rowles, M. & Murray-Parahi, P. (2022). The community nurse in Australia. Who are they? A rapid systematic review. *Journal of Nursing Management, 30*(1), 154–68. https://doi.org/10.1111/jonm.13493

Blotenberg, B., Seeling, S. & Büscher, A. (2023). Acceptance of preventive home visits by nurses – The user perspective. *Public Health Nursing, 40*(5), 662–71. https://doi.org/10.1111/phn.13217

Case Management Body of Knowledge. (n.d.). *Introduction to the Case Management Body of Knowledge*. Commission for Case Manager Certification. https://cmbodyofknowledge.com/content/introduction-case-management-body-knowledge

Dadich, A., Hodgins, M., Womsley, K. & Collier, A. (2023). 'When a patient chooses to die at home, that's what they want… comfort, home': Brilliance in community-based palliative care nursing. *Health Expectations: An International Journal of Public Participation in Health Care and Health Policy, 26*(4), 1716–25. https://doi.org/10.1111/hex.13780

Department of Health and Aged Care (2020). *National Strategic Framework for Chronic Conditions*. Commonwealth of Australia. www.health.gov.au/resources/publications/national-strategic-framework-for-chronic-conditions?language=en

——— (2023). *What is palliative care?* Commonwealth of Australia. https://www.health.gov.au/topics/palliative-care/about-palliative-care/what-is-palliative-care

——— (2024a). *Commonwealth Home Support Programme: Programme (CHSP): Program Manual 2024–2025*. Commonwealth of Australia.

——— (2024b). *Home Care Packages Program*. Commonwealth of Australia. www.health.gov.au/our-work/home-care-packages-program

Gasperini, G., Renzi, E., Longobucco, Y., et al. (2023). State of the art on family and community health nursing international theories, models and frameworks: A scoping review. *Healthcare, 11*(18). https://doi.org/10.3390/healthcare11182578

Gray, E., Currey, J. & Considine, J. (2018). Hospital in the home nurses' assessment decision making: An integrative review of the literature. *Contemporary Nurse: A Journal for the Australian Nursing Profession, 54*(6), 603–16. https://doi.org/10.1080/10376178.2018.1532802

Halcomb, E., Ashley, C., Dennis, S., et al. (2023). Telehealth use in Australian primary healthcare during COVID-19: A cross-sectional descriptive survey. *BMJ Open, 13*(1), e065478. https://doi.org/10.1136/bmjopen-2022-065478

Health New Zealand. (2024). *About the assisted dying service*. New Zealand Government. www.tewhatuora.govt.nz/for-the-health-sector/assisted-dying-service/about-the-assisted-dying-service/

Hecimovic, A., Matijasevic, V. & Frost, S.A. (2020). Characteristics and outcomes of patients receiving Hospital at Home Services in the South West of Sydney. *BMC Health Services Research, 20*(1), 1090–1090. https://doi.org/10.1186/s12913-020-05941-9

Hospital in the Home Society Australasia. (2015). *History of the HITH Society*. www.hithsociety.org
.au/Our-History

Joo, J.Y. & Liu, M.F. (2019). Case management effectiveness for managing chronic illness in Korea:
A systematic review. *International Nursing Review, 66*(1), 30–42. https://doi.org/10.1111/
inr.12472

Kelly, J., Stevenson, T., Arnold-Chamney, M., et al. (2022). Aboriginal patients driving kidney
and healthcare improvements: recommendations from South Australian community
consultations. *Australian and New Zealand Journal of Public Health, 46*(5), 622–9. https://doi
.org/10.1111/1753-6405.13279

Landefeld, J. & Incze, M.A. (2020). Advance care planning – What should I know? *JAMA Internal
Medicine, 180*(1), 172–2. https://doi.org/10.1001/jamainternmed.2019.0005

Madsen, W. (2013). Exploring the ethos of district nursing, 1885–1985. *Contemporary Nurse: A Journal
for the Australian Nursing Profession, 44*(2), 242–52. https://doi.org/10.5172/conu.2013.44.2.242

Marsh, P., Fuller, A. & Anderson, J. (2021). Can a Home Care Package deliver a meaningful life?:
Challenges for rural home care delivery. *Journal of Hospital Administration, 10*(2), 12–20.
https://doi.org/10.5430/jha.v10n2p12

McKinlay, E. (2021). Doing what it takes: A qualitative study of New Zealand carers' experiences of giving
home-based palliative care to loved ones. *New Zealand Medical Journal, 134*(1533), 21–32.

Mohammad, N., DiTommaso, M. & Jacobsen, S. (2020). Nurse practitioner-led Care Transitions
Program: Medication management from skilled nursing facility to home. *Journal for Nurse
Practitioners, 16*(8), 560–3. https://doi.org/10.1016/j.nurpra.2020.05.017

Moore, C.B. (2021). Consumer directed care aged care reforms in Australia since 2009:
A retrospective policy analysis. *Health Policy, 125*(5), 577–81. https://doi.org/10.1016/
j.healthpol.2021.03.012

New South Wales Health (NSW Health). (2018). *Last days of life home support services*. www.health
.nsw.gov.au/palliativecare/Pages/last-days-of-life-home-support-services.aspx

—— (2023). *What is voluntary assisted dying and who is eligible?* www.health.nsw.gov.au/
voluntary-assisted-dying/Pages/eligibility.aspx

Ministry of Health. (2023). *New Zealand Health Strategy*. New Zealand Government. www.health
.govt.nz/publications/new-zealand-health-strategy

—— (2024). *About the assisted Dying Service*. New Zealand Government. www.health.govt.nz/
our-work/regulation-health-and-disability-system/assisted-dying-service/about-assisted-dying-
service#:~:text=The%20Assisted%20Dying%20Service%20allows,Zealand%20on%207%20
November%202021

Montalto, M. & Ko, S.Q. (2022). Telling the difference and the telling differences between hospital in
the home and outpatient parenteral antibiotic therapy. *Internal Medicine Journal, 52*(5), 880–4.
https://doi.org/10.1111/imj.15780

Nix, E. & Altom, K. (2023). Safety concerns associated with home care nursing. *Home Healthcare
Now, 41*(3), 135–9. https://doi.org/10.1097/nhh.0000000000001161

Nursing and Midwifery Board of Australia (NMBA). (2016). *Registered Nurses Standards for
Practice*. NMBA.

Nursing Council of New Zealand (NCNZ). (2007). *Competencies for Registered Nurses*. NCNZ.

Palliative Care Australia. (2018). *National Palliative Care Standards* (5th ed.). Palliative Care Australia.

Polivka, B.J., Wills, C.E., Darragh, A., et al. (2015). Environmental health and safety hazards
experienced by home health care providers: A room-by-room analysis. *Workplace Health and
Safety, 63*(11), 512–22. https://doi.org/10.1177/2165079915595925

Putra, A.D.M. & Sandhi, A. (2021). Implementation of nursing case management to improve
community access to care: A scoping review. *Belitung Nursing Journal, 7*(3), 141–50.
https://doi.org/10.33546/bnj.1449

Rusli, K.D.B., Ong, S.F., Speed, S., et al. (2022). Home-based care nurses' lived experiences and
perceived competency needs: A phenomenological study. *Journal of Nursing Management,
30*(7), 2992–3004. https://doi.org/10.1111/jonm.13694

Safe Work Australia. (2024). *Managing risks*. www.safeworkaustralia.gov.au/safety-topic/managing-health-and-safety/identify-assess-and-control-hazards/managing-risks

Saurman, E., Wenham, S. & Cumming, M. (2021). A new model for a palliative approach to care in Australia. *Rural and Remote Health, 21*(4). https://doi.org/10.22605/RRH5947

Shahrestanaki, S.K., Rafii, F., Najafi Ghezeljeh, T., Farahani, M.A. & Majdabadi Kohne, Z.A. (2023). Patient safety in home health care: A grounded theory study. *BMC Health Services Research, 23*(1), 467–467. https://doi.org/10.1186/s12913-023-09458-9

Shang, J., Chastain, A.M., Perera, U.G.E., et al. (2021). The state of infection prevention and control at home health agencies in the United States prior to COVID-19: A cross-sectional study. *International Journal of Nursing Studies, 115*, 103841–103841. https://doi.org/10.1016/j.ijnurstu.2020.103841

Small, T.F. (2020). Home visiting safety for home healthcare clinicians. *Home Healthcare Now, 38*(3), 169–169. https://doi.org/10.1097/nhh.0000000000000880

Small, T.F., Gillespie, G.L., Kean, E.B. & Hutton, S. (2020). Workplace violence interventions used by home healthcare workers: An integrative review. *Home Healthcare Now, 38*(4), 193–201. https://doi.org/10.1097/nhh.0000000000000874

Somes, J. (2023). Agitated geriatric patients and violence in the workplace. *Journal of Emergency Nursing, 49*(3), 320–5. https://doi.org/10.1016/j.jen.2022.12.009

Wood, P. & Arcus, K. (2012). 'Sunless lives': District nurses' and journalists' co-construction of the 'sick poor' as a vulnerable population in early twentieth-century New Zealand. *Contemporary Nurse: A Journal for the Australian Nursing Profession, 42*(2), 145–55. https://doi.org/10.5172/conu.2012.42.2.145

Community mental health nursing

17

Caroline Picton and Christopher Patterson
With acknowledgement to Rhonda Brown

LEARNING OBJECTIVES

At the completion of this chapter, you should be able to:

- describe the context of mental health care in Australia and Aotearoa New Zealand.
- describe the recovery-oriented model of care.
- explain the role and key functions of community mental health nurses (CMHNs).
- explain the importance of promoting mental health.
- describe the role of community mental health nursing in addressing the social determinants of health.

Introduction

Mental illness continues to be a leading cause of illness in Australia and Aotearoa New Zealand. The effects of reduced mental health have significant consequences for individuals, families and the community. Prevention and early intervention are crucial to improve health outcomes. Much of the support and care for individuals and families experiencing mental health illness occurs within the community, and nurses are major providers of that care. This chapter focuses on the role of CMHNs in providing recovery-orientated care for individuals living with mental illness and their families.

The context of mental health care

There is a high prevalence of mental illness with around 43 per cent of Australians aged 16–85 experiencing a mental illness in their lifetime (Australian Bureau of Statistics (ABS), 2023). Around 22 per cent of the adult population aged 16–85 years will experience a common mental illness over a 12-month period (ABS, 2023). One in five Aotearoa New Zealanders aged 15 years and over are diagnosed with a mood and/or anxiety disorder (Wilson & Nicolson, 2020). Mental distress can be experienced in many ways and may be described as depression or anxiety, feeling isolated, being overwhelmed with stress or even in terms of physical symptoms. The use of terms, such as 'mental distress', 'mental health concerns' and 'psychological

Mental illness – a broad term for a range of illnesses and symptoms, sometimes referred to as a mental disorder, that significantly affect how a person thinks, feels and acts. Examples include depression, anxiety disorders, schizophrenia, post-traumatic stress disorder and bipolar disorder.

distress', recognise that people experience unpleasant and disruptive thoughts, feelings and other symptoms that are not necessarily related to a diagnosed mental illness. The use of these terms may sometimes be preferred by a person as the term 'mental illness' can be viewed as pathologising and having negative connotations.

The stigmatisation of mental illness within the community has had a significant and detrimental impact. People living with mental illness are among some of the most disadvantaged people in the community (Mental Health Coordinating Council (MHCC), 2022). Many live with psychosocial difficulties exacerbated by trauma, poverty and poor physical health. Often, they may encounter stigma as an inherent aspect of their daily life (MHCC, 2022).

Health professionals, including nurses, must be mindful of their own attitudes and language to avoid reinforcing stigma and negatively impacting those with mental distress and illness. Stigma can result in social isolation, social exclusion for those experiencing mental health issues and a reluctance to seek support (Kvalsvig, 2018). Fear of restrictive and traumatic interventions in mental health settings can also deter individuals from seeking help and following through with treatment (Kvalsvig, 2018).

Mental health – 'a state of well-being in which an individual realizes their own abilities, can cope with the normal stresses of life, can work productively and is able to make a contribution to his or her community' (World Health Organization (WHO), 2018).

Increasing awareness of **mental health** and mental illness in the community must be met with genuine, helpful support that is provided with hope and sensitivity to an individual's particular requirements (MHCC, 2022). No one should be defined by the mental health concerns, mental illness or psychosocial difficulties that they experience.

The recovery-oriented model of care

Since the 1990s, there has been a coordinated approach towards introducing a recovery model of care with an increasing shift away from institutional care (Ministry of Health, 2021; National Mental Health Commission (NMHC), 2023). National policy and funding have been redirected into delivering flexible and accessible community mental care services where people live and work. There is a greater emphasis on delivering comprehensive mental health care that includes the principles of primary health care (PHC) and health promotion. Over the last decade, a greater understanding of the impact of psychological trauma on mental health has led to incorporating trauma-informed approaches within service delivery. Complex models of care offer multiple options that are dynamic, collaborative and integrated, supporting prevention, treatment and recovery (Ministry of Health, 2021).

Mental health policies in Australia and Aotearoa New Zealand emphasise the prevention of suicide and stigma, early intervention and a recovery and trauma-informed culture (Department of Health, 2015; Ministry of Health, 2021). A whole-of-government approach is taken to collaborate with communities at a local level, with suicide prevention being central to policy reform (NMHC, 2023). From a recovery perspective, the lived experience of individuals and their families and carers is crucial to planning care. Recovery, unique for each individual, encompasses the capability to create and live a meaningful life. Recovery enhances participation and meaningful contribution at home, work, study and in the community, with or without the presence of mental health issues. In a recovery framework, mental health care is delivered through **recovery-oriented practice**.

Recovery-orientated practice – care that places the lived experience, skills and insights of individuals living with mental health issues, and their families, central to care. Individuals are supported to identify their strengths and determine their own paths to recovery.

Recovery-oriented practice emphasises hope, empowerment and social connection (Australian Health Ministers' Advisory Council, 2013). This way of working facilitates enhanced health and well-being and enables individuals to live self-directed and self-determined lives, self-manage symptoms and strive to reach their full potential (Australian Health Ministers' Advisory Council, 2013). In Australia, the Department of Health has outlined practice guidelines encompassing the promotion of a culture of instilling hope, person-centred and holistic care, personal support for recovery, organisational commitment and workplace development, and social inclusion (see Table 17.1).

Table 17.1 Recovery-orientated practice

Domains	Domain 1: Promoting a culture and language of hope and optimism (overarching domain) The culture and language of a recovery-oriented mental health service communicates positive expectations, promotes hope and optimism, and results in a person feeling valued, important, welcome and safe.			
	Domain 2: Person first and holistic	Domain 3: Supporting personal recovery	Domain 4: Organisational commitment and workforce development	Domain 5: Action on social inclusion and the social determinants of health, mental health and well-being
Capabilities	Holistic and person-centred service	Promoting autonomy and self-determination	Recovery vision, commitment and culture	Supporting social inclusion and advocacy on social determinants
	Responsive to Aboriginal and Torres Strait Islander peoples	Focusing on strengths and personal responsibility	Acknowledging, valuing and learning from lived experience	Challenging stigmatising attitudes and discrimination
	Responsive to people from immigrant and refugee backgrounds	Collaborative relationships and reflective practice	Recovery-promoting service partnerships	Partnerships with communities
	Responsive to gender, age, culture, spirituality and other diversity		Workforce development and planning	
	Responsive to lesbian, gay, bisexual, transgender and intersex people			
	Responsive to families, carers and support people			

Source: Australian Health Ministers' Advisory Council (2013, p. 5).

The attitudes of family, friends, and the broader community towards people living with a mental illness can exert a major influence on their quality of life. One of the main barriers to recovery is overcoming stigmatising attitudes that can cause isolation and discrimination. Nurses have a role in educating families and the community about mental illness and providing them with strategies to support individuals in their recovery. The CMHN may also need to advocate on behalf of the individual experiencing mental health issues or to support the community to call for changes in resources, policies and procedures to enhance community understanding of mental health, maintain safety in the community and improve service delivery (Keet et al., 2019). CMHNs can act as mediators and coordinate interactions between these different groups, who often have competing interests, in the pursuit of positive mental health outcomes for the individual and the community (NMHC, 2023).

Community mental health nursing

Community mental health nursing – nursing practice based on the social model of health focused on providing accessible and comprehensive mental health care within community settings.

The provision of mental health care in the community is a central focus of transforming mental health for all (WHO, 2022). Nursing is at the forefront of delivering this transformation. Though mental health care is the responsibility of all nurses (Halcomb et al., 2018), particularly in PHC, mental health nurses are highly specialised and possess postgraduate specialist qualifications (Buus et al., 2020). **Community mental health nursing** occurs outside the traditional confines of mental health inpatient settings, with community practice focused on the least restrictive care, that is, person-centred. Advances in medical care, newer and more effective pharmaceutical treatments, broader definitions of mental health and a deepening understanding of psychological trauma have driven significant developments in service delivery and have influenced the practice of mental health nurses. Central to the role of the CMHN is the emphasis on facilitating individuals' participation and collaboration with health care providers, and their families when appropriate, with a focus on empowerment and building of the strengths of the person living with a mental illness. Emphasis may also be on working to support a person experiencing social and economic consequences related to living with a mental illness or health concern. The term psychosocial difficulty is sometimes used to describe the social disruption, barriers, challenges or inequalities a person experiences in life to their mental health condition. However, it is important to remember that not everyone living with a mental health condition has psychosocial difficulty.

CMHNs practise in a range of settings including public and private mental health services, community health centres, schools, general practice, forensic services, community nursing programs, substance abuse programs, aged care and supportive residential care (see Table 17.2). The practice of nurses working in community mental health settings is founded on the principles of PHC, health promotion and public health. Central to their practice are principles of self-determination and empowerment, and the participation of individuals and families in identifying needs and planning care consistent with recovery-oriented practice (NMHC, 2023). CMHNs have a specific role with individuals and families, focusing on maintaining physical and mental health and wellness, minimising the impact of mental health issues, and improving health and well-being. CMHNs may work in independent advanced practice roles, such as nurse practitioners, or as registered nurses within nursing or multidisciplinary teams.

The practice of CMHNs is diverse and focuses on recovery involving advocacy, counselling, symptom and medication management, education, mental health and risk assessment, physical assessment and monitoring of individuals at home or in supportive residential programs. These nurses can act in a pivotal role as care coordinators working with individuals who have complex needs. In this role, they consult and liaise with other health professionals, particularly when working with challenging presentations, to help find effective management strategies for a range of mental health issues as well as concomitant social and physical health

Table 17.2 Examples of community mental health nursing practice settings

Organisation	Services
Child and adolescent mental health services	Supporting children and adolescents aged 0–18 with emotional, psychological, behavioural, social and family problems including family education, individual and family therapeutic interventions
Early psychosis prevention and intervention programs	Supporting young people aged 14–25 who are experiencing or recovering from their first episode of psychosis to reduce the frequency and severity of relapse including education, individual and group psychosocial and vocational support, case management, family and carer support, and medication management
Crisis assessment and treatment teams	Providing acute mental health services for individuals in the most appropriate and least restrictive setting including assessment, community-based treatment and support, and referral to prevent admission to hospital
Mobile support and treatment services	Providing intensive long-term support for individuals with severe mental illness including review and assessment, care planning, monitoring and medication management
Dual diagnosis programs	Supporting people with a mental illness and substance abuse problem including referral, education for individuals, families and communities, and individual and group therapeutic interventions
Homeless outreach services	Early identification, treatment and rehabilitation outreach for homeless individuals who may not otherwise engage with clinical and treatment services
Aged persons mental health services	Providing support for individuals aged over 65, including community assessment, care planning, case management, treatment and rehabilitation programs
Community care units	Providing medium- to long-term support for individuals in a supportive community-based residential program either by health professionals who work there or who visit regularly
Forensic and correctional services	Providing health care to individuals and their families in contact with the legal system including community and hospital forensic services, court and police systems, and correctional facilities
Migrant and refugee programs	Providing health and social needs assessments, advocacy and support that promotes social connection, integration and well-being of newly arrived people
Suicide Prevention Outreach Team	Providing assertive, mobile outreach support to people experiencing a situational crisis or suicidal distress. Peer workers with lived experience and clinicians work collaboratively with the person seeking help to provide recovery-oriented and trauma-informed support. This includes assertive follow-up, psychosocial support, safety planning and identification of community supports.

problems (Buus et al., 2020). They also provide support to carers and families through health education and supportive individual and family counselling. CMHNs teach personal, life and relationship skills for building healthy relations that enable individuals to recover within their own environment with the support of their own social networks (Keet et al., 2019). A significant development from a recovery perspective is the emphasis on and the recognition of the

Peer support – mental health, emotional and social support provided by individuals with a shared personal experience as consumers or carers, who are trained to use their experiences to support others in recovery (Mutschler et al., 2022).

value of the **peer support** workforce. Peer support workers, sometimes referred to as consumer consultants, have experienced mental illness and the use of the service system. They work collaboratively with CMHNs and other health professionals, using their experience to support others, adding value through empathy for lived experience and recovery (Ministry of Health, 2021). The Suicide Prevention Outreach Team (see Table 17.2) exemplifies this collaborative, person-centred and empathetic approach when supporting people who are experiencing psychosocial situational and/or suicidal distress.

CASE STUDY 17.1

Neave was first hospitalised for depression when she was 16. She remembers being happy as a child, having friends and loving school. In her second year of high school, she began to have episodes of dark moods and felt detached from those around her. She lost her sense of fun and would often withdraw, not wanting to go to school or see anyone. There were times when she felt it would be better 'not to be around'. During her teens, she had several admissions to an adolescent psychiatric unit. Her experiences of being an inpatient were not very positive, and she would always resist admission as 'they didn't get it; they didn't understand me'.

Despite this, she did well at school and got into university to do a bachelor of arts degree, with a particular interest in writing. Throughout her twenties, Neave continued to experience periods of depression but also had instances when she was happy, elated even, and energetic. During these times, she was always 'on the go' and often stayed up most of the night to write. It was during these periods that she believed her writing was the most creative and productive. But these times were often followed by deep despair and depression. Her parents did not understand what was happening or how best to support her.

Neave was eventually diagnosed with bipolar disorder when she was 29. She began taking mood stabiliser medication and started seeing Rachel, a psychiatrist with whom she really connected and was able to talk. With Rachel's support, and that of her friends and family, Neave has come to understand more about bipolar disorder and how it affects her. Over time, she has accepted her diagnosis and has learnt how to recognise and manage her symptoms. As part of Neave's recovery, she contacted a peer support and advocacy organisation where she met other people who had experienced living with mental illness. Here, she felt understood, accepted and able to be herself.

Three years on, Neave is now a peer support worker helping others who are experiencing mental distress and living with mental illness. She is also writing a book of short stories that she hopes will be published.

REFLECTION

1. Consider Neave's story. What do you believe contributed to her recovery?
2. How do you imagine the role of the peer support worker is similar or different to the role of the CMHN?
3. What are the advantages of having peer support workers or consumer consultants in mental health care?

For more information about the work of peer support workers, visit the website of the Aotearoa New Zealand-based Mental Health Advocacy and Peer Support (MHAPS) organisation (www.mhaps.org.nz).

To support individuals in planning their recovery, CMHNs need information and understanding of the factors affecting the individuals' health. This information is gained through comprehensive mental health assessment in collaboration with individuals and, where appropriate, their families and carers (Hungerford et al., 2020). Not only does assessment gather information about presenting mental health issues and personal and social circumstances, but it also identifies individual's goals, hopes, aspirations and the actions they can take to improve their health and recovery. Assessment is used to identify needs, provide a baseline of an individual's mental health, and plan and support recovery. There are many components of a comprehensive mental health assessment and aspects to consider (see Table 17.3). A strengths-based approach begins with an assessment emphasising the importance of the interpersonal relationship between the CMHN and the individual, and focuses on the strengths of the individual to achieve their own defined goals and recovery (Naidoo, 2017).

Table 17.3   Components of a comprehensive mental health assessment

Domain	Aspects to consider
Presenting issues	Recent difficulties
	Psychological symptoms
	Feelings
	Mental state
	Cognition
	Risks and vulnerability – suicide risk, physical risks
Personal	Expectations and priorities
	Current relationships and sexual partners
	Education
	Children
	Interests
	Spiritual beliefs and cultural influences
	Stress and coping skills
	Major life events (losses, transitions, change, trauma, abuse)
	Current or past dealings with the law
Physical and mental health	Previous and ongoing health problems, developmental history
	Previous admissions to hospital and community mental health services
	Ongoing physical and mental health problems
	Medications – past and present
	Use of alcohol and other drugs
	Understanding of health problems, medications and path to recovery (health literacy)
	Other health and community care providers involved

Table 17.3 (cont.)

Domain	Aspects to consider
Social	Living arrangements
	Relationships – past and present
	Work/study
	Employment
	Social networks
	Available support and/or carer involvement
	Current and past life events impacting mental health
Family	Childhood
	Adolescence
	Family members' medical and psychiatric condition and/or drug use
	Family violence
Personal strengths	Aspirations
	Hopes
	Goals
	Relationship skills
	Coping skills
	Resilience – strategies used to deal with adversity

Promoting mental health

Mental health promotion is work central to transforming the environments that influence our mental health (WHO, 2022). Mental health promotion works by identifying factors that influence mental health and intervening at individual, familial and community levels to positively influence mental health and well-being (WHO, 2022). There has been an increasing focus on **mental health promotion**, with opportunities for CMHNs to incorporate a health promotion framework into their practice. For example, CHMNs can be involved in providing individualised health education about symptoms and strategies for managing depression but can also work with community groups to build community capacity, raise awareness, develop support and education programs, or implement wellness programs that promote emotional health through physical activity.

Mental health promotion – involves actions that enable people to adopt and maintain healthy lifestyles and create living conditions and environments that support mental health (NMHC, 2023).

Health promotion and prevention is targeted across the lifespan beginning in childhood through to older adulthood. The interventions should be directed towards prevention, early intervention, the promotion of human rights and the impact of mental health issues (WHO, 2022). As such, CMHNs are involved in a range of health-promoting interventions including:

- raising public awareness and understanding of mental health to reduce stigma and discrimination
- creating suicide prevention strategies

- promoting the rights, opportunities and care for individuals and families experiencing mental illness
- supporting parents to build child-parent relationships through developing effective parenting skills
- promoting the mental health of children and adolescents through school-based personal development programs to build life skills, support diversity and acceptance, promote healthy lifestyles, counter bullying and violence, and promote early detection and intervention for mental health issues
- devising mental health interventions at work (for example, programs to reduce stress)
- supporting the elderly including promoting social connection (for example, through attending community-based day centres)
- screening, assessing and providing referral and intervention for family violence and hazardous alcohol and other drug use as well as raising awareness of its impact on mental health
- providing mental health promotion activities targeting vulnerable populations including Indigenous and Māori populations, refugees and migrants, and LGBTQIA+ populations (WHO, 2022).

REFLECTION

1. What mental health promotion programs are you aware of in your community?
2. How effective do you think these programs are in raising awareness of mental health and reducing the impact of mental illness?

The CMHN must recognise that promotion alone is insufficient. Depending on the psychosocial difficulties resulting from mental illness and their urgency, access to quality interventions for mental health improvement or recovery is crucial (WHO, 2022).

Addressing the social determinants of health

Mental health promotion interventions work by identifying the factors influencing mental health at the individual, social and structural levels. They aim to mitigate risks, enhance resilience and foster supportive environments conducive to mental health and well-being. There are many factors that contribute to mental health and, therefore, recovery. Among these, social determinants feature prominently, impacting mental health and also access to help and resources (NMHC, 2023). Not only do social determinants impact mental health, but mental health also impacts social determinants. For example, experiencing mental distress or mental illness can cause psychosocial difficulties and affect one's capacity to complete school or work, affecting economic security and potentially leading to homelessness. Therefore, there is a reciprocal relationship between mental health and determinants of health (Deferio et al., 2019). Integrating a social model of health alongside medical and psychological approaches enables CMHNs to work with individuals and communities more holistically. From this perspective, CMHNs are well placed to not only identify the impact of social determinants but also to identify and address the impact of mental distress on social determinants including housing, employment, relationships and social connectedness.

CMHNs work in partnership with individuals, their families, communities and other health and community care professionals in education, welfare, community health, general practice, employment, housing and legal and financial services to address identified psychological, social, economic and environmental issues that affect mental health and quality of life. Interventions focus on improving mental health and well-being by promoting:

- social inclusion and connectedness
- a feeling of safety
- a shared experience and peer connection
- resilience building
- empowerment through self-determination, agency, responsibility
- a sense of well-being
- self-esteem and self-worth
- optimism
- hope
- a sense of wellness
- regaining meaning and purpose
- meaningful participation in life family, community and schoolwork (Brown et al., 2019, p. 171).

Case manager – a term for an individual or team, who provides continuity of care, and plans and organises the coordination of health care services (Stretton, Chan & Wepa, 2023).

A CMHN often takes on the role of **case manager**. In this role, the CMHN works in collaboration with the individual and, where appropriate, the family or carer to coordinate assessment, facilitate access to services and support the development of and follow the individual's plan for recovery (Stretton, Chan & Wepa, 2023). In the case manager role, the CMHN works closely with individuals and other involved health professionals and community services – including GPs, PHC nurses, allied health professionals, peer workers and networks, mental health services, schools, employment agencies and support groups. Within this collaboration, the CMHN seeks to identify opportunities to source appropriate community-based resources and help individuals and their families/carers increase their health knowledge, skills and confidence in finding the support and resources that they need.

CASE STUDY 17.2

Lucas, aged 45, is married to Sara and they have two children aged 11 and 13. Lucas has a long history of depression and anxiety, which he remembers starting in his adolescence around the time his parents separated. Lucas didn't like school and didn't do very well. However, he later trained as a journalist but has only been able to work as a freelance writer due to long periods of depression requiring absences from work. He has also been hospitalised in the past for treatment of depression. Growing up, he remembers his mother working very hard but still struggling to provide for Lucas and his younger sister, with little support from Lucas' father, whom Lucas has not seen since he was 13. Lucas is close to his mother, who he sees regularly.

Twelve months ago, Lucas' sister died in a car accident when she was on her way to visit him, and he has struggled to come to terms with her death. Lucas has recently visited his GP, who prescribed a new course of antidepressants and suggested that he may benefit from some additional support. Lucas has agreed to see Megan – a CMHN working in their general practice.

In their first session, Megan asks Lucas what his main concerns are at present. Lucas reveals that he is feeling overwhelmed, is not sleeping very well, is worried 'about everything' and doesn't have much energy for the children or for writing. He doesn't believe that he is contributing enough to the family, particularly financially. Sara is pregnant with their third child, which was unplanned. Even though they have adjusted to the news and are happy to be having another child, Lucas is worried that this will be an added burden to their financial situation. Sara works part-time at a plant nursery, but Lucas worries that if he does not find more permanent work, they may not be able to meet the mortgage repayments. Sara is very supportive of Lucas, and tries to reassure him that everything will be OK and that things are not as bad as he thinks. He tells Megan that he finds exercise helpful to deal with stress but at the moment feels too tired and unmotivated to do it. This makes him feel worse about himself. Megan listens to Lucas and asks him what has worked to help improve his mood in the past. He struggles to answer but does say that if only he had the energy to exercise more regularly, he is sure he would feel better. He also says he misses contact with other writers since not having a regular job.

REFLECTION

1. What social determinants can you identify that potentially impact on Lucas' mental health?
2. What would you include in your assessment of Lucas?
3. From a recovery framework, what would your approach be to help Lucas?

Conclusion

With most mental health care now provided in community settings, CMHNs have a significant role in providing specialist support for people who experience mental health distress and who live with mental illness. This support emphasises empowerment, self-determination and recovery. Recovery-oriented practice is individualised and encompasses the ability for the person to create and live a meaningful life with or without mental illness. By integrating a social model with medical and psychological approaches, CMHNs can work with individuals and communities more holistically. They practise in diverse settings with individuals, groups and communities in enabling, advocating and mediating roles that promote and support recovery as defined by the individuals with whom they work. They work collaboratively with individuals, their families, carers and other health and community care providers to offer specialist nursing expertise to promote mental health and well-being.

CRITICAL THINKING ACTIVITIES

There are a growing number of community support and mental health promotion initiatives. Investigate and review one of the following examples using the questions below to guide your inquiry:

- Australian Indigenous Health*InfoNet* (https://healthinfonet.ecu.edu.au/)
- Beyond Blue (https://www.beyondblue.org.au/)
- Mental Health Foundation of New Zealand (https://mentalhealth.org.nz/)
- Waitematā DHB Whītiki Maurea – Māori Mental Health and Addiction Services (https://www.waitematadhb.govt.nz/hospitals-clinics/clinics-services/whitiki-maurea-maori-mental-health-and-addictions-service/)

1. Does your chosen initiative provide community-based mental health care? On what basis have you made this decision?
2. What strategies are used to promote mental health and well-being?
3. Do these strategies incorporate a recovery framework?

FURTHER READING

Hungerford, C., Hodgson, D., Clancy, R., et al. (2020). *Mental Health Care: An Introduction for Health Professionals*. John Wiley & Sons.

Mutschler, C., Bellamy, C., Davidson, L., Lichtenstein, S. & Kidd, S. (2022). Implementation of peer support in mental health services: A systematic review of the literature. *Psychological Services*, *19*(2), 360–74. https://doi.org/10.1037/ser0000531

Picton, C., Fernandez, R., Moxham, L. & Patterson, C. (2020). Experiences of outdoor nature-based therapeutic recreation programs for persons with a mental illness: A qualitative systematic review. *JBI Evidence Synthesis*, *18*(9), 1820–69. https://doi.org/10.11124/jbisrir-d-19-00263

REFERENCES

Australian Bureau of Statistics (ABS). (2023). *National Study of Mental Health and Wellbeing*. Australian Government. www.abs.gov.au/statistics/health/mental-health/national-study-mental-health-and-wellbeing/latest-release

Australian Health Ministers' Advisory Council. (2013). *A National Framework for Recovery-Oriented Mental Health Services: Guide for Practitioners and Providers*. Commonwealth of Australia. www.health.gov.au/sites/default/files/documents/2021/04/a-national-framework-for-recovery-oriented-mental-health-services-guide-for-practitioners-and-providers.pdf

Brown, R., McGarry, D., Kent, K., Miles, M. & Francis, M. (2019). Living with mental illness. In L. Deravin & J. Anderson (eds), *Chronic Care Nursing: A Framework for Practice* (2nd ed., pp. 162–83). Cambridge University Press.

Buus, N., Clifford, B., Isobel, S., et al. (2020). *Exploring the Role of Mental Health Nurses in a Successful Mental Health System*. www.researchgate.net/profile/Niels-Buus/publication/346932934_Exploring_the_role_of_Mental_Health_Nurses_in_a_successful_Mental_Health_System/links/5fd2ce2f92851c00f8662073/Exploring-the-role-of-Mental-Health-Nurses-in-a-successful-Mental-Health-System.pdf

Deferio, J.J., Breitinger, S., Khullar, D., Sheth, A. & Pathak, J. (2019). Social determinants of health in mental health care and research: A case for greater inclusion. *Journal of the American Medical Informatics Association*, *26*(8–9), 895–9. https://doi.org/10.1093/jamia/ocz049

Department of Health. (2015). *Australian Government Response to Contributing Lives, Thriving Communities – Review of Mental Health Programmes and Services*. Commonwealth of Australia. www.health.gov.au/sites/default/files/response-review-of-mental-health-programmes-and-services.pdf

Halcomb, E., McInnes, S., Moxham, L. & Patterson, C. (2018). *Mental Health Practice Standards for Nurses in Australian General Practice*. Australian College of Mental Health Nurses Inc.

Hungerford, C., Hodgson, D., Clancy, R., Murphy, G. & Doyle, K. (2020). *Mental Health Care: An Introduction for Health Professionals* (4th ed.). John Wiley & Sons.

Keet, R., deVetten-McMahon, M., Shields-Zeeman, L., et al. (2019). Recovery for all in the community. Position paper on principles and key elements of community-based mental health care. *BMC Psychiatry*, *19*, 174. https://doi.org/10.1186/s12888-019-2162-z

Kvalsvig, A. (2018). *Wellbeing and Mental Distress in Aotearoa New Zealand: Snapshot 2016*. Health Promotion Agency. www.hpa.org.nz/sites/default/files/Wellbeing-And-Mental-Distress-Snapshot-2016-Final-FEB2018.PDF

Mental Health Coordinating Council (MHCC). (2022). *Recovery Oriented Language Guide (3rd ed)*. MHCC NSW. https://mhcc.org.au/wp-content/uploads/2022/10/Recovery-Oriented-Language-Guide-3rd-edition.pdf

Ministry of Health. (2021). *Mental Health and Addiction Year in Review*. New Zealand Government. www.health.govt.nz/system/files/documents/publications/moh-mental-health-and-addiction-year-in-review-web.pdf

Mutschler, C., Bellamy, C., Davidson, L., Lichtenstein, S. & Kidd, S. (2022). Implementation of peer support in mental health services: A systematic review of the literature. *Psychological Services*, *19*(2), 360–74. https://doi.org/10.1037/ser0000531

Naidoo, V. (2017). Identifying strengths and formulating needs statements. In S. Trenoweth & N. Moone (eds), *Psychosocial Assessment in Mental Health* (pp. 144–84). SAGE Publications.

National Mental Health Commission (NMHC). (2023). *Vision 2030 for Mental Health and Suicide Prevention*. www.mentalhealthcommission.gov.au/projects/vision-2030

Stretton, C., Chan, W.-Y. & Wepa, D. (2023). Demystifying case management in Aotearoa New Zealand: A scoping and mapping review. *International Journal of Environmental Research and Public Health*, *20*(1), 784. https://doi.org/10.3390/ijerph20010784

Wilson, A. & Nicolson, M. (2020). *Mental Health in Aotearoa: Results from the 2018 Mental Health Monitor and the 2018/19 New Zealand Health Survey*. Te Hiringa Hauora/Health Promotion Agency. www.hpa.org.nz/sites/default/files/Mental_Health_Aotearoa_Insight_2020.pdf

World Health Organization (WHO). (2018). *Mental health: Strengthening our response. Fact Sheet 220*. www.who.int/news-room/fact-sheets/detail/mental-health-strengthening-our-response

——— (2022). *World Mental Health Report: Transforming Mental Health for All*. WHO. www.who.int/publications/i/item/9789240049338

18 Maternal, child and family health nursing

Catina Adams and Leesa Hooker
With acknowledgement to Anne Hepner,
Barbara Hanna and Kim Hyde

LEARNING OBJECTIVES

By the end of this chapter, you should be able to:

- understand the practice and policy context of maternal, child and family health nursing.
- describe the role of the maternal, child and family health nurse in primary care and primary health care (social justice, equity, and empowerment).
- identify the role of the enhanced maternal, child and family health and outreach service.
- describe the scope of maternal, child and family health nursing practice.

Introduction

The health and well-being of families is an important consideration for federal, state, and/or local levels of government. Family health policies based on recent knowledge of early child-hood development have evolved to emphasise the importance of providing every child with the best possible start to life (Center on the Developing Child, 2016). Childhood sets the foundation for future health and well-being and is recognised by the 1979 *United Nations Convention on the Rights of the Child* (United Nations Children's Fund (UNICEF), 2009). To impact health inequalities, government policies and services must address the social determinants of early child health, development and well-being (Marmot, 2010; World Health Organization (WHO), 2023). External factors directly influencing a child's health, such as maternal health and antenatal care during pregnancy, socio-economic gradients, food security, housing, child care and education, are emphasised (Marmot, 2010).

Nursing has a long history of working with families and promoting health. Nurses' and midwives' knowledge of families and health promotion are pivotal to the health and well-being of parents and children, given that pregnancy, birth and the early years are significant life events. The early years of life are critical in influencing future health and social outcomes across the lifespan (Crouch et al., 2020). **Epigenetic** studies show that early adversity, stress and poor development affect physical and mental health, behaviour and learning in later years (Janus et al., 2021). Investing in early childhood development

Epigenetics – the study of how our behaviours and environment can cause changes that affect how our genes work. Epigenetic changes affect gene expression, turning genes 'on' and 'off'. These changes are reversible and do not change our DNA sequence.

and early intervention is crucial, with returns far greater than the original investment (Jeong et al., 2021).

Developmental neurobiology studies indicate that every baby has billions of neurons representing lifelong potential (Shonkoff, Slopen & Williams, 2021). The more stimulating the environment, the greater the connection between neurons, which leads to increased potential for enhanced development in children. This is particularly important during the first three years of life (National Scientific Council on the Developing Child, 2020).

Families thrive with adequate antenatal care, universal access to child and family health services (Marmot, 2010; Schmied et al., 2015), and quality early childhood education, child care and preschool (Goldfeld et al., 2019). Children will grow into adults who, in turn, will have greater potential to contribute towards a rapidly changing global society.

This chapter introduces maternal, child and family health nursing and outlines the key functions of this crucial community nursing role. Foundational principles of primary health care practice are explored, and case studies are used to illustrate strengths-based, family-centred care (FCC).

Practice and policy context

Child health

In Australia and Aotearoa New Zealand, most children are healthy. A 50 per cent improvement in child mortality has occurred in Australia in the past 25 years with improvements in child morbidity (Australian Bureau of Statistics (ABS), 2024). A similar fall in child mortality rates can also be seen in Aotearoa New Zealand (Adams et al., 2022). There is room for improvement, however, with differences in child development according to where the family resides and their socio-economic status, reflecting the social gradient in 'all-cause mortality' (Adams et al., 2022; Chen et al., 2018). Almost one-quarter of Australian children have been classified as developmentally vulnerable (Australian Institute of Health and Welfare (AIHW), 2024). In addition, one in four children (aged 5–14 years) are overweight or obese, and Indigenous Australian children have significantly poorer health compared with non-Indigenous Australian children (AIHW, 2024). Similarly, Māori and Pacifica children and young people have significantly poorer health outcomes than other ethnic groups (Adams et al., 2022).

Universal health care services

Many countries, including Australia and Aotearoa New Zealand, provide universal community maternal, **child and family health services** free to all families. These services are based on core primary health care principles such as equity, access and empowerment, and intersectoral collaboration (Department of Health, 2022; New Zealand Guidelines Group, 2012) and aim to promote maternal, child and family health and well-being.

Community-based services are staffed by nurses who are educated in maternal, child and family health and who can provide a range of primary prevention and early intervention programs designed to support families in their parenting role (Department of Health, 2019b). In Australia, nurses who provide these services have different titles. This chapter uses the term 'maternal, child and family health nurse'. In Aotearoa New Zealand, Plunket or Well Child

Universal child and family health services – services offered to all families within the community through health promotion and preventative health initiatives. These may include immunisation programs, nurse home visits, centre consultations, telephone support and parenting groups (Department of Health, 2019a).

Tamariki Ora nurses are experts in child health and growth, supporting families to protect and improve child health (Health New Zealand, 2018).

Maternal, family and child health services differ in each state and territory in Australia and Aotearoa New Zealand (Schmied et al., 2015). The length of service provision varies between jurisdictions. Services most commonly include home visits, health centre-based consultations, telephone support, group education and health promotion sessions (Schmied et al., 2015). In most jurisdictions, the delivery of an equitable '**progressive universalism**' approach sees families offered universal access to services with more support provided proportionate to need (Collier et al., 2020).

Progressive universalism – a service-based response to address inequities, providing a universal service base that adds levels of support progressively for those with additional needs (Marmot, 2010; Schmied et al., 2015).

Service delivery

First contact with families is usually within two weeks of birth and attended in the home. Subsequent services are commonly provided in a health centre/clinic environment. In some jurisdictions, services may be available until a child is three and a half years old or extend to school entry age and beyond (Department of Health and Ageing, 2011). Aotearoa New Zealand's The Well Child Tamariki Ora Program is similar to Australia's maternal, child and family health nursing services. It is delivered nationally to families with children under five (Health New Zealand, 2018).

Flexible service delivery by some maternal, child and family health services allows additional consultations, drop-in sessions and outreach services (Department of Health, 2019a). After the initial home visit, subsequent visits are usually centre-based and involve assessments, health promotion and education. Depending on the age and stage of the child and family, discussions may include breastfeeding, sleep and settling, maternal health, family violence, child behaviour, communication, oral health, safety and play. The child health record is held by the parents, and provides information about the child's birth, immunisations, growth and development.

Maternal, child and family health nurses are registered nurses with postgraduate qualifications in midwifery and/or child and family health nursing. Postgraduate qualification requirements, length of study and nomenclature differ across states and territories (Schmied et al., 2015). Although many maternal, child and family health nurses are midwives, Victoria is the only state that requires these nurses to be registered as both a registered nurse and registered midwife in order to practise. Other Australian states and territories allow a single registered nurse or midwifery qualification (Schmied et al., 2015).

Continuity of care – the ability to provide uninterrupted care or service across programs, practitioners and levels over time (AIHW, 2024).

Continuity of care is provided following birth through hospital and/or midwife liaison with the maternal, child and family health nurse and continued through centre visits when possible. However, there is often inadequate information transfer from maternity to maternal, child and family health services, and improvements in communication and electronic data collection are needed (Schmied et al., 2015).

The role of the maternal, child and family health nurse

While experience and education levels may vary, maternal, child and family health nurses practise in a similar way (Fraser, Grant & Mannix, 2016). Working in partnership, maternal, child and family health services aim to promote healthy outcomes for children and their families by providing comprehensive primary health care. According to the Australian *National*

Framework for Universal Child and Family Health Services, the principles underpinning the maternal, child and family health service are:

- access
- equity
- health promotion and prevention
- working in partnership with families
- diversity
- collaboration and continuity
- evidence-based service (Department of Health and Ageing, 2011).

The maternal, child and family health nurse offers health promotion, education and support to families within local communities while providing early detection and referral for any developmental or health concerns (Department of Health, 2019a). This includes primary prevention (child safety), health promotion and education (sudden infant death syndrome prevention), anticipatory guidance, parenting skill development and support for parents (Department of Health, 2019a). Nurses participate in community capacity building and work collaboratively with families, other health professionals and other sectors of the community – such as early childhood educators, housing services and community police – to enable the best outcomes for families.

Across Australia, the timing and coverage of services offered by maternal, child and family health nurses differ (Schmied et al., 2015). In Victoria, the universal service is scheduled using a framework that delivers 10 free visits at key developmental ages and stages. These include a home visit soon after the infant is born, at 2, 4 and 8 weeks; 4, 8, 12 and 18 months; and 2 years and 3 and a half years (Department of Health, 2019b). Almost 90 per cent of 12-month-olds and 64 per cent of 3-and-a-half-year-olds are seen by maternal, child and family health nurses (Department of Health 2019c).

In Aotearoa New Zealand, the Well Child Tamariki Ora program consists of a series of health visits and support free to all families for children from around six weeks up to five years. The first visit is when the baby is four–six weeks. Visits are then scheduled at 8–10 weeks, 3–4 months, 5–7 months, 9–12 months, 15–18 months, 2–3 years, and then a before-school check (Health New Zealand, 2018).

The initial home visit enables the maternal, child and family health nurses to observe and gather information related to the family and the infant's feeding and sleeping patterns in a more relaxed atmosphere. Key areas of health promotion are addressed at each visit, and this is augmented with written educational information. According to local laws and within the context of practice, the maternal, child and family health nurse is mandated to report child abuse and neglect and is required to act on professional judgement regarding any child abuse concern under the Victorian government's *Children, Youth and Families Act 2005* (Victorian Government, 2005). Similar legislation and requirements apply in other states, and in Aotearoa New Zealand, the Oranga Tamariki Act 1989/Children's and Young People's Well-Being Act 1989 (Parliamentary Counsel Office, 1989) applies.

Many maternal, child and family health nurses provide maternal psychosocial health and well-being assessments. This includes supporting women recovering from birth, providing education and promotion of breastfeeding, contraception advice, and physical and emotional health assessments including routine screening for perinatal mental health disorders (for example, using the Edinburgh Postnatal Depression Scale) (Fraser, Grant & Mannix, 2016) and family violence screening (Hooker, Small & Taft, 2016). Women face significant morbidity in the postnatal period that is not being addressed by general practice; maternal, child and family health nurses are ideally placed to address this public health issue (Adams, Hooker & Taft, 2021; Hooker et al., 2016). Maternal, child and family health nursing is a complex and advanced clinical role that continues to evolve.

Equity and access

The social determinants inform health service delivery. Maternal, child and family health services informed by 'progressive universalism' seek to ensure improvements in the whole population and those with additional needs by providing additional resources and services. Some families require more support to access services or benefit from culturally appropriate support groups (Pokharel et al., 2021). Providing this service enhances access to maternal, child and family health services and prevents further disadvantage (Talbot & Verrinder, 2018).

To ensure ease of access, maternal, child and family health services are often co-located alongside other children's services. In remote settings, the maternal, child and family health nurse may travel to the community or arrange transport for families to the health service. For example, Queensland Health's Deadly Ears Program promotes ear and hearing health for Indigenous rural and remote children. Ear and hearing health is a major public health concern as hearing loss affects how a person interacts, understands and communicates with the world around them (Children's Health Queensland, 2020).

This free public health outreach program involves ready access to care from an interdisciplinary team of medical/nursing and allied health professionals and early childhood educators, all working collaboratively to prevent hearing loss and its consequences. Through equitable access, culturally safe practices and accessible health information, all children – regardless of their social, economic or cultural background – are provided with the chance to achieve and maintain optimal growth and development.

Community engagement and participation

Maternal, child and family health nurses work with parents and their children as well as community groups and agencies. Nurses hold community awareness campaigns on child accident prevention and encourage and support women to begin their children's playgroups or walking groups. Such self-sustaining support networks may lead directly to greater self-efficacy and personal empowerment for participating women (Schmied et al., 2015). Community participation is far more than simply engaging, consulting and informing. It involves ownership by the community with shared planning and decision-making.

REFLECTION

1. How do maternal, child and family health nursing principles and practices compare with other community nursing roles you are familiar with, or have read about in this text?
2. What personal attributes are important to have and to develop in this community work?

Practice approach

There have been significant changes to maternal, child and family health practice to provide a family-centred, **strengths-based approach** (Fraser et al., 2016). The strength-based approach requires service providers to view families through a lens of possibilities and potential rather than incapacities and deficits, to facilitate necessary change (Williams, 2019). Strengths-based practice involves assisting people to identify and appreciate their strengths and resources. It is 'based upon principles of respect, self-determination, empowerment, social justice and the sharing of power' (Fenton et al., 2015, p. 31).

FCC is a strengths-based relational approach to working in partnership with families (Ridgway et al., 2020). The family-centred approach may be implemented by using an evaluation tool known as the Parents' Evaluation of Developmental Status (PEDS) (Glascoe, 2013), which allows the maternal, child and family health nurse to discuss parental concerns related to the child's development. Conversation may progress towards anticipatory guidance of normal behavioural or developmental expectations. A secondary process, using developmental screening materials such as Brigance screening, is completed if developmental concerns are identified. The maternal, child and family health nurse uses professional judgement to guide parents to have developmentally appropriate expectations of their children and refer them to other services as necessary (Department of Health, 2019b).

> **Strengths-based approach** – based upon the principles of primary health care and the sharing of power, it works with and builds on people's strengths and capacities rather than focusing on their deficits or problems (McCashen, 2017).

CASE STUDY 18.1

The nurse, Sue, arrives at Yuan and Dave's home following the birth of their first baby, Ruben, seven days ago. Yuan had an unexpectedly difficult birth and is finding breastfeeding painful. Yuan and Dave are emotional and tired. Their families live interstate and overseas. Sue quietly sits with them and listens to their concerns, comforting them as to the normality of their emotions. She explains the maternal, child and family health service and the help available. Ruben awakes, and Sue observes Yuan's breastfeeding, offering simple ideas to improve her comfort. She offers reassurance and anticipatory guidance on normal infant behaviour and expectations and discusses safe infant sleeping positions. Sue writes the next few visit times, which have been arranged prior to this visit, in the child record book and shows Yuan and Dave the phone number of the 24-hour maternal and child health phone line. She provides educational information. Yuan and Dave appear to be comforted by Sue's presence.

REFLECTION

1. Consider the actions taken by Sue. Which of them could be considered health promotion?
2. How did Sue engage with Yuan and Dave?
3. What immediate, short-term and long-term needs were addressed through this visit?

Enhanced maternal, child and family health and outreach services

Throughout Australia and Aotearoa New Zealand, enhanced and/or outreach services are available for families identified as vulnerable and who require additional assistance (Department of Health, 2019a; Ministry of Social Development, 2015). Maternal, child and family health nurses see families with complex needs, including young parents, migrant and refugee families, parents with alcohol and other drug problems, and those involved with child protection (Rossiter et al., 2017). Enhanced services are often conducted in the home environment and have the flexibility of more frequent and longer visits than centre-based services. Outreach service teams may include a range of personnel such as maternal, child and family health nurses, family/parenting support workers, mental health nurses, social workers and psychologists (Adams, Hooker & Taft, 2022).

Enhanced nurse home visiting programs aim to prevent child abuse and neglect and are frequently targeted towards vulnerable, first-time parents. While the evidence is mixed, some intensive home visiting programs (for example, programs working with families prenatally until their children are two years old) have shown improvements in socio-economic, parenting and educational outcomes for family members (Goldfeld et al., 2019; Van Assen et al., 2020). Families may only require outreach services for a short time, or they may require them for many months. In Victoria, an evaluation of enhanced maternal, child and family health services showed significant diversity with variations in referral and intake criteria, service models and delivery modes (Adams, Hooker & Taft, 2019). Enhanced outreach service provision varies by service provider to suit local community requirements, for example, a focus on teenage parenting or Indigenous families. One example is the Australian Nurse-Family Partnership Program (ANFPP) for Indigenous Australian families delivered by community-controlled Aboriginal health services in the Northern Territory, New South Wales and Queensland (Zarnowiecki et al., 2018). This program aims to improve pregnancy, child health and development outcomes through enhanced parenting skills, parental education and work opportunities (ANFPP National Support Service, 2021).

Exploring maternal, child and family health nursing scope of practice

This case study provides an opportunity to explore some of the differences in the delivery of selective and comprehensive primary health care.

CASE STUDY 18.2

Kim, a maternal, child and family health nurse, is working with Tracee, who is a single parent with two children aged 8 weeks and 18 months. Tracee is thinking of weaning the eight-week-old baby from the breast so she can return to work, as she is having trouble making ends meet. The 18-month-old child has an eczema-type rash, and his behaviour has become increasingly challenging. Tracee is unwell, with an infection in her left breast (mastitis). She is feeling overwhelmed and tired and rarely goes out except to go to the supermarket. The family is new to the community and does not have any relatives or friends living nearby.

REFLECTION

1. What are the main issues that Tracee has identified?
2. What are the main concerns for Kim to address?
3. Care may be delivered using a primary care or primary health care approach. Consider both approaches for this family. What would each include?

A primary care approach

Within a primary care model, Kim will visit the family and assess Tracee's needs. She will advise on how to manage the mastitis and continue breastfeeding if this is Tracee's wish. Kim will assess the baby and enquire about possible causes of the toddler's rash. She may refer the child to a doctor. Kim may identify that Tracee needs extra support and will share information about how to recognise postnatal depression and contraceptive options and may offer additional visits with the family. In this model, the maternal, child and family health nurse provides medically focused, selective primary health care or primary care. However, within this service, there are some elements of a comprehensive primary health care approach as it is essential, free (affordable) and ongoing (available), culturally appropriate, easy to access and equitable.

A primary health care approach

Along with this medical care and advice, the primary health care approach to Tracee's care will be more comprehensive, working together to address the social determinants of health and improve outcomes for her and her children. Kim might encourage Tracee to contact a free financial services agency, to determine her eligibility for any financial support and connect with a local breastfeeding support group. Kim may also provide Tracee with details of a parenting class to assist with her toddler's challenging behaviour. Kim might discuss low-cost daycare options through the local council. Tracee is keen to continue breastfeeding, so Kim can encourage her to make enquiries at the daycare centre to determine how they can support her to maintain breastfeeding. With the support of her new friends at her local breastfeeding support group, Kim and Tracee might decide to approach other places, like the local cafe, about becoming accredited as 'breastfeeding friendly'.

Here, we can see Kim working with her client and other sectors of the community. Kim can offer encouragement and support. Tracee may feel more empowered discussing her options with someone who is familiar with the community, so she can make informed choices to improve her and her family's health. Respectful and non-discriminatory approaches enable and empower families to link with and strengthen community resources and may lead to economically productive and healthy lives.

REFLECTION

1. Has Kim used a strengths-based approach?
2. If so, how is this demonstrated?
3. What do you think the benefits and pitfalls of a strengths-based approach may be?

Conclusion

Maternal, child and family health nurses work with communities to provide primary health care services for infants, parents and families. Pregnancy, birth and the early years of parenting are significant transitional life events that influence child health and well-being into the future (Marmot, 2010). Service provision has changed over the years in response to the social needs of contemporary families. Maternal, child and family health nurses work collaboratively with other sectors and disciplines; engage with women, families and the community; and deliver primary health care services that are available, acceptable and sustainable as well as culturally safe. They work with families and in collaboration with other services to ensure that all 'children transition to school with the necessary skills for life and learning' (Department of Health and Ageing, 2011, p. 3).

CRITICAL THINKING ACTIVITIES

1. Locate the Primary Health Network in your area. What is its emphasis? Is this primary care or primary health care? How is maternal, child and family health nursing practice included?
2. Consider the written health promotion information provided to families at each consultation. How useful do you think it is for families? What other sources of information do families use? What can we do better to improve the health literacy of clients?
3. Consider the importance of involving the community in the design and delivery of services.

FURTHER READING

Ministry of Social Development. (n.d.). *Child and Youth Wellbeing.* New Zealand Government. https://www.msd.govt.nz/documents/about-msd-and-our-work/child-youth-wellbeing/reports/final-monitoring-of-child-and-youth-wellbeing-strategy-implementation.pdf

Moore, T., McDonald, M., McHugh-Dillon, H. & West, S (2016). *Community engagement: A key strategy for improving outcomes for Australian families.* (CFCA Paper no. 39.) Child Family Community Australia information exchange, Australian Institute of Family Studies.

Zarnowiecki, D., Nguyen, H., Catherine, H., Boffa, J. & Segal, L. (2018). The Australian Nurse-Family Partnership Program for aboriginal mothers and babies: Describing client complexity and implications for program delivery. *Midwifery, 65,* 72–81. https://doi.org/10.1016/j.midw.2018.06.019

REFERENCES

Adams, C., Hooker, L. & Taft, A. (2019). The Enhanced Maternal and Child Health nursing program in Victoria: A cross-sectional study of clinical practice. *Australian Journal of Primary Health, 25*(3), 281–7. https://doi.org/10.1071/PY18156

———— (2021). Threads of practice: Enhanced maternal and child health nurses working with women experiencing family violence. *Global Qualitative Nursing Research, 8*. https://doi.org/10.1177/23333936211051703

———— (2022). The characteristics of Australian Maternal and Child Health home visiting nurses undertaking family violence work: An interpretive description study. *Journal of Advanced Nursing, 79*(4), 1314–28. https://doi.org/10.1111/jan.15160

Adams, J., Duncanson, M., Oben, G., et al. (2022). *Indicators of Child and Youth Health Status in Aotearoa 2021 (Commissioned Report for External Body)*. New Zealand Child and Youth Epidemiology Service. http://hdl.handle.net/10523/14853

Australian Bureau of Statistics (ABS). (2024). *Births, Australia*. Government of Australia. www.abs.gov.au/statistics/people/population/births-australia/latest-release

Australian Institute of Health and Welfare (AIHW). (2024) *Australia's Health performance framework*. Government of Australia. https://www.aihw.gov.au/reports-data/australias-health-performance-v1/australias-health-performance-framework

Australian Nurse-Family Partnership Program (ANFPP) National Support Service. (2021). *Australian Nurse-Family Partnership Program*. Molly Wardaguga Research Centre and Charles Darwin University.

Center on the Developing Child. (2016). *From Best Practices to Breakthrough Impacts: A Science-Based Approach to Building a More Promising Future for Young Children and Families*. Harvard University. https://developingchild.harvard.edu/resources/from-best-practices-to-breakthrough-impacts/

Chen, Q., Kong, Y., Gao, W. & Mo, L. (2018). Effects of socioeconomic status, parent–child relationship, and learning motivation on reading ability. *Frontiers in Psychology, 9*. https://doi.org/10.3389/fpsyg.2018.01297

Collier, L.R., Gregory, T., Harman-Smith, Y., Gialamas, A. & Brinkman, S.A. (2020). Inequalities in child development at school entry: A repeated cross-sectional analysis of the Australian Early Development Census 2009–2018. *The Lancet Regional Health–Western Pacific, 4*. https://doi.org/10.1016/j.lanwpc.2020.100057

Crouch, E., Jones, J., Strompolis, M. & Merrick, M. (2020). Examining the association between ACEs, childhood poverty and neglect, and physical and mental health: Data from two state samples. *Children and Youth Services Review, 116*, 105155. https://doi.org/10.1016/j.childyouth.2020.105155

Children's Health Queensland. (2020). *Queensland Minimum Standards of Practice: Early Intervention for Children who are Deaf or Hard of Hearing and their Families*. Queensland Government. https://www.childrens.health.qld.gov.au/__data/assets/pdf_file/0025/174805/hh-min-stds-prac-qld.pdf

Department of Health. (2019a). *Maternal and Child Health Service Guidelines*. Victorian Government. www.health.vic.gov.au/publications/maternal-and-child-health-service-guidelines

———— (2019b). *Maternal and Child Health Service Practice Guidelines 2009. Revised 2019*. Victorian Government. www2.health.vic.gov.au/about/publications/policiesandguidelines/maternal-child-health-service-practice-guidelines

———— (2019c). *Enhanced Maternal and Child Health Program Guidelines*. Victorian Government. www.health.vic.gov.au/publications/enhanced-maternal-and-child-health-program-guidelines

Department of Health. (2022). *Future Focused Primary Health Care: Australia's Primary Health Care 10 Year Plan 2022–2032*. Commonwealth of Australia. https://www.health.gov.au/sites/default/files/documents/2022/03/australia-s-primary-health-care-10-year-plan-2022-2032.pdf

Department of Health and Ageing. (2011). *National Framework for Universal Child and Family Health Services*. Commonwealth of Australia. Commonwealth of Australia. www.health .gov.au/resources/publications/national-framework-for-universal-child-and-family-health-services?language=en

Fenton, A., Walsh, K., Wong, S. & Cumming, T. (2015). Using strengths-based approaches in early years practice and research. *International Journal of Early Childhood, 47*(1), 27–52. https://doi .org/10.1007/s13158-014-0115-8

Fraser, S., Grant, J. & Mannix, T. (2016). Maternal child and family health nurses: Delivering a unique nursing speciality. *Maternal and Child Health Journal, 20*(12), 2557–64. https://doi.org/10.1007/ s10995-016-2081-2

Glascoe, F. (2013). *Parents' Evaluation of Developmental Status – Revised (PEDS-R)*. https://www.rch .org.au/ccch/peds/For_Practitioners/

Goldfeld, S., Price, A., Smith, C., et al. (2019). Nurse home visiting for families experiencing adversity: A randomized trial. *Pediatrics, 143*(1), e20181206. https://doi.org/10.1542/ peds.2018-1206

Health New Zealand. (2018). *Well Child Tamariki Ora visits*. New Zealand Government. www.health .govt.nz/your-health/pregnancy-and-kids/services-and-support-you-and-your-child/well-child-tamariki-ora-visits?icn=promo-wellchild

Hooker, L., Small, R. & Taft, A. (2016). Reflections on maternal health care within the Victorian Maternal and Child Health Service. *Australian Journal of Primary Health, 22*(2), 77–80. https://doi.org/10.1071/PY15096

Janus, M., Reid-Westoby, C., Raiter, N., Forer, B. & Guhn, M. (2021). Population-level data on child development at school entry reflecting social determinants of health: A narrative review of studies using the Early Development Instrument. *International Journal of Environmental Research and Public Health, 18*(7), 3397. https://doi.org/10.3390/ijerph18073397

Jeong, J., Franchett, E.E., Ramos de Oliveira, C.V., Rehmani, K. & Yousafzai, A.K. (2021). Parenting interventions to promote early child development in the first three years of life: A global systematic review and meta-analysis. *PLoS Medicine, 18*(5), e1003602. https://doi .org/10.1371/journal.pmed.1003602

Marmot, M. (2010). *Fair Society, Healthy Lives: (The Marmot Review)*. www.instituteofhealthequity .org/resources-reports/fair-society-healthy-lives-the-marmot-review

McCashen, W. (2017). *The Strengths Approach: A Strengths-Based Resource for Sharing Power and Creating Change* (2nd ed.). St Lukes Innovative Resources.

Ministry of Social Development. (2015). *Investing in New Zealand's Children and their Families*. New Zealand Government. www.msd.govt.nz/about-msd-and-our-work/work-programmes/ investing-in-children/eap-report.html

National Scientific Council on the Developing Child. (2020). *Connecting the brain to the rest of the body: Early childhood development and lifelong health are deeply intertwined*. (Working Paper No. 15.) www.developingchild.harvard.edu

New Zealand Guidelines Group. (2012). *New Zealand Primary Care Handbook* (3rd ed.). New Zealand Guidelines Group. https://www.tewhatuora.govt.nz/publications/new-zealand-primary-care-handbook-2012

Parliamentary Counsel Office. (1989). *Oranga Tamariki Act 1989/Children's and Young People's Well-Being Act 1989*. New Zealand Government. www.legislation.govt.nz/act/public/1989/0024/ latest/whole.html

Pokharel, B., Yelland, J., Hooker, L. & Taft, A. (2021). A systematic review of culturally competent family violence responses to women in primary care. *Trauma, Violence, & Abuse, 0*(0), 1–18. https://doi.org/10.1177/15248380211046968

Ridgway, L., Hackworth, N., Nicholson, J.M. & McKenna, L. (2020). Working with families: A systematic scoping review of family-centred care in universal, community-based maternal, child, and family health services. *Journal of Child Health Care, 0*(0), 1–22. https://doi .org/10.1177/1367493520930172

Rossiter, C., Schmied, V., Kemp, L., et al. (2017). Responding to families with complex needs: A national survey of child and family health nurses. *Journal of Advanced Nursing, 73*(2), 386–98. https://doi.org/10.1111/jan.13146

Schmied, V., Homer, C., Fowler, C., et al. (2015). Implementing a national approach to universal child and family health services in Australia: Professionals' views of the challenges and opportunities. *Health & Social Care in the Community, 23*(2), 159–70. https://doi.org/10.1111/hsc.12129

Shonkoff, J.P., Slopen, N. & Williams, D.R. (2021). Early childhood adversity, toxic stress, and the impacts of racism on the foundations of health. *Annual Review of Public Health, 42*, 115–34. https://doi.org/10.1146/annurev-publhealth-090419-101940

Talbot, L. & Verrinder, G. (2017). *Promoting health: The primary health care approach*. Elsevier Health Sciences.

United Nations Children's Fund (UNICEF). (2009). *The State of the World's Children – Special Edition: Celebrating 20 Years of the Convention on the Rights of the Child*. UNICEF. www.unicef.org/media/61751/file/SOWC%20Spec.%20Ed.%20CRC%20Main%20Report_EN_090409.pdf

Van Assen, A.G., Knot-Dickscheit, J., Post, W.J. & Grietens, H. (2020). Home-visiting interventions for families with complex and multiple problems: A systematic review and meta-analysis of out-of-home placement and child outcomes. *Children and Youth Services Review, 114*(2020), 1–14. https://doi.org/10.1016/j.childyouth.2020.104994

Victorian Government. (2005). *Children, Youth and Families Act 2005*. State Government of Victoria. www.legislation.vic.gov.au/in-force/acts/children-youth-and-families-act-2005/137

Williams, A. (2019). Family support services delivered using a restorative approach: A framework for relationship and strengths-based whole-family practice. *Child & Family Social Work, 24*(4), 555–64. https://doi.org/10.1111/cfs.12636

World Health Organization (WHO). (2023). *Social determinants of health*. www.who.int/health-topics/social-determinants-of-health

Zarnowiecki, D., Nguyen, H., Catherine, H., Boffa, J. & Segal, L. (2018). The Australian Nurse-Family Partnership Program for aboriginal mothers and babies: Describing client complexity and implications for program delivery. *Midwifery, 65*, 72–81. https://doi.org/10.1016/j.midw.2018.06.019

19 School and youth health nursing

Elizabeth Halcomb and Lisa Chalmers
With acknowledgement to Diana Guzys, Leona Evans,
Andrea Scott, Marisa Monagle and Christine Ashley

LEARNING OBJECTIVES

At the completion of this chapter, you should be able to:

- describe the purpose and key functions of the school and youth health nurses across various settings.
- identify how school and youth health nurses provide a primary health care (PHC) focus.
- explain the common issues faced when nursing adolescents and young adults.

Introduction

School nurse – a registered nurse who is employed within an educational setting. These settings span various age groups, public and private organisations, and include day and boarding facilities (ANMF, 2019).

Youth health nurse – a registered nurse employed to provide nursing services specifically to young people aged 12–25 years in a youth-friendly setting.

The **school nurse** is a nurse who works in a range of education settings across all age groups (Australian Nursing and Midwifery Federation (ANMF), 2019; Ministry of Health, 2009). While Australia does not have a formal national school health service, nurses have worked in schools for over a century (Moyes, McGough, & Wynaden, 2024b). Today, they are employed in various independent schools, colleges and fragmented programs within government schools (Moyes et al., 2024b; Sanford et al., 2020). There has been interest in recent years in growing the presence of nurses in Australian schools to facilitate access to health care for students from disadvantaged backgrounds (Jones et al., 2020; Sanford et al., 2020).

A **youth health nurse** provides health care specifically to young people aged 12–25 years in community settings. Most often, this role requires a combination of mental and physical health care, although greater emphasis on one or the other may be apparent in some settings. Regardless of the focus of care provided, what is most important is that the service is youth-friendly, flexible and safe for young people to access.

Youth health and school nurses are recognised internationally as playing an important part in contributing to the prevention of health risks among children and young people (World Health Organization (WHO), 2015). This chapter commences with consideration of the school nurse. Similarities of working in a school environment and the differences experienced between issues faced when working with primary- and secondary-school aged students are noted. Similar client issues are addressed by secondary school nurses and youth health nurses, and the difference in settings between these two roles is explored.

The role of the school nurse

School nurses have a pivotal role in the health system. They are often the initial point of contact for students needing health care and offer invaluable support to students, families and the broader school community (Jones et al., 2020; McCluskey, Kendall & Burns, 2019). Nurses are important members of the school team as they can support the physical and mental health needs of students (Moyes et al., 2024b). Their contributions to preventative health and building health literacy can significantly influence students' long-term educational and health outcomes. The WHO (2015) describes school health programs as 'one of the most cost-effective investments a nation can make to simultaneously improve education and health'. The WHO views school health programs as a strategy to reduce health risks and facilitate engagement of the education sector in changing the range of educational, social, economic and political factors that affect risk in young people (WHO, 2021).

Given the importance of school health programs, school nurses must be experts in their field, have a broad knowledge and understanding of PHC principles, and understand and can apply evidence-based practice. While the specific tasks undertaken by school nurses may vary across geographic regions and the individual needs of the school community, there are many commonalities.

The school nurse works not only with individual students, families or specific student groups, but they also engage with diverse stakeholders across the school and broader community to respond to local community needs and national health priorities (ANMF, 2019). School nurses play an important role in identifying and addressing physical and mental health issues among students, as well as assisting students and their families to navigate educational and medical systems to optimise health and educational outcomes (Jones et al., 2020; Sanford et al., 2020). The activities of the school nurse can broadly be categorised into four areas:

1. Addressing health care needs
2. Health assessments, screenings and referrals
3. Health promotion and education
4. Creating a safe environment.

Addressing health care needs

Regardless of the age of students or the type of school, providing clinical care to address health care needs is a key part of the school nurse's role (Jones et al., 2020). When an injury occurs, or a student becomes unwell, nursing care may consist of assessing and intervening, or care may involve the ongoing management of chronic conditions. The nurse will also need to communicate with parents/caregivers and, if necessary, refer to or liaise with outside health services and advocate for the student's needs (Sanford et al., 2020).

Students with chronic conditions, such as diabetes, or with potential health issues, such as significant allergies, epilepsy or asthma, may be referred to the school nurse to develop an individual health care plan to assist them in managing their condition and reducing the risk of harm while at school (Sanford et al., 2020). The nurse will also need to ensure that teachers are provided with the appropriate information, training and equipment to understand and respond appropriately to the health issues of students with specific health needs.

The school nurse may also provide mental health assessment, first aid and psychosocial intervention if students present with social, emotional or mental health concerns such as bullying, family/friendship conflict, low self-esteem, gender- or drug-related issues or are in a crisis (Moyes et al., 2024b). The importance of mental health in young people is being increasingly recognised (Kaskoun & McCabe, 2022; Moyes et al., 2024b). Indeed, one in seven young people aged between 4 and 17 years old have experienced a mental health disorder, some 23 per cent of 15–19-year-olds experience a probable serious mental illness, and suicide is the leading cause of death among Australian children and young people (Australian Child Rights Taskforce, 2018). Similarly, in Aotearoa New Zealand, rates of psychological distress and mental illness are on the rise, particularly among minority groups (Mental Health Foundation of New Zealand, 2023). The Aotearoa New Zealand suicide rate for people aged between 15–19 years in 2013–15 was the second highest across the European Union and OECD countries (McKinlay et al., 2021). This is even more concerning considering these data are largely from before the COVID-19 pandemic, which has since seen a decline in mental health among young people (Moyes, McGough & Wynaden, 2024a). The nurse can play a vital role in listening, providing support and intervention, referring to local services and reporting to authorities as required by law.

Health assessments, screening and referrals

Health assessments, screening and referrals are another aspect of the school nurses' role, however, the types of assessment and screening will vary according to the student's age (Jones et al., 2020; WHO, 2021). A key part of health assessment by school nurses is input from the teachers who work with the students on a day-to-day basis (Marrapese, Gormley & Deschene, 2021). Developing trusting relationships and good communication between teachers and school nurses can greatly assist in identifying students with health issues early, prompting early intervention to reduce the impact on education and improve health outcomes.

The primary school nurse is often focused on issues relating to developmental, behavioural and sensory concerns. School nurses must use evidence-informed assessment and screening tools and follow established guidelines for diagnosis and assessment so that students' progress can be monitored over time and the assessment findings understood by other health professionals. At this age, care is very much 'family-centred', with the assessment incorporating confidential and personal conversations with the parent and child. Problems that are identified may be dealt with directly by the nurse, or parents may be given information about or referrals to local health services such as general practice, optometry, physiotherapy, occupational therapy, speech pathology, psychology and family counsellors (Ministry of Health, 2009). In some cases, the school nurse may need to advocate on the young person or family's behalf to ensure their needs are met and must be aware of mandated reporting legislation should there be concerns regarding the risk of harm.

Nurses working with students in secondary schools may assess and screen students for developmental, behavioural and sensory concerns. However, they will also be involved in general health checks including blood pressure, weight management and mental health assessments. Young people in this age group may experience the onset of a range of mental health issues, such as eating disorders, schizophrenia, anxiety and depression, as well as gender identity issues and sexual health concerns. Schools are important settings for the early identification of these issues to promote early intervention and health literacy (Moyes et al., 2024b). Health issues may be impacted by factors such as poor social support, family dysfunction, financial concerns and bullying or harassment. To assist in appropriate management, the school nurse must have a thorough knowledge of the scope of locally available services, referral pathways and costs of service provision (Sanford et al., 2020).

In some areas, immunisation programs or immunisation catch-ups are offered within schools. The school nurse may coordinate these programs, taking responsibility for providing advice to parents and students, liaising with school staff and maintaining documentation. These programs must be established following *The Australian Immunisation Handbook* (Department of Health and Aged Care, 2018) and the New Zealand Ministry of Health (2024) *Immunisation Handbook* that outlines current best practices. Such programs enhance uptake and vaccination rates (Altinoluk-Davis, Gray & Bray, 2020; Guarinoni & Dignani, 2021).

Health promotion and education

Health promotion and education are integrated into all aspects of the school nurse's practice (ANMF, 2019; WHO, 2021), although the focus of the activities will vary according to the nurse's position, student age ranges and individual school needs (Jones et al., 2020). This may involve working with other school staff to develop plans for health promotion and prevention, responding to school violence, bullying or suicide, or managing major grief events such as the sudden death or serious illness of a student or staff member.

Primary school nurses are likely to focus education activities on advising families and teachers about condition-specific health problems, addressing issues like puberty and body image, and promoting a healthy school environment. Education may be provided in group or individual sessions involving children and/or parents and teachers. Such sessions enable the primary school nurse to positively influence parent-child communication by promoting health discussions to promote better health outcomes.

In secondary schools, adolescents often face a range of issues that affect their health including chronic conditions, eating disorders, sexual and gender issues, mental health challenges, and smoking and substance abuse. Social issues, such as bullying, family breakdown, homelessness, immigration, poverty and violence, escalate their physical and mental health needs (Australian Child Rights Taskforce, 2018; Blakemore, 2019). Secondary school nurses perform a critical role, working directly with students on a one-to-one basis, in tailored group activities and through long-term follow-up to enhance health literacy, promote healthy lifestyles, encourage acceptance of diversity, as well as offering confidential support and advice.

CASE STUDY 19.1

The school nurse is asked to assist Gaby, a child in Year 3 who has autism and associated severe behavioural issues and is experiencing the early onset of puberty. Gaby's mother feels unable to explain puberty changes and menstruation to her daughter. The nurse meets Gaby and her mother in school and provides developmentally appropriate resources. While Gaby is difficult to engage, the nurse can assist her mother to ensure that Gaby has a basic understanding of what to expect by using a combination of pictures, words and suggestions. The nurse also liaises with Gaby's teacher, and together, they explore other support networks within the school and Gaby's community.

REFLECTION
1. How appropriate are the nurse's actions in dealing with this issue?
2. What else could she have done to assist Gaby, her family and the school?
3. What follow-up should the nurse put in place?

Creating a safe environment

The school environment has the potential to be unsafe for students for a range of reasons. Physical safety can be impacted by numerous factors such as environmental factors that create high injury risk, unhealthy canteen foods that encourage poor dietary choices, and violence and aggression that can lead to physical injury and negative mental well-being. Similarly, issues such as bullying and marginalisation of groups such as particular cultural groups and LGBTQIA+ youth are also key risks to psychological safety.

School bullying and violence in the school setting is not a new phenomenon; however, it has received renewed attention as the negative impacts of bullying have become more apparent (Ahmad et al., 2023; Jadambaa et al., 2019). Research reports about one in seven Australian children experience bullying (Jadambaa et al., 2019). Internationally, some 67 per cent of children report having been bullied, with 41 per cent reporting having been bullied for a year or more (Australian Child Rights Taskforce, 2018).

The growth of the Internet, mobile phones and social media has created a new medium by which bullying can occur with the bully interacting with the victim in their own environment (Jadambaa et al., 2019). Cyberbullying is particularly pervasive as social media provides a continuous platform to rapidly disseminate humiliating or malevolent information. Self-expression and validation are important during adolescence, in particular, and sites that encourage competition via the number of 'friends' or 'likes' a person receives may influence the person's sense of self-worth (Fryt, Szczygiel & Duell, 2021; Sabik, Falat & Magagnos, 2019). Limited self-regulation and judgement skills may lead to online disinhibition. Personal details and private information may be shared far more easily online than if interacting in person. Such information can then be used against the person or shared more widely than the individual intended. Cyberbullying is a form of relational aggression that attempts to damage a person's social relationships and has been linked to depression, anxiety and poor self-esteem (Jadambaa et al., 2019). Websites such as eSafety Commissioner in Australia (www.esafety .gov.au/) and Keep It Real Online in New Zealand (www.keepitrealonline.govt.nz/) provide valuable resources for school nurses to assist in educating and supporting students, parents and teachers around cyber safety issues.

Those who experience bullying are more likely to exhibit more physical and psychosomatic symptoms (e.g. headaches, nausea, problems sleeping), develop mental illness and are at greater risk of suicide than their peers who are not bullied (Arango et al., 2018). Additionally, a relationship has been demonstrated between bullying and substance misuse, delinquency and adult criminality (Pichel et al., 2022). Often, adolescents may be reluctant to report bullying or cyberbullying, but as with other adolescent health issues, building rapport and a non-judgemental attitude increases the likelihood of disclosure.

School nurses have an important role in promoting a positive and safe environment in which children and adolescents can grow and develop. Students attending schools where there is a negative environment are more likely to experience bullying than those who attend schools with positive environments (Miranda, Oriol & Amutio, 2019). A positive environment is welcoming and conducive to learning for all students. This means that the environment is inclusive of all, including those from priority groups (e.g. ethnic or racial backgrounds, LGBTQIA+ or special needs). Additionally, for those who perpetrate bullying, positive environments have negative repercussions (Miranda et al., 2019). The school nurse can play a role in facilitating a positive culture within the school by promoting inclusion, providing education regarding relevant minority groups and promoting positive engagement in the school culture.

The school nurse is often seen as a trusted person that students can turn to for support (Harding et al., 2019). Students may present with a range of minor complaints or symptoms, such as neck, shoulder and back pain; stomachaches; fatigue; insomnia; weight loss and dizziness (Kaskoun & McCabe, 2022), rather than overtly identifying that they are being bullied. Careful questioning by the school nurse and the reassurance that they will be safe to disclose their concerns can assist in revealing if bullying or violence is present. Given the potential serious and long-term sequelae related to bullying, the school nurse should ensure that students who have experienced bullying are appropriately referred for specialist support. Depending on the nature and context of the situation, referrals may be to GPs, counsellors, psychologists, psychiatrists, local mental health services or support groups. Consideration should be given to encourage parental involvement, if appropriate, to facilitate long-term support. The school nurse also must be cognisant of the mandatory reporting requirements of nurses in their jurisdiction and the professional responsibility to report illegal activity (for example, actual or threatened assault) to local law enforcement.

Challenges for the school nurse

Working as a school nurse is exciting and challenging, as school nurses often work autonomously. While many school nurses enjoy the opportunity to work independently, there is the potential for **professional isolation** (ANMF, 2019; McCluskey et al., 2019; Ministry of Health, 2009). Indeed, Aotearoa New Zealand's Ministry of Health (2009) reports that around one-third of school nurses did not participate in clinical supervision due to isolation. This highlights the need for nurses to continuously critically reflect on and evaluate their practice. Many school nurses find involvement in professional organisations, local school nurse support groups and online communities of practice to be invaluable in providing debriefing, clinical supervision/mentorship, professional development opportunities and networking (McCluskey et al., 2019). Nurses must also be aware of their professional responsibilities in meeting the practice standards and continuing professional development requirements of the Nursing and Midwifery Board of Australia (2016) and the Nursing Council of New Zealand (2016).

Another challenge faced in the school environment is promoting the service and maintaining support within the teaching and student population. Schools are busy places, where education is the core business. Engaging people in health programs within a hectic school timetable requires perseverance and commitment, as well as the ability to develop respectful and collaborative relationships (WHO, 2021). In their review, Best and colleagues (2018) highlight how school nurse interventions improve student health and education outcomes. However, Bayik Temel and colleagues (2017) highlight the range of literature that demonstrates a poor understanding of the school nurse role by parents, teachers and school leaders. Such poor understanding of the role of the school nurse is a key challenge for school nurses as it means that they may not be engaged to the extent of their practice scope and this may create role conflict. This highlights the need for nurses to work closely with their school community in defining and developing their role to ensure that it meets the health needs of the students, their families and the community (Bayik Temel et al., 2017; McCluskey et al., 2019; Moyes et al., 2024b).

Professional isolation – individuals working in any environment where they are apart from their own professional peers. This isolation may occur as the result of a remote geographical location or simply where a professional works autonomously in a setting without professional peers.

The COVID-19 pandemic has intensified the emergence of mental health issues among young people and created challenges in schooling internationally (Cook et al., 2023). School nurses have an important role to play in supporting mental health through supporting health promotion and education as well as early intervention and referral (Moyes et al., 2024b). However, a growing need for mental health support by students may not be able to be addressed by the currently under-resourced system (McCluskey et al., 2019). Investment in the school nursing workforce and its infrastructure has the potential to enhance access to services and health outcomes (Cook et al., 2023; McCluskey et al., 2019). In Australia and Aotearoa New Zealand, this means building well-defined and consistent school health services to ensure equitable access to this health care service.

REFLECTION

Consider the challenges of working in an environment where you are the only nurse.

1. How could you educate school colleagues and the school community about your role?
2. What actions could you take to minimise your professional isolation?

Youth-focused health services

Whether employed in an educational or community setting, a youth-focused health nurse needs to provide adequate, non-judgemental information and support to young people, enabling them to make informed choices. Youth-friendly environments provide care in a way that is accessible (affordable), acceptable (by being responsive to ethnic, gender and social diversity), appropriate in the kinds of services it provides and effective in providing care that improves health outcomes (McKinlay et al., 2021). If young people believe that you are not interested in them or feel that you are making judgements, it is difficult to develop the rapport required to identify health concerns, discuss treatments and provide health education. Ensuring that young people can access health care is vital as poor health outcomes have lifelong impacts on the young person, their family and the wider community (McKinlay et al., 2021).

Adolescence – a transitional stage of physical, cognitive, social and emotional development that is generally accepted to occur between the ages of 12 until an individual is in their early twenties. Social, cultural and legal differences impact on how adolescence is defined.

Puberty – a hormone-induced process of sexual development of the gonads and maturation of the reproductive organs of a young person enabling the physical capability of sexual reproduction.

Adolescence and youth health

For many years, adolescents were included in the infant and child caring framework as differences and the specific needs related to this part of the lifespan were not acknowledged. Historically, **adolescence** is a relatively new social construction. In the past, you were a child and then, once you were physically developed enough to work or reproduce, you became an adult. However, the time between childhood and adulthood has expanded as lifespan has increased and the threats to survival have diminished. Cultural values and laws have shaped a distinct time of transition, expectation and psychological adjustment that we refer to as 'adolescence'. **Puberty** has generally been considered the beginning of adolescence, however, when it ends is less clear. Legal definitions relating to adulthood vary between, as well as within, countries. Adult rights such as the right to vote, drink alcohol, smoke, drive a car and get married are often used as markers for the end of adolescence. Yet technological advances have provided evidence that physiological and psychological maturation continues into the early to mid-third decade of life. There has been limited emphasis on understanding how young people transition from receiving child health services to independently seeking health care as adolescents or adults (McKinlay et al., 2021).

Adolescence is a significant period of psychological and biological change as puberty, brain maturation and social development, including identity formation, occur. The need to form an identity is a major task of adolescence that is strongly associated with experimentation with different behaviours (Blakemore, 2019). Young people are usually considered a healthy group, however, experimentation with alcohol, tobacco and other drug misuse; unsafe sex; risky and unsafe driving; as well as associated risks of violence and mental health problems influence short-term or long-term morbidity and mortality (Fryt et al., 2021; Tomova, Andrews & Blakemore, 2021). This is a period of self-consciousness, mood variability, exploration and risk-taking, as well as the development of skills that will enable young people to lead independent adult lives (Blakemore, 2019).

Social reorientation occurs during adolescence, with the desire to be accepted by peers and avoid social rejection. There is also a shift in social interaction from predominately parents and family to peers, and this tends to make the opinions of peers more important than those of family (Blakemore, 2019; Tomova et al., 2021; Van Hoorn, Crone & Van Leijenhorst, 2017). A key developmental task in early adolescence is to establish strong peer relationships. This coincides with an increased sensitivity to the opinion of peers that can positively or negatively influence young people's health (Fryt et al., 2021; Tomova et al., 2021; Van Hoorn et al., 2017). The emotion associated with making decisions in exciting or stressful situations is intensified in the presence of peers, which influences experimentation with health-related behaviours during adolescence (Van Hoorn et al., 2017). The likelihood of experiencing depression or participating in antisocial and illegal activities (e.g. substance misuse, unsafe sex and dangerous driving) increases with poor peer relationships such as feeling isolated or bullied (Blakemore, 2019; Van Hoorn et al., 2017) and lower perceived family support (Fryt et al., 2021).

Family **connectedness** remains one of the most important **protective factors** against poor health outcomes during adolescence despite the reduced influence of parents or caregivers. Adolescents who feel connected to their families are less likely to participate in substance use or engage in violence and are more likely to delay becoming sexually active (Tomova et al., 2021). Adolescents commonly identify that their families are the most influential source of health information and crucial to their sense of well-being (Tomova et al., 2021). However, young people are more likely to adopt negative health behaviours if these are modelled by their parents such as smoking, drinking alcohol or engaging in violence. Safe and supportive families, schools, peers and communities assist young people transition into healthy adulthood. The vulnerability or resilience of young people when exposed to health-compromising experiences is influenced by connectedness with family, school, the community and their peers (Tomova et al., 2021).

Connectedness – the quality and quantity of relationships between people and their interactions with each other that are necessary for a person's well-being.

Protective factors – the skills, resources, coping strategies and conditions that enhance the likelihood of positive outcomes and help people deal more effectively with stressful events or lessen the risk of negative consequences or socially undesirable outcomes caused by exposure to risk.

Working with young people

A youth-focused health nurse may be situated within a school or hospital, attached to a primary care service or work within a community health service. The practice setting often influences the range of activities undertaken. Youth-friendly services usually allow clients to either make an appointment or simply drop by to see the nurse. As adolescents often present with complex issues that affect their relationships with their families, friends and schooling, the nurse must ensure that enough time is set aside for each appointment. The most common issues young people present with include mental health concerns, stress and anxiety, sexual health issues, substance use, housing problems, relationship problems, as well as general health concerns. Approximately half of all lifelong mental health problems begin around 14 years of age or earlier (WHO, 2024), and 75 per cent of all adult mental health disorders appear before the age of 24 years (Tomova et al., 2021). The youth-focused nurse must be up to date with the latest information about these issues and the local services and referral pathways that may further assist clients.

Confidentiality

It is extremely important to always be clear about what can and cannot be kept confidential before providing care to a young person. The young person should be reassured that the nurse will provide confidential care within the parameters of local and national legal requirements regarding child protection (Grilo et al., 2019). Generally, these rules apply to young people under the age of 18, and relate to threats of self-harm, harming someone else or experiencing harm from someone else. Being clear about what this means enables the young person to understand this from the beginning.

Advocacy

Youth health nurses are often required to advocate on behalf of young people. This may mean attending meetings and appointments with, or on behalf of, a young person or arranging referrals and advocating for access to services. For example, a young person may need to be referred for a medical assessment. The nurse may assist by arranging an appointment with a youth-friendly GP and, if necessary, accompany the young person to the appointment. The nurse may also guide the young person through what they need to do, such as talking to the receptionist or guiding them through the medical consultation itself. The aim of this is to help build the young person's capacity to do this independently the next time medical treatment is needed. Introducing the young person to a youth-friendly GP is also a means of helping them to overcome barriers.

Networking – purposeful interactions that assist in the creation and maintenance of professional and social relationships.

Networking with the medical service and developing protocols between services about how they address the needs and provide services to young people demonstrates a further level of advocacy. This may also allow the youth health nurse to negotiate services free of charge for a young person.

CASE STUDY 19.2

Seventeen-year-old Cassie, a Year 12 student, is concerned that a wound on her inner thigh might be infected so she visits the nurse. She is also seeking advice on anxiety and housing options.

By explaining what services can be provided, and the limitations of confidentiality and record-keeping, the nurse helps Cassie feel physically and emotionally comfortable. A full health history is then taken, including how the injury occurred. Cassie admits that the wound is self-inflicted and that she frequently cuts herself to release the stress that she feels. Several faint scars and healing cuts are visible on Cassie's legs and arms. The nurse cleans and dresses the wound that Cassie is concerned about. While attending to the wound, the nurse discusses the underlying issues that contribute to Cassie's stress and the potential problems relating to her current coping strategies.

Cassie also says that she is feeling extremely anxious. Cassie reveals that she has a difficult relationship with her mother, who is constantly threatening to have her removed from the family home. This creates a difficult atmosphere for Cassie at home and has made it almost impossible for her to study for her Year 12 exams. After taking a further history on Cassie's circumstances and, with her consent, the nurse refers Cassie for a mental health assessment and education on stress and anxiety management.

The constant threat of becoming homeless is incredibly stressful for Cassie and she is fearful of what will happen should her mother follow through with her threat. After consultation with Cassie, it is decided that a referral to the youth housing support worker may assist Cassie to understand her options should she find herself homeless.

Following advice from the nurse, Cassie asks to see a GP to discuss her anxiety and the possible need for antibiotics. The nurse explains the options available to Cassie, who chooses to have the nurse attend the appointment with her.

An appointment is made for Cassie with a youth-friendly GP with whom the nurse has formed a professional partnership. The appointment is free of charge and long enough for Cassie to discuss her needs. The nurse introduces Cassie to the reception staff and then the doctor. Cassie can attend the appointment without the worry of having to pay, or the worry about whom she is seeing and how she might explain what she needs. This is the only time the youth nurse attends the doctor with Cassie, as she feels capable of attending follow-up appointments on her own.

Cassie also asks the nurse to speak to the Year 12 coordinator to explain the difficult situation she is in with her living arrangements. As a result of this discussion, the nurse and Year 12 teachers support an application for Cassie to be considered disadvantaged during her exam period because of her family and living situations.

Cassie's mother decides to have her removed from the family home. Although this is emotionally traumatic for Cassie, she has somewhere to go and live immediately, as this has been organised as a result of her referral to housing support.

REFLECTION

Consider the complex range of issues experienced by Cassie.

1. How would you prioritise responding to Cassie's needs?
2. Do you consider all of Cassie's problems to be health issues?
3. What did the nurse provide in the way of health care for Cassie?
4. What were the possible consequences for Cassie if she had not visited the youth-focused nurse?

Building capacity

Often, there are highly complex needs to be addressed in assisting a young person to maintain positive health and well-being. Case study 19.2 illustrates how important it is to provide a youth-friendly service (Cassie would not have told her story if she did not feel comfortable) and to have a complete understanding of local referral pathways. Developing strong professional relationships within schools and their local medical and health services helps to ensure the best outcomes for young people. Networking also allows local people who work with young people to consolidate their knowledge and gain an understanding of what other services are available. One of the most important outcomes of belonging to a youth network is that it enables the development of a local, united health professionals' voice to promote the needs and issues that affect the young people within their community. Such networks add weight to applications for funding and strengthen the argument for service expansion, as well as provide useful information to the local adult community, all levels of government and the health system.

Barriers to accessing health services

Several individual, social and systemic barriers to young people accessing general health services have been identified. Young people consistently indicate that they are often unwilling to attend health services due to the fear of being judged or asked difficult questions by health professionals and fear of a lack of confidentiality (McKinlay et al., 2021; Radez et al., 2021). Being recognised in the waiting room of a health service is a particular concern for young people who live in small communities. Other common barriers include a lack of knowledge of the services available for young people, the distance to the service, limited transport and inconvenient opening hours (McKinlay et al., 2021; Radez et al., 2021).

Breaking down barriers

The nurse needs to understand how to provide a space that is youth-friendly and non-threatening. Strategies to inform and encourage young people to attend the service include giving talks at school assemblies and assisting in health education classes and/or any youth events within the area covered by the clinic. It is useful to work with local schools to invite students to visit the health service and to meet the staff, including the nurse. Young people are less likely to feel threatened by entering a building that they have previously visited, so this type of activity reduces perceived barriers to accessing health services. It is also valuable to ask some young people to decorate the space to increase the likelihood of the area being attractive to their peers. Consulting with young people in the community about the best time to open the service and who to liaise with will help ensure that the service provided is the service that they want.

Promotional material, such as brochures, posters and appointment cards, is also important. Having young people design the logo is an effective activity that helps raise awareness of the service and makes the advertising material age-appropriate. Another important consideration in promoting services to young people is through social networking. Many young people use social networking in their everyday lives to connect with friends and to find information. Numerous youth services are turning to the Internet to promote what they offer through social networking sites that are linked to other youth services in the local community. Such sites usually explain what the clinic does, how to access it and provide contact details. Social networking sites are particularly useful for sharing information that adolescents may not feel comfortable discussing face-to-face, particularly sexual health.

REFLECTION

Consider health care services you are familiar with.

1. Could these be described as being 'youth-friendly'?
2. What criteria would you use to make this decision?

Conclusion

School nurses are expert PHC nurses who play important roles in educational settings providing clinical care, screening and assessment, health promotion, and health education. Youth-focused health nursing provides appropriately specialised care tailored to meet the needs of young people. This group has identifiable and specific needs that require knowledgeable health care professionals to address them. As well as high-level clinical skills, the nurse needs to have excellent written and verbal communication and liaison skills to develop good relationships with families, teachers and other school staff, and with service providers in the community. The health concerns targeted by such nurses are diverse, reflecting the life issues and multiple areas of decision-making faced by young people as they grow and develop. The behaviours of adulthood are most often formed during this period of life, so the promotion of healthy behaviours and the development of confidence in engaging with health care services need to be considered priorities in addressing future health issues. The importance of youth-focused nursing services cannot be underestimated. However, limited resources and fragmented health programs often mean that nurses need to be realistic about the level of service they can provide and prioritise their activities appropriately.

CRITICAL THINKING ACTIVITIES

Consider the following quote:

Promoting healthy behaviours during adolescence, and taking steps to better protect young people from health risks are critical for the prevention of health problems in adulthood, and for countries' future health and ability to develop and thrive. (YouthPower2, 2019)

1. Why would the YouthPower2 consider the health of adolescents to be critical to the future of a country's health and social infrastructure?
2. How can youth-focused health nurses best address the needs of young people?
3. Which adolescent behaviours do you believe are most amenable to intervention?
4. What actions or activities would support or improve the connectedness of young people with their families, neighbourhood and school?

FURTHER READING

Australian Nursing and Midwifery Federation (ANMF). (2019). *National School Nursing Standards for Practice: Registered Nurse.* www.anmf.org.au/media/x1gaxvbj/anmf_national_school_nursing_standards_for_practice_rn_2019.pdf

McKinlay, E., Morgan, S., Garrett, S., Dunlop, A. & Pullon, S. (2021). Young peoples' perspectives about care in a youth-friendly general practice. *Journal of Primary Health Care, 13*(2), 157–64. https://doi.org/10.1071/HC20134

Ministry of Health. (2009). *Nursing Services in New Zealand Secondary Schools: A Summary.* New Zealand Government. www.wgtn.ac.nz/health/centres/health-services-research-centre/docs/ reports/downloads/School-Nursing-Summary.pdf

World Health Organization (WHO). (2024). *Adolescent and young adult health – Fact sheet.* www.who.int/news-room/fact-sheets/detail/adolescents-health-risks-and-solutions

REFERENCES

Ahmad, K., Beatson, A., Campbell, M., et al. (2023). The impact of gender and age on bullying role, self-harm and suicide: Evidence from a cohort study of Australian children. *PLoS ONE, 18*(1), e0278446. https://doi.org/10.1371/journal.pone.0278446

Altinoluk-Davis, F., Gray, S. & Bray, I. (2020). Measuring the effectiveness of catch-up MMR delivered by school nurses compared to signposting to general practice on improving MMR coverage. *Journal of Public Health 42*(2), 416–22. https://doi.org/10.1093/pubmed/fdaa004

Arango, C., Diaz-Caneja, C.M., McGorry, P.D., et al. (2018). Preventive strategies for mental health. *Lancet Psychiatry, 5*(7), 591–604. https://doi.org/10.1016/S2215-0366(18)30057-9

Australian Child Rights Taskforce. (2018). *The Children's Report: Australia's NGO Coalition Report to the United Nations Committee on the Rights of the Child.* https://childrightstaskforce.org.au/ the-childrens-report-2019/

Australian Nursing and Midwifery Federation (ANMF). (2019). *National School Nursing Standards for Practice: Registered Nurse.* www.anmf.org.au/media/x1gaxvbj/anmf_national_school_nursing_ standards_for_practice_rn_2019.pdf

Bayik Temel, A., Yildirim, J.G., Kalkim, A., Muslu, L. & Yildirim, N. (2017). Parents' and teachers' expectations of school nurse roles: A scale development study. *International Journal of Nursing Sciences, 4*(3), 303–10. https://doi.org/10.1016/j.ijnss.2017.05.002

Best, N.C., Oppewal, S. & Travers, D. (2018). Exploring school nurse interventions and health and education outcomes: An integrative review. *Journal of School Nursing, 34*(1), 14–27. https://doi.org/10.1177/1059840517745359

Blakemore, S.J. (2019). Adolescence and mental health. *Lancet, 393*(10185), 2030–1. https://doi .org/10.1016/S0140-6736(19)31013-X

Cook, G., Appleton, J.V., Bekaert, S., et al. (2023). School nursing: New ways of working with children and young people during the Covid-19 pandemic: A scoping review. *Journal of Advanced Nursing, 79*(2), 471–501. www.ncbi.nlm.nih.gov/pmc/articles/PMC9877849/pdf/ JAN-79-471.pdf

Department of Health and Aged Care. (2018). *The Australian Immunisation Handbook.* Australian Government. https://www.health.gov.au/resources/publications/the-australian-immunisation- handbook?language=en

Fryt, J., Szczygiel, M. & Duell, N. (2021). Positive and negative risk taking in adolescence: Age patterns and relations to social environment. *New Directions in Child and Adolescent Development, 2021*(179), 127–46. https://doi.org/10.1002/cad.20431

Grilo, S.A., Catallozzi, M., Santelli, J.S., et al. (2019). Confidentiality discussions and private time with a health-care provider for youth, United States, 2016. *Journal of Adolescent Health, 64*(3), 311–18. https://doi.org/10.1016/j.jadohealth.2018.10.301

Guarinoni, M.G. & Dignani, L. (2021). Effectiveness of the school nurse role in increasing the vaccination coverage rate: A narrative review. *Annali di Igiene, 33*(1), 55–66. https://doi .org/10.7416/ai.2021.2408

Harding, L., Davison-Fischer, J., Bekaert, S. & Appleton, J.V. (2019). The role of the school nurse in protecting children and young people from maltreatment: An integrative review of the literature. *International Journal of Nursing Studies, 92*, 60–72. https://doi.org/10.1016/ j.ijnurstu.2018.12.017

Jadambaa, A., Thomas, H.J., Scott, J.G., et al. (2019). Prevalence of traditional bullying and cyberbullying among children and adolescents in Australia: A systematic review and meta-analysis. *Australian and New Zealand Journal of Psychiatry, 53*(9), 878–88. https://doi .org/10.1177/0004867419846393

Jones, D., Randall, S., White, D., et al. (2020). Embedding public health advocacy into the role of school-based nurses: Addressing the health inequities confronted by vulnerable Australian children and adolescent populations. *Australian Journal of Primary Health, 27*(2), 67–70. https://doi.org/10.1071/PY20155

Kaskoun, J. & McCabe, E. (2022). Perceptions of school nurses in addressing student mental health concerns: An integrative review. *Journal of School Nursing, 38*(1), 35–47. https://doi .org/10.1177/10598405211046223

Marrapese, B., Gormley, J.M. & Deschene, K. (2021). Reimagining school nursing: Lessons learned from a virtual school nurse. *NASN School Nursing, 36*(4), 218–25. https://doi.org/10.1177/1942 602X21996432

McCluskey, A., Kendall, G. & Burns, S. (2019). Students', parents' and teachers' views about the resources required by school nurses in Perth, Western Australia. *Journal of Research in Nursing, 24*(7), 515–26. https://doi.org/10.1177/1744987118807250

McKinlay, E., Morgan, S., Garrett, S., Dunlop, A. & Pullon, S. (2021). Young peoples' perspectives about care in a youth-friendly general practice. *Journal of Primary Health Care, 13*(2), 157–64. https://doi.org/10.1071/HC20134

Mental Health Foundation of New Zealand. (2023). *Statistics on Mental Health in Schools in New Zealand.* https://mentalhealth.org.nz/statistics-on-schools-and-youth-mental-health

Ministry of Health. (2009). *Nursing Services in New Zealand Secondary Schools: A summary.* New Zealand Government. www.wgtn.ac.nz/health/centres/health-services-research-centre/docs/ reports/downloads/School-Nursing-Summary.pdf

—— (2024). *Immunisation Handbook, Version 6.* New Zealand Government. https://www .tewhatuora.govt.nz/for-health-professionals/clinical-guidance/immunisation-handbook

Miranda, R., Oriol, X. & Amutio, A. (2019). Risk and protective factors at school: Reducing bullies and promoting positive bystanders' behaviors in adolescence. *Scandinavian Journal of Psychology, 60*(2), 106–15. https://doi.org/10.1111/sjop.12513

Moyes, A., McGough, S. & Wynaden, D. (2024a). An untenable burden: Exploring experiences of secondary school nurses who encounter young people with mental health problems. *Journal of School Nursing, 40*(3), 10598405221088957. https://doi.org/10.1177/10598405221088957

—— (2024b). Hidden and unacknowledged: The mental health and psychosocial interventions delivered by school nurses in Western Australia. *International Journal of Mental Health Nursing, 33*(2), 463–72. https://doi.org/10.1111/inm.13261

Nursing and Midwifery Board of Australia. (2016). *Registered Nurse Standards for Practice.* Australian Health Practitioner Regulation Agency. https://www.nursingmidwiferyboard.gov.au/Codes-Guidelines-Statements/Professional-standards/registered-nurse-standards-for-practice.aspx

Nursing Council of New Zealand. (2016). *Standards and Guidelines for Nurses.* https://www .nursingcouncil.org.nz/Public/NCNZ/nursing-section/Standards_and_guidelines_for_nurses .aspx?hkey=9fc06ae7-a853-4d10-b5fe-992cd44ba3de

Pichel, R., Feijóo, S., Isorna, M., Varela, J. & Rial, A. (2022). Analysis of the relationship between school bullying, cyberbullying, and substance use. *Children and Youth Services Review, 134*, 106369. https://doi.org/10.1016/j.childyouth.2022.106369

Radez, J., Reardon, T., Creswell, C., et al. (2021). Why do children and adolescents (not) seek and access professional help for their mental health problems? A systematic review of quantitative and qualitative studies. *European Child and Adolescent Psychiatry, 30*(2), 183–211. https://doi.org/10.1007/s00787-019-01469-4

Sabik, N.J., Falat, J. & Magagnos, J. (2019). When self-worth depends on social media feedback: Associations with psychological well-being. *Sex Roles*, *82*(7–8), 411–21. https://doi.org/10.1007/s11199-019-01062-8

Sanford, C., Saurman, E., Dennis, S. & Lyle, D. (2020). 'We're definitely that link': The role of school-based primary health care registered nurses in a rural community. *Australian Journal of Primary Health*, *27*(2), 76–82. https://doi.org/10.1071/PY20149

Tomova, L., Andrews, J.L. & Blakemore, S.-J. (2021). The importance of belonging and the avoidance of social risk taking in adolescence. *Developmental Review*, *61*, 100981. https://doi.org/10.1016/j.dr.2021.100981

Van Hoorn, J., Crone, E.A. & Van Leijenhorst, L. (2017). Hanging out with the right crowd: Peer influence on risk-taking behavior in adolescence. *Journal of Research on Adolescence*, *27*(1), 189–200. https://doi.org/10.1111/jora.12265

World Health Organization (WHO). (2015). *Global School Health Initiative*. https://www.who.int/publications/i/item/global-school-health-initiatives-achieving-health-and-education-outcomes

——— (2021). *WHO Guideline on School Health Services: Web Annex B: Brief Exploratory Review of School Health Services Globally: Methodology and Select Findings*. https://iris.who.int/handle/10665/343784

——— (2024). *Adolescent and young adult health*. www.who.int/news-room/fact-sheets/detail/adolescents-health-risks-and-solutions

YouthPower2. (2019). *Adolescents: Health risks and solutions*. www.youthpower.org/resources/adolescents-health-risks-and-solutions

Sexual health nursing

Leah East, Sharon James and Ruth Mursa
With acknowledgement to Diana Guzys

20

LEARNING OBJECTIVES

At the completion of this chapter, you should be able to:

- describe the role of a sexual health nurse in primary health care (PHC) settings.
- discuss the key components of sexual health care.
- explain why nurses need to practice in a non-judgemental and culturally sensitive manner.
- discuss a range of reproductive and sexual health issues relevant to the provision of nursing care.

Introduction

Sexual health nurses are employed to work in a range of practice settings and work with diverse population groups. Sexual and reproductive health care is considered a human right and is fundamental to positive well-being (World Health Organization (WHO), 2024a). The nurse's role in sexual and reproductive health varies between settings within and across different jurisdictions. Work settings include dedicated sexual health clinics, family planning services, community health centres, women's health services, correctional services, general practices and tertiary education settings. In some jurisdictions, nurses also provide care in publicly funded sexual health clinics aimed at providing services to specific priority population groups to increase their access to services and reduce the prevalence of adverse sexual and reproductive health outcomes, including sexually transmitted infections (STIs) and unplanned pregnancy. Priority populations can include young people, travellers, men who have sex with men, people in custodial settings, culturally and linguistically diverse people, Indigenous peoples, pregnant women, trans and gender diverse people, and sex workers (Department of Health, 2018; NSW Health, 2022). Sexual health nurses work with people of any gender identity and sexual orientation. As there is variability in role expectations and settings, this chapter explores a range of activities that may be undertaken by nurses working in sexual and reproductive health roles.

The role of the sexual health nurse

Sexual and reproductive health care addresses the needs of people across their lifespan, not simply during their years of reproduction. Furthermore, sexual and reproductive health is influenced by psychosocial, cultural and political constructs that can impact availability, access and service provision (WHO, 2022). Despite this, sexual health care services can address a range of health care needs and often focus on two key areas: reproductive health and sexual well-being, including the prevention and management of STIs. Most sexual health nursing practice involves seeing people individually for screening, assessment, treatment and/or health education (Cappiello, Levi & Nothnagle, 2016). Importantly and fundamentally, the role of the sexual health nurse is to support and promote individuals to achieve positive sexual and reproductive well-being and provide person-centred care.

Taking a sexual health history

People who attend sexual health services may be symptomatic or asymptomatic for sexual ill health. However, taking a sexual history should occur in either circumstance to thoroughly assess the needs of the individual. Discussing sexual health can be difficult for individuals due to an array of factors such as embarrassment, stigma and the personal nature of such conversations. Therefore, nurses need to create a positive sexual health discussion, reassure clients of privacy and explain confidentiality, including who has access to their personal information (Rubin et al., 2018). During the consultation, the nurse needs to advise the client that although confidentiality is to be maintained, there are circumstances (as with any consultation) when health care professionals are required to report information. An example is if there are serious concerns about an individual's safety (NSW Health, 2023b) and in the instance of a positive STI where there is a need for contact tracing (discussed later in this chapter).

Sexual health history questions

Sexual orientation – who an individual is attracted to, emotionally, romantically or sexually.

Gender identity – an individual's concept of who they are and how they refer to themselves. This might be as a male, female, non-binary, a combination of both or gender fluid.

Sexual behaviour – a person's sexual practices.

An essential component of positive communication is to not make assumptions about a person's **sexual orientation, gender identity**, relationship status, and/or **sexual behaviour**. The nurse should not assume that every person is a cisgender woman or man and/or in a traditional dyadic partnership. It is less threatening to start the consultation by asking about preferred pronouns and with some basic closed questions such as 'Are you currently sexually active?' People who feel comfortable are likely to expand beyond simple 'yes' or 'no' answers. With people who are less comfortable, a 'yes' or 'no' answer will provide direction for following questions, but the ice will have been broken in a non-threatening manner.

In addition to taking a general health history, sexual history questions include sexual practices and behaviours, inclusive of sexual partners and the presence of physical symptoms or previous history of STIs. Behaviours associated with drug and alcohol use may be asked about, and women should be asked about their menstrual cycle and the possibility of pregnancy.

Rubin and colleagues (2018) provide a helpful mnemonic that outlines the important elements of a sexual health assessment, which is inclusive of sexual orientation and gender identity. The six Ps approach includes:

1. Partners – the number of partners and when they last had a sexual relationship
2. Practices – the methods of sexual engagement
3. Protection from STIs – practices and barrier methods used
4. Past history of STIs – past diagnoses, symptoms (if present), treatment
5. Prevention of pregnancy – contraceptive use and adherence
6. Plus – assessment of trauma, violence, sexual satisfaction, sexual health concerns/problems and support for gender identity and sexual orientation (Rubin et al., 2018).

REFLECTION

1. What biases or assumptions impact you when discussing sexual health?
2. What processes would you follow if you were concerned about someone's safety?
3. What are some other questions you could ask when taking a sexual history that are in line with the six Ps mnemonic?

Culture and sexual well-being

Cultural safety is especially relevant to sexual health as attitudes and sexual practices are often strongly influenced by culture. Culture refers to a set of practices and norms that are shared by members of a group. Beyond simply ethnic cultures, consideration should be given to other groups such as religious culture and youth culture. Culture includes the traditions, symbols, gestures, language, values, norms and rituals that add richness and meaning to our lives and that we use to understand the world in which we live (Woodman & Threadgold, 2021). Consideration of cultures is essential as these may all influence individuals' beliefs and choices about their sexual health.

CASE STUDY 20.1

Te Puāwai Tapu is an established kaupapa Māori primary health organisation that specialises in sexual and reproductive health promotion, education and research. Te Puāwai Tapu agrees that the voices of young Māori residing in urban and semi-urban regions throughout Aotearoa New Zealand are essential for the preparation of national STI online sites.

REFLECTION
What cultural considerations would be key in targeting Māori youth and young adults about sexual health, particularly STIs?

Working in a culturally safe manner means that nurses need to be conscious of their own assumptions and culture. 'Nurses engage with people as individuals in a culturally safe and respectful way, foster open and honest professional relationships, and adhere to their obligations about privacy and confidentiality' (Nursing and Midwifery Board of Australia, 2018, p. 8). Nurses should also be aware that people may be experiencing cultural conflict about their sexuality and may need assistance to work through personal cultural issues. Many **LGBTQIA+** individuals experience discrimination and may feel that their identity and sexual orientation are not respected (Davies et al., 2021; Hill et al., 2020). When health care interactions are based within a culturally safe framework, individualised care that caters to the unique needs of all people can be provided, enhancing health care engagement and improving health outcomes for LGBTQIA+ people (Tan & Sai Ang, 2022).

LGBTQIA+ – an acronym for lesbian, gay, bisexual, transgender, queer, intersex, asexual and people questioning their sexuality, sex and gender, who may self-identify using a non-conforming term.

'Sexuality' is dynamic, diverse and personal, and includes many aspects that make us the individual we are such as our beliefs and values, relationships, gender, desires and feelings. However, 'sexual orientation' refers to a person's emotional, romantic or sexual attraction to other people and is independent of their gender identity (Human Rights Campaign, 2023).

People's sexual behaviour includes not just what they choose to do sexually, but also encompasses their attitudes, desires, experiences and preferences. Sexual behaviour in humans involves more than reproduction and refers to the way we experience and express our own sexuality. Sometimes, people's sexual identity, how people see themselves and how they present themselves to others can be different to their sexual orientation and sexual behaviour (Geary et al., 2018).

Examinations and investigations

Preventive screening

Sexually active people should be encouraged to have a sexual health check-up on a regular basis. This check-up provides an opportunity to discuss any sexual health concerns that the person may have while providing an opportunity for a sexual health history to be taken, STI testing to be undertaken as indicated and ongoing management and education provided. A standard asymptomatic sexual health check should be undertaken in people who request STI testing when there has been a change of sexual partners and when the person has had a known exposure to an STI or a history of an STI in the past 12 months. Asymptomatic STI testing is also recommended in people who have a partner who is pregnant, sex workers and in men who have sex with men (Ong et al., 2023).

Some people may be considered at a greater risk of sexual health issues if they are within a population group that has a high prevalence of STIs. For example, men who have sex with men are advised to have three-monthly testing for gonorrhoea, chlamydia, hepatitis A, hepatitis B, syphilis and human immunodeficiency virus (HIV) (Australasian Society for HIV, Viral Hepatitis and Sexual Health Medicine (ASHM), 2024). Testing for HIV, hepatitis C, hepatitis B (if not immune), syphilis, chlamydia and gonorrhoea should be offered to all people who inject drugs and all people who participate in sexual activity under the influence of substances (ASHM, 2024). Although there is no current evidence that sex workers in Australia have higher rates of STIs, regular testing for STIs and blood-borne viruses, such as hepatitis B, hepatitis C and HIV, is recommended., However, the testing frequency is guided by judicial-based legislation and guidelines (Ong et al., 2023). Opportunistically testing all sexually active young people aged 15–29 years for chlamydia is currently recommended (The Royal Australian College of General Practitioners, 2016), as well as offering chlamydia and other STI screening to all young people at least annually (Ong et al., 2023).

Physical examinations may involve examination of the cervix, vagina, penis or rectum. In addition, a cervical screening test (CST) may also be undertaken in women. This simple test is used to detect potential abnormalities of the cervix caused by the human papillomavirus (HPV), and the test can be undertaken by a clinician, or self-collected (Department of Health and Aged Care, 2022).

STI screening

STI screening is also important when people suspect that they may have an STI, have had a known exposure or have genital symptoms such as pain, discharge or itching (NSW Health, 2019). There are several swabs that may be self-collected by patients including vaginal, ano-rectal and throat swabs (Ong et al., 2023). Blood and urine tests may also be required to check for STIs. Patients need to be made aware of what is being tested for and why, and their consent must be obtained before testing.

When any investigations are undertaken, it is essential to stress the importance of following up to get the results. This may be done in several ways depending on the policy of the health care service. It may be possible to get the results over the telephone or the patient may be required to attend the clinic. If symptoms are present at the time of screening, the person should be asked to return so that the effectiveness of treatment can be monitored. Being informed that someone has an STI can be extremely upsetting. However, although some require ongoing monitoring and management, many STIs can be easily treated. It is important that the STI is not spread to sexual partners, therefore the options for protecting and maintaining the health of sexual partners must be discussed. This may involve abstaining from sex while being treated or for a designated period of time. The follow-up review also allows for further sexual health education and prevention counselling to be provided.

Contact tracing

Contact tracing is the process of identifying people who have been in sexual contact with a person diagnosed with an STI. Once diagnosed, it is important to work out who else the individual has engaged in sexual activity with, allowing these people the opportunity to be tested and treated as necessary to reduce the continual spread of the infection and avoid future medical complications (Ong et al., 2023). Notifiable STIs include chlamydia, gonor-rhea, *Mycoplasma genitalium*, syphilis, trichomonas, hepatitis and HIV (Melbourne Sexual Health Centre, 2023). Clinicians have a legal responsibility to ensure contact tracing takes place in most jurisdictions (ASHM, 2022a). The need to contact one or more sexual partners depends on a number of factors, including which STI is involved and even whether it is possible to trace the sexual partners.

Contact tracing should be undertaken respecting the individual's needs. The patient must be fully informed about why contact tracing is required while providing assistance in identifying who needs to be informed (i.e. how far back to trace) and explaining the notification options available, including patient- or provider-initiated contact tracing. For patient-initiated contact tracing, the options include in-person, anonymously or via apps such as The Drama Downunder, Let Them Know and Better to Know (ASHM, 2022).

Health promotion activities

Health education relating to sexuality and sexual health is the major focus of health promotion activity for sexual health nurses. Assumptions should not be made that all adults are literate about sexual health. Nurses should also not assume that because an individual has sexual health knowledge they are able to protect themselves against sexual adversity, such as sexual assault or reproductive coercion (Silva et al., 2022). Sexual and reproductive education is diverse and varies across the globe and within communities. For example, consider women who may not have received formal sexual and reproductive education and may follow specific cultural practices or have been exposed to female genital mutilation (FGM). People may also have some knowledge from school or social media but may have misperceptions about contraception or ways to support fertility. These two examples highlight the importance of the nurse considering individual backgrounds and tailoring care and activities to best support individual needs.

Sexuality is an important aspect of an individual's well-being and is about a person's feelings, thoughts, attractions and behaviours to other people (Bolin et al., 2021). Sexual health incorporates physical, emotional, intellectual and social components with sexuality and sexual activity generally being positive and life-enhancing experiences for people (WHO, 2024a). Sexual health nurses promote attitudes and behaviours that support positive sexual health. Health education may be aimed at individuals, specific groups or the wider community. The three key areas of health education that sexual health nurses focus on are safer sex, reproductive choices and consent and domestic violence.

Safer sex

Safer sex – practices that minimise the risk of spreading an STI or an unplanned pregnancy as well as ensuring the emotional health of those involved (True Relationships and Reproductive Health, 2022).

Safer sex refers to practices that minimise the risk of spreading STIs or an unplanned pregnancy and ensure the emotional health of those involved (True Relationships and Reproductive Health, 2022). It is, therefore, very important to establish a shared understanding of this concept and the related implications when asking whether someone is practising safer sex.

Raising awareness of the range of STIs, possible symptoms and the asymptomatic nature of many STIs is useful. STIs can be transmitted through sexual contact including vaginal, anal and oral sex as well as from mother to child during pregnancy, childbirth or during breastfeeding (WHO, 2024b). Barrier methods support the prevention of body fluid exchange during sexual contact, such as blood, pre-ejaculatory fluid, semen, vaginal or oral secretions, via direct contact or objects (Jean Hailes for Women's Health, 2023). Placing too great an emphasis on the signs and symptoms of individual STIs may reinforce the belief that STIs are only present when a person has symptoms; this undermines the safer sex message. A standard asymptomatic STI check-up should occur:

- in special subpopulations with increased risk or poor outcomes from infection
- if someone requests testing

- if someone has had an exposure or history of STIs in the last year
- if someone has a partner from a special subpopulation
- if someone has had a new sexual partner or lived in/travelled to areas with increased prevalence of STIs (ASHM, 2024).

These will include tests for HIV antigen/antibodies, syphilis serology, hepatitis B, gonorrhea and chlamydia (ASHM, 2024).

The purpose of safer-sex education is to encourage the use of barrier methods such as male/female condoms and dental dams when engaging in sexual activity. These barriers are usually made from latex and create a physical barrier between the people having sex – reducing the exchange of bodily fluids and the subsequent risk of STI transmission. Individuals need to understand the risks associated with acquiring an STI and to be motivated to use these barriers to protect themselves and others from the risk of infection. As well as motivation to adopt safer-sex practices, good safer-sex education will provide the opportunity for a person to become familiar and comfortable with handling condoms and dental dams.

Pre-Exposure Prophylaxis (PrEP) is an antiretroviral medication used to reduce the transmission of HIV. PrEP is used to protect people who do not have a diagnosis of HIV but are at risk of contracting it. The medication is highly effective at preventing HIV infection; however, it does not protect against other STIs (ASHM, 2021). PrEP is recommended for all people who are at risk of HIV, that is, men who have sex with men, transgender people, and people who inject drugs (ASHM, 2021). For people whose sexual and/or intravenous drug use indicates the necessity for PrEP, a clinical assessment, including blood tests, is required to ensure the medication is indicated and safe for use. PrEP can be taken orally, daily or 'on demand', and is also available as a long-acting intramuscular injection. GPs, medical specialists and authorised nurse practitioners can prescribe PrEP (ASHM, 2021).

Reproductive choices

The prevention of unplanned, or unintended, pregnancy generally involves discussion of a wide range of contraceptive options that are available, including barriers (e.g. condoms), chemicals (e.g. spermicides) and hormones (e.g. contraceptive pill or implant). Most options provide temporary pregnancy prevention, while others, such as vasectomy and tubal ligation, are considered permanent. To support informed consent about contraceptive options, the effectiveness of each contraceptive type should be explored, as well as any specific possible side effects or limitations. For example, while temporary options, such as male condoms, are an effective barrier method for STI prevention, contraceptive benefit varies between 88–98 per cent efficacy depending on typical to perfect use (ASHM, 2022b). In contrast, long-acting reversible contraceptive methods, such as intrauterine devices, are 99.95 per cent effective and a 'set and forget' contraceptive method for 5–10 years but do not prevent STIs (ASHM, 2022b). It should be noted that in instances where unprotected sex has occurred in the previous five days, and the individual does not want to be pregnant, the emergency contraceptive pill or non-hormonal copper intrauterine device may be used (ASHM, 2022b).

A pregnancy may be confirmed through a urine and blood test and often an ultrasound. The sexual health nurse may be in a position where the patient wants to discuss pregnancy options. Not all pregnant people want or need pregnancy options counselling. However, for others, the availability of unbiased and non-directive counselling is essential. Pregnancy options counselling considers the individual's concerns about the pregnancy and the impact of these issues on their health, the things they have been unable to talk to others about regarding the pregnancy, and what would help them make decisions about the pregnancy (The Royal Women's Hospital, 2022). Pregnancy options include continuing the pregnancy and adoption or foster care, continuing the pregnancy and parenting, or abortion (Sexual Health Victoria, 2021a). Medication abortion can be provided in Australian primary care up to nine weeks gestation, and procedural abortion can be provided in clinics or hospitals, commonly up to 12 weeks gestation (Sexual Health Victoria, 2021b).

Consent and violence

Health education relating to sexuality and sexual health also considers the impacts of issues, such as consent and violence, on the overall health of the individual. Sexual violence can occur to any individual (East & Hutchinson, 2023). The sexual health nurse must reinforce what consent entails, namely that each person feels safe and comfortable during intimacy (Family Planning Australia, n.d.). Consent specifically involves the agreement of actions, what this involves, consequences and having a choice to say 'no' (Family Planning Australia, n.d.). The presence of drugs and alcohol can also influence someone's ability to consent to intimacy and/or sexual activity (Family Planning Australia, n.d.). During consultations where sexual assault has taken place, nurses need to consider the individual's safety, supports, whether the individual would like to make a complaint to police, sexual health and pregnancy screening, psychosocial health, counselling referral and mandatory reporting requirements (ASHM, 2022; Department of Families, Fairness and Housing, 2023).

Reproductive coercion and abuse (RCA) is a form of sexual violence, generally perpetrated against women by male intimate partners or other family members (Tarzia & Hegarty, 2021). It involves pregnancy coercion, contraceptive sabotage or controlling pregnancy outcomes (Grace & Anderson, 2018). Non-consensual sex and RCA can have ongoing implications for the emotional and physical health of the individual through poor mental health, unwanted pregnancies and increased STI risks (NSW Health, 2023b, Tarzia & Hegarty, 2021). RCA is also associated with intimate partner violence and decreased contraceptive self-efficacy (Tarzia & Hegarty, 2021). Understanding the overlay between consent, violence, STIs, contraceptive use and unplanned pregnancy will support a comprehensive sexual assessment.

CASE STUDY 20.2

Joel (cisgender male) presents at the sexual health clinic as he is concerned that he may have acquired an STI. When providing his sexual health history, Joel says that he has been going out with Sarah for almost a year and they have been having sex for the past six months. Before they had sex together for the first time, they were tested for STIs and were clear. They chose not to use condoms as Sarah is taking the pill. During the discussion, Joel also reveals that before he started seeing Sarah, he had been dating Bianca, who had left to live overseas. Bianca has recently returned home, and Joel has started seeing her again, although Sarah is unaware of this.

REFLECTION
1. What other information might be useful to ask Joel?
2. What are your priorities of care?
3. How should this situation be best managed?

Conclusion

This chapter acknowledges the range of settings and activities that may be undertaken by sexual health nurses in Australia and Aotearoa New Zealand. The core activities of practice have been identified and discussed, and pertinent issues highlighted. The need to avoid assumptions and provide culturally safe care has been emphasised as the best strategy to optimise care quality and health outcomes.

CRITICAL THINKING ACTIVITIES

Identify sexual health care providers/services in your local area.

1. How did you identify these services?
2. Are these services advertised?
3. Are sexual health care providers usually housed with other service providers? What are the advantages or disadvantages of such an arrangement?
4. How would you describe the role of the sexual health nurse in terms of providing PHC?

FURTHER READING

Aotearoa New Zealand STI Management Guidelines for Use in Primary Care. (n.d.). *Home page.* https://sti.guidelines.org.nz

Australasian Society for HIV Viral Hepatitis and Sexual Health Medicine (ASHM). (2022a). *Decision making in contraception.* https://ashm.org.au/resources/decision-making-in-contraception-consultation-essentials/

———. (2022b). *Australasian Contact Tracing Guidelines 2022.* https://contacttracing.ashm.org.au/

Australasian STI Management Guidelines for Use in Primary Care. (2024). *Standard asymptomatic check-up.* https://sti.guidelines.org.au/standard-asymptomatic-checkup/

Ministry of Health. (2020). *New Zealand Aotearoa's Guidance on Contraception.* New Zealand Government. https://www.health.govt.nz/publications/new-zealand-aotearoas-guidance-on-contraception

New Zealand Sexual Health Society. (2023). *PrEP and PEP Guidelines for Aotearoa New Zealand.* https://az659834.vo.msecnd.net/eventsairaueprod/production-forumpoint2-public/c8e6e4cf56014739aa2d9cb16ccfb4f6

The Royal Australian and New Zealand College of Obstetricians and Gynaecologists. (2023). *Abortion Decision Aid.* https://ranzcog.edu.au/wp-content/uploads/2023/10/Abortion-Decision-Aid.pdf

REFERENCES

Australasian Society for HIV Viral Hepatitis and Sexual Health Medicine (ASHM). (2021). *Prevent HIV by Prescribing PrEP.* https://prepguidelines.com.au/wp-content/uploads/2021/11/ASHM-National-PrEP-Guidelines.pdf

——— (2022a). *Australasian Contact Tracing Guidelines 2022.* https://contacttracing.ashm.org.au/

——— (2022b). *Decision making in contraception.* https://ashm.org.au/resources/decision-making-in-contraception-consultation-essentials/

——— (2024a). *Standard asymptomatic check-up.* https://sti.guidelines.org.au/standard-asymptomatic-checkup/

———— (2024b). *Australian STI management guidelines for use in primary care*. https://sti .guidelines.org.au/

Bolin, A., Whelehan, P., Vernon, M. & Antoine, K. (2021). *Human Sexuality: Biological, Psychological, and Cultural Perspectives*. Taylor & Francis Group. https://doi.org/10.4324/9780429269158

Cappiello, J., Levi, A. & Nothnagle, M. (2016). Core competencies in sexual and reproductive health for the interprofessional primary care team. *Contraception, 93*(5), 438–45. https://doi .org/10.1016/j.contraception.2015.12.013

Davies, C., Robinson, K.H., Metcalf, A., et al. (2021). Australians of diverse sexual orientations and gender identities. In T. Dune, K. McLeod & R. Williams (eds), *Culture, Diversity and Health in Australia: Towards Culturally Safe Health Care* (pp. 213–31). Routledge.

Department of Families, Fairness and Housing. (2023). *Mandatory reporting*. State Government of Victoria. https://providers.dffh.vic.gov.au/mandatory-reporting

Department of Health. (2018). *Fourth national sexually transmitted infections strategy*. Commonwealth of Australia.

Department of Health and Aged Care. (2022). *About the National Cervical Screening program*. Commonwealth of Australia. www.health.gov.au/our-work/national-cervical-screening-program/about-the-national-cervical-screening-program

East, L. & Hutchinson, M. (2023). Sexual violence matters: Nurses must respond. *Journal of Advanced Nursing, 79*(2), e10–e11. https://doi.org/10.1111/jan.15495

Family Planning Australia. (n.d.). *Consent and sex*. www.fpnsw.org.au/health-information/consent-and-sex/consent-and-sex

Geary, R.S., Tanton, C., Erens, B., et al. (2018). Sexual identity, attraction and behaviour in Britain: The implications of using different dimensions of sexual orientation to estimate the size of sexual minority populations and inform public health interventions. *PloS ONE, 13*(1), e0189607. https://doi.org/10.1371/journal.pone.0189607

Grace, K.T. & Anderson, J.C. (2018). Reproductive coercion. *Trauma, Violence & Abuse, 19*(4), 371–90. https://doi.org/10.1177/1524838016663935

Hill, A.O., Bourne, A., McNair, R., Carman, M. & Lyons, A. (2020). *Private Lives 3: The Health and Wellbeing of LGBTIQ People in Australia*. (ARCSHS Monograph Series no. 122.) Australian Research Centre in Sex, Health and Society, La Trobe University.

Human Rights Campaign. (2023). *Sexual orientation and gender identity definitions*. www.hrc.org/resources/sexual-orientation-and-gender-identity-terminology-and-definitions

Jean Hailes for Women's Health. (2023). *Safer sex and sexually transmitted infections (STIs)*. www.jeanhailes.org.au/health-a-z/sex-sexual-health/safer-sex-stis#what-is-safer-sex

Melbourne Sexual Health Centre. (2023). *Contact tracing & partner notification*. www.mshc.org.au/health-professionals/contact-tracing-notification

NSW Health. (2019). *Sexual health check-up*. NSW Government. www.health.nsw.gov.au/sexualhealth/Pages/sexual-health-check-up.aspx

———— (2022). *NSW Sexually Transmissible Infections Strategy 2022–2026*. NSW Government. www .health.nsw.gov.au/sexualhealth/Publications/nsw-sti-strategy.pdf

———— (2023b). *Information for victims of sexual assault*. NSW Government. www.health.nsw.gov.au/parvan/sexualassault/Pages/default.aspx

———— (n.d.). *Home page*. NSW Government. www.health.nsw.gov.au/Pages/default.aspx

Nursing and Midwifery Board of Australia. (2018). *Joint statement – cultural safety: Nurses and midwives leading the way for safer healthcare*. www.nursingmidwiferyboard.gov.au/codes-guidelines-statements/position-statements/leading-the-way.aspx

Ong, J.J., Bourne, C., Dean, J.A., et al. (2023). Australian sexually transmitted infection (STI) management guidelines for use in primary care 2022 update. *Sexual Health, 20*(1), 1–8. https://doi.org/10.1071/SH22134

Rubin, E.S., Rullo, J., Tsai, P., et al. (2018). Best practices in North American pre-clinical medical education in sexual history taking: Consensus from the summits in medical education in sexual health. *The Journal of Sexual Medicine, 15*(10), 1414–25. https://doi.org/10.1071/SH22134

Sexual Health Victoria. (2021a). *Unplanned pregnancy.* https://shvic.org.au/for-you/pregnancy/unplanned-pregnancy

—— (2021b). *Types of abortions.* https://shvic.org.au/for-you/abortion/abortion-overview

Silva, M., Kassegne, S., Nagbe, R.-H.Y., et al. (2022). Changing the script: Intergenerational communication about sexual and reproductive health in Niamey, Niger. *Journal of Health Communication, 27*(10), 755–63. https://doi.org/10.1080/10810730.2022.2160527

Tan, K.K.H. & Sai Ang, L. (2022). Cultural safety for LGBTQIA+ people: A narrative review and implications for health care in Malaysia. *Sexes, 3*(3), 385–95. https://doi.org/10.3390/sexes3030029

Tarzia, L. & Hegarty, K. (2021). A conceptual re-evaluation of reproductive coercion: Centring intent, fear and control. *Reproductive Health, 18*(1), 87–87. https://doi.org/10.1186/s12978-021-01143-6

The Royal Australian College of General Practitioners (RACGP). (2016). *Guidelines for preventive Activities in General practice* (9th ed.). RACGP. www.racgp.org.au/download/Documents/Guidelines/Redbook9/17048-Red-Book-9th-Edition.pdf

The Royal Women's Hospital. (2022). *Unplanned pregnancy: options counselling.* https://thewomens.r.worldssl.net/images/uploads/fact-sheets/UnplannedPreg_OptionsCounselling.pdf

True Relationships and Reproductive Health. (2022). *Safer sex.* www.true.org.au/education/programs-resources/for-communities/safer-sex

Woodman, D. & Threadgold, S. (2021). *This is Sociology: A Short Introduction.* SAGE Publications.

World Health Organization (WHO). (2022). *Critical considerations and actions for achieving universal access to sexual and reproductive health in the context of universal health coverage through a primary health care approach.* WHO.

—— (2024a). *Sexual health.* www.who.int/health-topics/sexual-health#tab=tab_1

—— (2024b). *Sexually transmitted infections (STIs).* www.who.int/news-room/fact-sheets/detail/sexually-transmitted-infections-(stis)

21 Drug and alcohol nursing

Ravina Raidu and Rebecca Bosworth
With acknowledgement to Rhonda Brown,
Dean Hyland and Eileen Petrie

> I became an Alcohol and Other Drug (AOD) nurse in 2007 and remained one since because in the chaotic stigmatised life that my AOD clients have, I can provide a space that is client-centered, trauma informed, free from discrimination with a non-judgemental environment my AOD clients can interact in.
>
> *Ravina Raidu, registered nurse (RN)*

LEARNING OBJECTIVES

At the completion of this chapter, you should be able to:

- explain the context of drug and alcohol nursing.
- recognise the effect of substance use and drug-related harms on overall health and well-being.
- identify how a harm minimisation approach may support people to reduce the risk of substance-related harms.
- explain the role of the community AOD nurse.
- explain how nurses contribute to the holistic physical and mental health care of people who use drugs.

Introduction

This chapter focuses on the theory, skills and professional role of a drug and alcohol nurse in community settings. It describes substance use and drug-related harms and provides a brief overview of the guiding principles and professional practice drug and alcohol nurses follow when providing care for people who use AOD. The chapter also describes the considerations for co-occurring needs and integrated care. Reflective activities throughout the chapter will guide the reader to consider how they can support people living with AOD in their nursing practice.

The context of drug and alcohol nursing

Understanding substance use

People use substances for various reasons. Substance use can be a normal part of a person's life, with many people in developed countries consuming alcohol at some point during their lives. However, only a minority of people may consume illicit (illegal or controlled) drugs (National Center for Health Statistics, 2023).

Prevalence of substance use

Globally, an estimated 296 million people used drugs in 2021 (United Nations Office on Drugs and Crime (UNODC), 2023). Although this represents an increase of 23 per cent over the previous decade, fewer than 20 per cent of people worldwide living with a **substance use disorder** were in treatment (UNODC, 2023). The *National Drug Strategy Household Survey 2022–2023* reports 31 per cent of Australians drank alcohol in ways that placed their health at risk, 8.3 per cent smoked tobacco daily, 7 per cent used electronic cigarettes and vapes, and greater than one in two have used an illicit drug during their lifetime (Australian Institute of Health and Welfare (AIHW), 2024b). Additionally, an estimated 5.3 per cent of Australians used a pharmaceutical drug for non-medical purposes (AIHW, 2024b), and one in five Australians will experience problems with AOD (Turning Point, 2024b). Similarly, in Aotearoa New Zealand, current data shows that some 18.8 per cent of adults have a hazardous drinking pattern, 8 per cent of adults are daily smokers and 49 per cent use recreational drugs in their lifetime (Ministry of Health, 2022). An estimated 1.3 million New Zealanders are at moderate or high risk of problematic substance use, with the drugs causing the most harm being alcohol and tobacco (New Zealand Drug Foundation, 2024a). The most commonly consumed substances in Australia and Aotearoa New Zealand are alcohol, followed by cannabis and tobacco (AIHW, 2024b; New Zealand Drug Foundation, 2024a). However, the usage of e-cigarettes and vape use is growing exponentially (AIHW, 2024b).

Drug and alcohol nurses play a vital role in prevention, brief and early intervention and harm reduction, contributing directly to achieving the United Nations' Sustainable Development Goals (SDG3), target 3.5 to strengthen the prevention and treatment of substance use (United Nations (UN), n.d.). Drug and alcohol nurses can also reach and deliver care to people underserved by the health care system experiencing significant health inequalities (Drug & Alcohol Nurses of Australasia (DANA), 2021).

> **REFLECTION**
>
> Given what you have read so far about AOD, what role do you think drug and alcohol nurses have in providing care and support for people consuming AOD at harmful levels?

Spectrum of substance use

Alcohol and other drug use may not always cause harm to a person's physical or mental health (**harmful use**) and the impact of addiction on people's lives may differ (NSW Health,

Substance use disorder – '…a cluster of cognitive, behavioral, and physiological symptoms indicating that the individual continues to use the substance despite significant substance-related problems.' (Note: Beyond detoxification, substance-use disorders cause an underlying change in the brain circuits which may cause repeated relapses and intense drug cravings when an individual is exposed to drug-related stimuli (American Psychiatric Association (APA), 2023)).

Harmful use – a pattern of use that causes damage to a person's physical or mental health or has resulted in behaviour leading to harm to the health of others (World Health Organization (WHO), 2024c).

Tolerance –
' …requiring a markedly
increased dose of a
substance to achieve
the desired effect or a
markedly reduced effect
when the usual dose is
consumed' (APA, 2023).

Withdrawal – '…a
syndrome that occurs
when blood or tissue
concentrations of a
substance decline
in an individual who
has maintained
prolonged, heavy use
of the substance.
After developing
withdrawal symptoms,
the individual is likely to
consume the substance
to relieve the symptoms'
(APA, 2023).

2023) (Figure 21.1). Regular drug use may lead to increased **tolerance** and may also lead to either physical and/or psychological dependence (Department of Health and Aged Care, 2019). Ceasing AOD use may lead a person to experience **withdrawal** symptoms, which can be physically and mentally unpleasant (Department of Health and Aged Care, 2019).

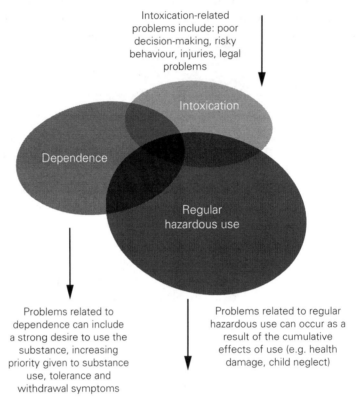

Figure 21.1 Domains of intoxication, regular use and dependence
Source: Adapted from Thorley (1982).

Dependence is a risk associated with all psychoactive substances (e.g. substances that result in perception, mood, cognition and behaviour alterations) (Darke, Lappin & Farrell, 2019). The dependence syndrome for all drugs now is simply referred to as substance use disorder, for example, Cannabis Use Disorder, Opioid Use Disorder (APA, 2013). The dependence syndrome may relate to a specific substance (e.g. nicotine, alcohol, diazepam), a class of substances (e.g. opioids), or a wider range of pharmacologically diverse substances (Darke et al., 2019). The diagnostic criteria for substance use disorders are defined in both the *Diagnostic and Statistical Manual of Mental Disorders* 5th edition (DSM-5) (APA, 2013) and the *International Classification of Diseases* 11th edition (ICD-11) (WHO, 2024c), and range in severity from mild to severe. It is important to recognise that AOD use occurs across a continuum, with each point requiring a different approach to health care and support, as observed in Figure 21.1 (Department of Health, 2017; National Centre for Education and Training on Addiction (NCETA), 2023b).

Consider the model in Figure 21.1 demonstrating how regular hazardous use represents the greatest harm for society. For some individuals, there may be some overlap and they may experience problems in all three domains (Thorley, 1982).

People use substances for different reasons

People may be living with or develop substance use disorders due to various factors. Understanding why a person is using AOD rather than solely focusing on the substance itself is vital (NSW Health, 2020). Reasons may include pleasure, curiosity, boredom or peer influences; to enhance performance, lifestyle factors, family environment, nature and nurture impacts; to alleviate physical or emotional pain, complex trauma, genetic factors; as well as long-lasting neuroadaptive changes from repetitive exposure to substances, brain chemistry and neurotransmitter levels (Mosel, 2024; NCETA, 2023a;).

Priority populations who are at an increased risk of experiencing disproportionate harms (indirect and direct) associated with AOD include Aboriginal and Torres Strait Islander and Māori peoples, people living with co-occurring mental health conditions, those in contact with the criminal justice system, young people, older people, culturally and linguistically diverse populations and people identifying as LGBTQIA+ (Department of Health, 2017).

The impact of substance use on health and well-being

Drug-related harms

Substance use is associated with significant health risks, contributing to a huge burden of disease (WHO, 2024b). Substance use disorders are considered the leading preventable cause of injury, illness and death (Turning Point, 2024b). A range of risks and harms may be associated with substance use, the most prominent being fatal and non-fatal, drug toxicity ('overdose') (Darke et al., 2019). In Australia, one fatal overdose is reported to occur every four hours. This equates to some 2231 drug-induced deaths annually, of which 75 per cent were unintentional (Penington Institute, 2023). Table 21.1 provides an insight into Australia's common drugs of concern, treatment and associated burden.

The burden of drug-related harm extends far beyond fatalities, as illustrated in Table 21.1. AOD-related harms may lead to decreased quality of life and impair personal, family, social, educational and occupational aspects of a person's life (WHO, 2024a). Understanding the risks and harms allows drug and alcohol nurses to work with people to implement targeted, person-centred interventions, to minimise the harms (Table 21.2).

REFLECTION

A 55-year-old male presents to the local medical centre with an injecting-related abscess. What are the main clinical concerns for this man?

Harm minimisation

Australia's *National Drug Strategy 2017–2026* provides a national framework, identifying national priorities related to alcohol, tobacco and other drugs, guides action and provides a national commitment to harm minimisation (Department of Health, 2017). Australia's

Table 21.1 Australia's common drugs of concern, treatment and associated burden

Substance	Principal drug of concern (2021–2)	Treatment (2021–2)	Burden of disease (2018)	Deaths (2022)	Geographic differences (2019)
Alcohol	Most common principal drug of concern (PDOC): 42% of all treatment episodes	48 400 received treatment 3 in 5 were male, 1 in 6 were Indigenous	Fifth highest risk factor contributing to burden of disease (4.5%)	1742 alcohol-induced deaths	People living in *regional and remote* areas more likely to exceed risk guidelines
Amphetamines	Second most common PDOC: 24% of treatment episodes	27 490 received treatment 3 in 5 were male, 1 in 5 were Indigenous 80% of amphetamine-treatment episodes were for methamphetamine as the PDOC	0.7% of the total burden of disease	Rapid increase in deaths involving methamphetamine and other stimulants, 2021 death rate almost 4 times higher than 2000	Similar proportions of people used meth/amphetamine regardless of location
Cannabis	Most widely used drug Third most common PDOC: 19% of treatment episodes	25 989 received treatment 3 in 5 were male, 1 in 5 were Indigenous	0.3% of the total burden of disease	Cannabinoids were present in 4.5% of all drug-induced deaths (2021)	People living in *regional and remote* areas more likely to have used cannabis in the past year
Heroin	Fourth most common PDOC 4.5% of treatment episodes	5242 received treatment 2 in 3 were male, 1 in 5 were Indigenous	0.9% of the total burden of disease	18% drug-induced deaths were heroin-related (2021)	Heroin consumption is higher in *capital cities*
Pharmaceuticals	PDOC in 5% of treatment episodes for client's own AOD use Opioids and benzodiazepines accounted for 3 in 4 treatment episodes	6155 received treatment for any pharmaceutical drug as the PDOC 3 in 5 were male, 1 in 7 were Indigenous		Rate of benzodiazepine-related deaths increased from 1.9 per 100 000 to 2.9 per 100 000 between 1997–2021.	People in *remote and very remote* areas 1.5 times more likely to have recently used painkillers/pain-relievers and opioids (excluding over-the-counter) for non-medical purposes
Tobacco	PDOC in 1.2% of treatment episodes for client's own AOD use	1820 received treatment 1 in 2 were male, 1 in 5 were Indigenous	8.6% of the total burden of disease and the leading cause of cancer (44% of cancer burden)	Leading cause of preventable morbidity and mortality	*People living in remote and very remote* areas of Australia are more likely to smoke daily

Source: Adapted from AIHW (2024b).

Table 21.2 Harm associated with substance use

Harms	Description
Physical	Infectious diseases (blood-borne viruses HIV/AIDS and hepatitis B and C), vascular disease, abscesses, bacterial infections (e.g. endocarditis), vein damage, skin lesions and infections, weakened immune system, regular colds and flu, chronic sleeping problems, menstrual problems, respiratory problems – lung damage and disease, sinus problems and damage to nose, poor oral health, hospitalisation from injury, malnutrition, weight loss, psychomotor deficits and Parkinson's disease, organ damage and disease (brain, heart, kidney, liver, lungs), heart attack and stroke, cancer, overdose and mortality
Psychological	Anxiety, depression, psychosis, disorientation, confusion, apathy, agitation and aggression, neurocognitive impairment, increased risk of self-harm and suicide
Social	Impairment in social cognition and occupational functioning, increased stress on relationships, loss of family support, housing instability, financial insecurity, poverty, unemployment, increased risk of violence and crime, risk of incarceration, unhealthy child development and trauma

Source: Adapted from Darke et al. (2019); Department of Health and Aged Care (2019); NSW Health (2021).

balanced approach rests on the three pillars of demand reduction, supply reduction and harm reduction (Department of Health, 2017). Demand reduction aims to prevent the uptake, as well as delay and decrease the use of AOD, and uses evidence-based treatment to support people to recover from substance use disorders (Department of Health, 2017). Supply reduction involves preventing, ceasing and disrupting illegal drug supply as well as legal drug regulation (Department of Health, 2017). Finally, harm reduction involves supporting people and their families to minimise substance-related harms including the health, social and economic impacts (Department of Health, 2017). Similarly, Aotearoa New Zealand drug policies are also underpinned by a harm minimisation philosophy (New Zealand Drug Foundation, 2024b). In adopting this approach, a person's choice to continue to use AOD is recognised while the person receives education and information to reduce drug-related harms (NSW Health, 2023; Turning Point, 2018).

REFLECTION

One-quarter to one-half of people using methamphetamine, who were seeking treatment, advised they would like to *reduce* use *not* abstain or completely stop (Turning Point, 2018). Considering the physical, psychological and social drug-related harms, can you think of any harm reduction interventions you might recommend to support someone to minimise drug-related harms?

Evidence-based harm reduction strategies

Drug and alcohol nurses play an important part in providing harm-reduction messages, as well as brief and early interventions (NSW Health, 2023). A wide body of evidence demonstrates that harm reduction approaches do not increase drug use, rather they support people to reduce the harms of drug use to individuals, and the wider community (Harm Reduction Australia, 2024).

Harm reduction may include providing education on safer drug administration, reduction in quantity/frequency of substance use and lifestyle improvements (Turning Point, 2018). Interventions may include access to needle and syringe programs (NSP), supervised injecting centres, pharmacotherapy treatment (methadone or buprenorphine for opioid dependence), take-home naloxone (THN), nicotine replacement therapy (NRT), withdrawal services and rehabilitation (Alcohol and Drug Foundation, 2023a, 2023b; Harm Reduction International, 2022; North Richmond Community Health, 2023). In Australia, the THN program makes naloxone (for opioid overdose reversal) free to people who may experience, witness, or are at risk of an opioid overdose (Monds et al., 2022). Naloxone may be accessed over the counter in community pharmacies, prescribed by a doctor and dispensed at a pharmacy, and supplied by AOD and NSP services (Department of Health and Aged Care, 2024; Monds et al., 2022). Pill testing (also referred to as drug checking) is available in 20 countries globally, including Australia and Aotearoa New Zealand (ACT Government, 2023; Alcohol and Drug Foundation, 2023c), although its role remains debated in many communities.

The role of the community drug and alcohol nurse

Drug and alcohol nurses work in various community- and hospital-based services, with the setting determining the nature of their role. Services may include drug and alcohol services, withdrawal services, specialist programs (chemical use in pregnancy, court diversion programs, cannabis clinics, pharmaceutical opioid clinics, psychiatric comorbidity clinics), shared care (supporting GPs), needle and syringe services, medically supervised injecting centres and opioid treatment centres (Health South Eastern Sydney Local Health District, 2023). The specialist drug and alcohol nurse must have comprehensive knowledge and skills to respond to complex problems among people living with AOD disorders or those using AOD at harmful levels (DANA, 2024).

DANA is the peak nursing body representing drug and alcohol nurses across Australia and Aotearoa New Zealand (DANA, 2021). DANA advocates that all nurses require a basic level of knowledge and skills to assess, identify and respond to individuals whose health and well-being is affected by AOD use and their families (DANA, 2024). In some cases, a generalist nurse may conduct initial AOD screening, deliver brief interventions within their scope of practice, and then refer to a specialist nurse or treatment provider for comprehensive assessment and intervention (NSW Health, 2020).

The Drug and Alcohol Specialist Nursing model covers the continuum of health, spanning primary and secondary prevention, early interventions and treatment, including intensive therapeutic interventions and support, as well as broader public health and community health promotion (DANA, 2024). The purpose of the role is to support and improve the health and well-being of people who use AOD and reduce any drug-related harms, while adopting a holistic, person-centred approach. Beyond specialist registered nurses, nurse practitioners can also specialise in drug and alcohol services (DANA, 2021).

Guiding principles and professional practice

Underpinning the drug and alcohol nurse's practice are strong advocacy skills and the important values of respect, compassion, commitment to human rights, autonomy and self-determination in a culturally safe manner (DANA, 2024). These qualities are particularly important for drug and alcohol nurses, given the care they provide is often delivered to people who are underserved by the current health system. There are often competing moral and ethical dilemmas for health professionals caring for people who use drugs, however, there remains an ethical obligation to uphold the bioethical principles of autonomy, non-maleficence, beneficence and justice (Williamson, 2021). A key role of nurses is supporting individuals to reduce their vulnerability and drug-related risk (NSW Health, 2021).

Addressing the experience of stigma and discrimination

> Attitudes are contagious. Are yours worth catching? (Mannering & Mannering, 1999)

Negative attitudes held by the public and health care professionals are barriers that deter people from seeking treatment (Turning Point, 2024b). Stigma and discrimination increase the risk of people leaving treatment prematurely and contribute to poorer treatment outcomes (Substance Abuse and Mental Health Services Administration, 2021). Drug and alcohol nurses are leaders in the field, promoting person-centred language when supporting people who use AOD. Stigmatising terms such as junkie, druggie or drug abuser should be replaced with neutral terms, including, but not limited to, a person who uses drugs, a person who injects drugs or a person living with a substance use disorder (Alcohol and Drug Foundation, 2019).

REFLECTION

The phrase 'drug addiction' has been omitted from the DSM-5-TR (text revision) as a diagnostic term in the classification of substance-related and addictive disorders. Instead, the more neutral term 'substance use disorder' is used due to the uncertain definition of 'drug addiction' and to avoid its potentially negative connotation (APA, 2023).

1. What is your experience of language related to AOD use?
2. What impact has this had on those around you?

Holistic physical and mental health care

Considerations for co-occurring needs: integrated care

In Australia, more than one-third of people living with an AOD use disorder are estimated to be living with at least one mental health condition (Marel et al., 2022). This is known as dual diagnosis. Given the high prevalence of people living with dual diagnosis, drug and alcohol nurses often need to manage complex psychiatric conditions while treating AOD use necessitating an integrated approach to treatment (Marel et al., 2022). However, current health systems often provide either sequential (one treatment, e.g. psychiatric treatment, followed by the other, e.g. substance use treatment) or parallel treatments. Other co-occurring needs to consider may include physical health (e.g. pain, blood-borne viruses, sleep and diet, sexual and reproductive health) or cognitive impairments (NSW Health, 2023). Where possible, the nurse should seek to understand the nature of all care being sought/received to support the person in best navigating the health system.

REFLECTION

1. The management of co-occurring conditions is part of the drug and alcohol nurse's core business. What could you do to build skills about the symptoms and evidence-based management of common coexisting conditions?
2. What might the impact of parallel rather than integrated health services be on the person receiving services? How might this affect their engagement with services?

CASE STUDY 21.1

Sebastian, a 34-year-old who identifies as male, was transferred into his local AOD service's opioid treatment program following his recent release from prison. Sebastian was living with an opioid use disorder prior to entering custody and commenced opioid agonist therapy during incarceration. As a drug and alcohol nurse working at the AOD service, you encounter Sebastian during his first visit. Sebastian has a few concerns that he would like to discuss with you. Firstly, he discloses there were times he needed to 'top up' his dose of prescribed methadone in prison by injecting illicit buprenorphine using shared injecting equipment. Sebastian is worried as he was diagnosed with hepatitis C virus (HCV) in prison. Although he was treated in prison and successfully cleared the virus, Sebastian knows re-infection can occur. Secondly, Sebastian is also worried about his increased risk of overdosing following release from prison. Sebastian is aware that he has a decreased tolerance and acknowledges that if he continues to 'top up', his risk of overdose increases. Sebastian has previously overdosed and has also witnessed an overdose in a friend. Sebastian expresses many feelings of regret, self-blame, and worthlessness as he shares that he did not respond effectively to opioid agonist therapy in the past. He mentions that when in prison, he heard of a new version of naloxone, stating they were giving it out to people upon release from prison in the form of a nasal spray, something called 'Nyxoid', he says. He thinks he may need this 'just in case'.

REFLECTION
1. Considering Sebastian's history of opioid overdose, his decreased tolerance and his interest in having access to naloxone upon release, as a drug and alcohol nurse, how can you support Sebastian to co-develop a comprehensive overdose prevention plan?
2. What factors would be important to include in this plan?

Coordinating care planning

The goal of a drug and alcohol nurse is to improve a person's health and well-being across all domains, while adopting a collaborative approach with the person and other services (Figure 21.2). This means focusing on the person and not the illness (e.g. not the mental health condition or level of dependence) (Marel et al., 2022). Care should also be tailored to align with the diverse needs and preferences of priority populations and to promote equity for these groups (NSW Health, 2020).

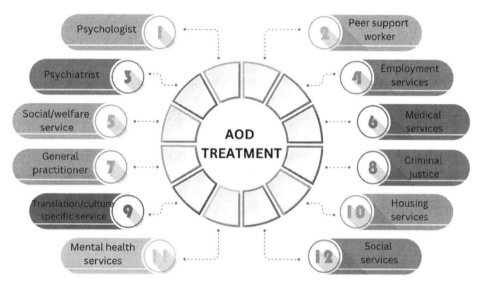

Figure 21.2   Services that drug and alcohol nurses may need to engage in person-centred care
Source: Adapted from Marel et al. (2022).

Case management

Drug and alcohol nurses are involved in person-centred case management for people who use AOD, which is considered comprehensive, tailored support, as illustrated in Figure 21.3. Case management also aims to provide a holistic approach to addressing physical, mental, socio-economic, psychosocial and legal aspects for the person and encompasses assessment, planning, linking and monitoring (AIHW, 2024a; Association of Alcohol and Other Drug Agencies, 2015). This collaborative approach comprises working alongside the person and planning for changes in their AOD use towards a more therapeutic, less harmful level.

Psychosocial approaches used in treatment

Drug and alcohol nurses may be involved in the delivery of psychological approaches, including acceptance and commitment therapy, behavioural activation, cognitive behavioural therapy, contingency management, dialectical behavioural therapy, exposure therapy, mindfulness training, psychosocial group therapy, motivational interviewing or relapse prevention (Marel et al., 2022; WHO, 2020). The choice and use of specific approaches are dependent on the individual nurse's scope of practice, the model of care in which they are working and local health policy.

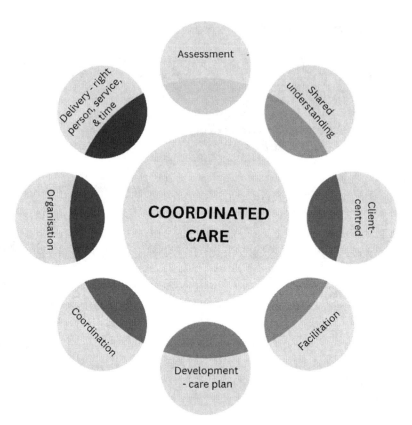

Figure 21.3 Coordinated care
Source: Adapted from Marel et al. (2022).

Drug and alcohol nurses provide brief interventions to deliver time-limited, short extracts of early advice or information regarding AOD use (Rodgers, 2018). These 5–20-minute intervention opportunities allow clinicians to assist in reducing substance-related harms, yet they should not be focused on a single session but rather repeated whenever possible (Rodgers, 2018).

Relapse prevention

Returning to substance use is described as a relapse, and most people will experience relapse as they progress through the change process (Figure 21.4) (Turning Point, 2024a). Relapses will help people learn what works for them and what does not. Therefore, it is important to help the person identify their individual strengths and weaknesses (Alcohol and Drug Foundation, 2024). Relapse prevention strategies help to identify environmental situations, interpersonal/intrapersonal variables and cues linked with use and returning to AOD. Relapse prevention also includes preparing individuals for managing a lapse or slip, to prevent the progression into a relapse (Alcohol and Drug Foundation, 2024). Factors to consider in relapse prevention are the strength of the person's resolution, their degree of attachment to the AOD, their control and coping mechanisms in high-risk situations plus the support and resources available for the individual on their recovery journey (Alcohol and Drug Foundation, 2024). Drug and alcohol nurses are prepared for this and are there to welcome people back into treatment when they are ready.

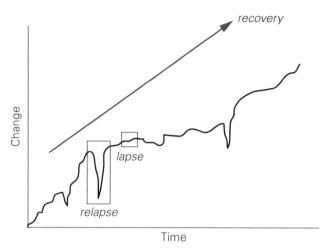

Figure 21.4   Lapse and relapse
Source: Turning Point (2024a).

Pharmacological approaches

Pharmacotherapy

Pharmacotherapies are common in the treatment of AOD disorders, and it is recommended that they be delivered as a package with psychosocial interventions (WHO, 2020). Substance-related disorders are chronic, treatable health conditions which often require continuing care rather than acute, episodic treatment (Substance Abuse and Mental Health Services Administration, 2021). Medications are used to treat cravings and withdrawal symptoms and to prevent relapse. Treatment services should be available, accessible, evidence-based, affordable and diversified (WHO, 2020). There is no 'one size fits all' approach, with many people benefiting from lifelong treatment (Substance Abuse and Mental Health Services Administration, 2021). A range of pharmacotherapies are available for different substances. Acamprosate, disulfiram or naltrexone may support a person to reduce or cease their alcohol use. Methadone, buprenorphine, buprenorphine/naloxone or naltrexone may support a reduction or cessation of opioid use. Medications to treat methamphetamine dependence are still being explored and some are currently prescribed in clinical trials, including dexamphetamine, lisdexamphetmine and modafinil (NSW Health, 2023). A collaborative approach between the person and the multidisciplinary health team is essential in assessing a person's suitability for pharmacotherapy (NSW Health, 2023).

Conclusion

This chapter offers valuable insights into the role of drug and alcohol nursing and its impact on those who use AOD at harmful levels. This chapter has provided a comprehensive understanding of the impact of AOD use and drug-related harms on an individual's overall health and well-being, as well as the potential benefits of harm minimisation strategies. Furthermore, it provides an opportunity to gain an improved understanding of the pivotal role of community drug and alcohol nurses in supporting and providing holistic care, both physical and mental, for individuals who use AOD.

CRITICAL THINKING ACTIVITIES

'Harm minimisation' is the stated policy in relation to substance use in Australia and Aotearoa New Zealand.

1. Alcohol continues to be the most commonly used substance in Australia and Aotearoa New Zealand, with drinking very much part of the cultural and social norms. The harm associated with excessive drinking is significant for individuals, families and the wider community. Do you think there is a need for cultural change regarding alcohol use in our society? If so, what else could be done to challenge attitudes?
2. What is your opinion of a harm minimisation approach to alcohol and other drug misuse?
3. Needle exchange programs have been found to be effective in reducing the harm associated with drugs, and there is increasing interest in scaling up the availability of medically supervised injecting centres for people who inject drugs. What are some of the barriers to opening medically supervised injecting centres?

FURTHER READING

Department of Health and Aged Care. (2019). *National Framework for Alcohol, Tobacco and Other Drug Treatment 2019–2029*. Australian Government. www.health.gov.au/resources/publications/national-framework-for-alcohol-tobacco-and-other-drug-treatment-2019-29?language=en

Drug & Alcohol Nurses of Australasia (DANA). (2024). *Home page*. www.danaonline.org

Marel, C., Siedlecka, E., Fisher, A., et al. (2022). *Guidelines on the Management of Co-occurring Alcohol and Other Drug and Mental Health Conditions in Alcohol and Other Drug Treatment Settings* (3rd ed.). Matilda Centre for Research in Mental Health and Substance Use, The University of Sydney. https://comorbidityguidelines.org.au/pdf/comorbidity-guideline.pdf

SBS. (2020). *Addicted Australia*. www.sbs.com.au/ondemand/tv-series/addicted-australia

REFERENCES

ACT Government. (2023). *Canberra's drug checking service extended*. ACT Government. www.cmtedd.act.gov.au/open_government/inform/act_government_media_releases/rachel-stephen-smith-mla-media-releases

Alcohol and Drug Foundation. (2019). *The Power of Words: Having conversations about alcohol and other drugs: A Quick Guide*. http://anyflip.com/line/fqdv/

—— (2023a). *Medically supervised injecting centres save lives*. https://adf.org.au/insights/medically-supervised-injecting-centres/

—— (2023b). *Supervised injecting facilities*. https://adf.org.au/reducing-risk/supervised-injecting-facilities/

—— (2023c). *Pill testing in Australia*. https://adf.org.au/insights/pill-testing-australia/

—— (2024). *Relapse*. https://adf.org.au/reducing-risk/relapse/

American Psychiatric Association (APA). (2013). *Diagnostic and Statistical Manual of Mental Disorders* (5th ed.). APA.

—— (2023). *Diagnostic and Statistical Manual of Mental Disorders; Substance-Related and Addictive Disorders*. www.psychiatry.org/file%20library/psychiatrists/practice/dsm/apa_dsm-5-substance-use-disorder.pdf

Association of Alcohol and Other Drug Agencies. (2015). *Case Management in Non-Government Alcohol and Other Drugs Service: A Practical Toolkit*. Northern Territory Government. www.aadant.org.au/sites/default/files/uploads/files/aadant-case-managing-in-non-government-aod-services-a-practical-toolkit.pdf

Australian Institute of Health and Welfare (AIHW). (2024a). *Alcohol and Other Drug Treatment Services in Australia Annual Report.* Australian Government. www.aihw.gov.au/reports/alcohol-other-drug-treatment-services/alcohol-other-drug-treatment-services-australia/contents/about

—— (2024b). *National Drug Strategy Household Survey 2022–2023.* Australian Government. www.aihw.gov.au/reports/illicit-use-of-drugs/national-drug-strategy-household-survey/contents/about

Darke, S., Lappin, J. & Farrell, M.P. (2019). *The Clinician's Guide to Illicit Drugs and Health.* Silverback Publishing.

Department of Health. (2017). *National Drug Strategy 2017–2026.* Commonwealth of Australia. www.health.gov.au/sites/default/files/national-drug-strategy-2017-2026.pdf

Department of Health and Aged Care. (2019). *What are the effects of taking drugs? Commonwealth of Australia.* www.health.gov.au/topics/drugs/about-drugs/what-are-the-effects-of-taking-drugs

—— (2024). *About the Take Home Naloxone program.* Commonwealth of Australia. www.health.gov.au/our-work/take-home-naloxone-program/about-the-take-home-naloxone-program

Drug & Alcohol Nurses of Australasia (DANA). (2021). *Specialist Nursing Standards and Competencies for Drug and Alcohol Nurses.* www.danaonline.org/public/188/files/Resources/DANA-nursing-standards-handbook.pdf

—— (2024). *DANA standards & competencies.* www.danaonline.org/publications/specialist-nursing-standards-and-competencies-for-drug-and-alcohol-nurses/

Harm Reduction Australia. (2024). *What is harm reduction?* www.harmreductionaustralia.org.au/what-is-harm-reduction/

Harm Reduction International. (2022). *The Global State of Harm Reduction 2022.* https://hri.global/flagship-research/the-global-state-of-harm-reduction/

Health South Eastern Sydney Local Health District. (2023). *Drug and alcohol services.* NSW Government. www.seslhd.health.nsw.gov.au/services-clinics/directory/drug-and-alcohol-services

Mannering, D.E. & Mannering, W.K. (1999). *Attitudes are Contagious: Are Yours Worth Catching?* Options Unltd.

Marel, C.S.E., Fisher, A., Gournay, K., et al. (2022). *Guidelines on the Management of Co-occurring Alcohol and Other Drug and Mental Health Conditions in Alcohol and Other Drug Treatment Settings.* Matilda Centre for Research in Mental Health and Substance Use, The University of Sydney. https://comorbidityguidelines.org.au/pdf/comorbidity-guideline.pdf

Ministry of Health. (2022). *Annual Update of Key Results 2021/22: New Zealand Health Survey.* New Zealand Government. www.health.govt.nz/publication/annual-update-key-results-2021-22-new-zealand-health-survey

Monds, L.A., Bravo, M., Mills, L., et al. (2022). The Overdose Response with Take Home Naloxone (ORTHN) project: Evaluation of health worker training, attitudes and perceptions. *Drug and Alcohol Review, 41*(5), 1085–94.

Mosel, S. (2024). *Is drug addiction genetic?* American Addiction Centers https://americanaddictioncenters.org/rehab-guide/addiction-genetic

National Center for Health Statistics. (2023). *Illicit drug use.* U.S. Department of Health & Human Services. www.cdc.gov/nchs/hus/sources-definitions/illicit-drug-use.htm

National Centre for Education and Training on Addiction (NCETA). (2023a). *Alcohol & drugs in society.* https://nceta.flinders.edu.au/society

—— (2023b). *Conceptualising alcohol and other drug issues.* https://nceta.flinders.edu.au/society/conceptualising-alcohol-and-other-drug-issues

New South Wales (NSW) Health. (2020). *Policy Directive: Nursing and Midwifery Management of Drug and Alcohol Use in the Delivery of Health Care.* NSW Ministry of Health. www1.health.nsw.gov.au/pds/ActivePDSDocuments/PD2020_032.pdf

—— (2021). *Handbook for Nurses and Midwives: Responding Effectively to People Who Use Alcohol and Other Drugs.* NSW Ministry of Health. www.health.nsw.gov.au/aod/professionals/Publications/handbook-nurses-aod.pdf

———— (2023). *Alcohol and Other Drugs Psychosocial Interventions Practice Guide*. NSW Ministry of Health. www.health.nsw.gov.au/aod/resources/Publications/nsw-health-psychosocial-interventions.pdf

New Zealand Drug Foundation. (2024a). *Drugs in Aotearoa – an overview*. https://drugfoundation.org.nz/topics/policy-and-advocacy/drugs-in-aotearoa-an-overview

———— (2024b). *Policy and advocacy*. https://drugfoundation.org.nz/topics/policy-and-advocacy

North Richmond Community Health. (2023). *Medically supervised injecting room*. Victorian Government. https://nrch.com.au/services/medically-supervised-injecting-room/

Penington Institute. (2023). *Australia's Annual Overdose Report*. www.penington.org.au/australias-annual-overdose-report/

Rodgers, C. (2018). Brief interventions for alcohol and other drug use. *Australian Prescriber*, *41*(4), 117. https://doi.org/10.18773/austprescr.2018.031

Substance Abuse and Mental Health Services Administration. (2021). *Medications for Opioid Use Disorder for Healthcare and Addiction Professionals, Policymakers, Patients, and Families*. www.ncbi.nlm.nih.gov/books/NBK574910/

Thorley, A. (1982). *The effects of alcohol. In* M.A. Plant (ed.), *Drinking and Problem Drinking*. Junction Books.

Turning Point. (2018). *Methamphetamine Treatment Guidelines*. http://s3-ap-southeast-2.amazonaws.com/turning-point-website-prod/drupal/2019-05/Turning-Point-Methamphetamine-Treatment-Guidelines.pdf

———— (2024a). *Lapse and relapse*. www.turningpoint.org.au/treatment/about-addiction/treating-addiction/lapse-and-relapse

———— (2024b). *Time to rethink addiction*. www.turningpoint.org.au/

United Nations (UN). (n.d.). *The 17 goals*. https://sdgs.un.org/goals

United Nations Office on Drugs and Crime (UNODC). (2023). *World Drug Report 2023*. www.unodc.org/res/WDR-2023/WDR23_Exsum_fin_SP.pdf

Williamson, L. (2021). Creating an ethical culture to support recovery from substance use disorders. *Journal of Medical Ethics*, *47*(12), e9–e9. https://doi.org/10.1136/medethics-2020-106661

World Health Organization (WHO). (2020). *International standards for the treatment of drug use disorders: revised edition incorporating results of field-testing*. www.who.int/publications/i/item/international-standards-for-the-treatment-of-drug-use-disorders

———— (2024a). *Alcohol, drugs and Addictive Behaviours Unit*. www.who.int/teams/mental-health-and-substance-use/alcohol-drugs-and-addictive-behaviours/alcohol/governance/sdgs

———— (2024b). *Drug (psychoactive)s*. www.who.int/health-topics/drugs-psychoactive#tab=tab_2

———— (2024c). *International Classification of Diseases, 11th Revision (ICD-11)*. www.who.int/standards/classifications/classification-of-diseases

Refugee health nursing

Bronwen Blake and Sandy Eagar

22

LEARNING OBJECTIVES

At the completion of this chapter, you should be able to:

- describe the difference between a refugee and a person seeking asylum.
- explain the impact of the refugee experience on current health status and needs.
- identify major health issues in refugee populations.
- apply acquired knowledge to formulate a refugee health assessment.

Introduction

> If ongoing conflicts remain unresolved and the risks of new ones erupting are not reigned in, one aspect that will define the twenty-first century will be the continuously growing numbers of people forced to flee and the increasingly dire options available to them. (United Nations High Commissioner for Refugees (UNHCR), 2022)

The world is facing an unprecedented number of forcibly displaced people as a result of war, conflict, human rights violations and natural disasters (UNHCR, 2023a). Conflicts have become more protracted, often lasting for years, and displacement as a short-term option is unrealistic.

The recent UNHCR annual global trends report shows an ever-increasing number of people displaced (see Figure 22.1) (UNHCR, 2023b). The UNHCR has estimated it will be supporting an expected 130 million people who are either stateless or forcibly displaced by the end of 2024 (UNHCR, 2024). Around half of the world's **refugees** and displaced people are children. Permanent resettlement is no solution as less than 1 per cent of the displaced people are ever resettled (UNHCR, 2023b).

Refugees are forced to flee their homes because of the consequences of war, violence and persecution. People need to leave their country of origin to be recognised under the international legal framework as a refugee. Refugees are sometimes referred to as migrants, however a migrant voluntarily chooses to leave their country to make a new life in another country (International Organisation for Migration (IOM), 2024).

Asylum seekers, like refugees, are people who have fled their own country due to fear of persecution and have applied for legal and physical protection in another country but their claim for protection has not yet been assessed. Seeking asylum is legal under international law (Philips, 2017).

Refugees – first defined in the *1951 Refugee Convention*, a refugee is 'someone who is unable or unwilling to return to their country of origin owing to a well-founded fear of being persecuted for reasons of race, religion, nationality, membership of a particular social group, or political opinion' (UNHCR, 2010, p. 3).

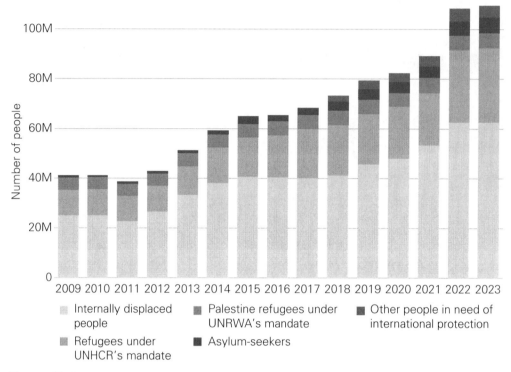

Figure 22.1   UNHCR's mid-year trends 2023
Source: UNHCR (2023b).

Since the end of World War II, Australia has resettled approximately 950 000 refugees from around the world (Department of Home Affairs, 2024b) and Aotearoa New Zealand has resettled approximately 35 000 (New Zealand Immigration, 2022).

The health of refugees is impacted by many social determinants, which may include the pre-displacement situation in their homelands, displacement in a first country and resettlement. Most refugees arrive from countries where health services have been severely disrupted or destroyed, and where access to health care, such as immunization or disease surveillance (e.g. polio or tuberculosis (TB)) programs, is limited or non-existent (Abbara et al., 2020). Therefore, refugees may arrive in their new host countries with injuries, diseases or conditions that have been inadequately managed in their home country or during displacement. Common health conditions in displaced populations include nutritional deficiencies like anaemia (especially in women of child-bearing years) and vitamin deficiency (especially vitamin D), poorly managed chronic diseases (like hypertension and diabetes), parasitic infections (schistosomiasis, strongyloidiasis), poor dental hygiene, underimmunisation, psychological grief and post-traumatic stress disorder (PTSD) (Ngo et al., 2018; Rehr et al., 2018).

Although specialist refugee health nurses are employed in all Australian states and territories (Refugee Nurses of Australia, 2017) and across Aotearoa New Zealand, nurses in both countries may encounter patients from a refugee background across all areas of the health system. Nurses employed in primary health and community settings, particularly in general practice, may be caring for refugees, both newly arrived and those who have been resettled for decades.

This chapter provides readers with a general overview of the impact of war and displacement on health, and an insight into the current Australian and Aotearoa New Zealand humanitarian programs for refugees arriving, including the offshore medical assessment and onshore settlement programs.

War, displacement and health

Wars and forced migration impact health in many ways. Essential public health infrastructure like water supply, sanitation, food supplies and transportation systems are targeted along with health-supporting infrastructure such as hospitals and medical care (Levy & Sidel, 2016). 90 per cent of war-time casualties are civilians (United Nations (UN), 2022) and, disproportionately, children aged under five years (Jawad et al., 2020).

The direct impact of war includes physical war-related injuries, for example, penetrating wounds, burns, and fractures (Levy & Sidel, 2016). Additionally, rape and other forms of sexual violence have been used as a tactic of warfare (Kapp, 2022; United Nations Development Fund for Women (UNIFEM), 2022). War can be systematic and destroy individuals, families and communities with long-lasting effects. Conflict can also have a long-term impact on mental health, including PTSD, anxiety and depression, and substance misuse (Rozanov et al., 2019).

The indirect impacts of war on communities include lack of access to health care and inadequate food and shelter, overcrowding and poor-quality water and sanitation. These factors lead to an increase in morbidity and mortality from preventable diseases, including both infectious (for example, measles and dysentery) and non-communicable diseases, malnutrition and untreated chronic conditions (Garry & Checchi, 2021). Chronic disease management in complex humanitarian emergencies is made more difficult by the loss of medical histories and records, limited infrastructure and a lack of access to ongoing health care, follow-up and treatment, including access to medication (Bausch et al., 2021).

REFLECTION

It can be difficult, in politically stable countries like Australia or Aotearoa New Zealand, to imagine the circumstances that force people to flee their country and seek safety elsewhere. Imagine that you have just two minutes to pack a bag for your family before you are forced to run and leave your home and community.

1. What would you take?
2. What is left behind?

Australia and Aotearoa New Zealand's Humanitarian Settlement Programs

In Australia, refugees arrive under the government's Refugee and Humanitarian Program, known as the 'Offshore Humanitarian Program' (Department of Home Affairs, 2023). This program has an annual refugee quota (Department of Home Affairs, 2024b). In 2023–4, this quota was 20 000 refugees per year (Department of Home Affairs, 2024b). Refugees are resettled across all Australian states and territories; however, the highest numbers of refugees arrive and are resettled in New South Wales and Victoria (Refugee Council of Australia (RCOA), 2023). Other refugees who have a link to Australia may apply for the Special Humanitarian Program (Department of Home Affairs, 2023).

Aotearoa New Zealand settles approximately 1500 refugees a year (New Zealand Government, 2023) and unlike the Australian program (whereby people are accommodated in the private rental market) refugees arriving in Aotearoa New Zealand are accommodated at a joint facility in Auckland for the first six weeks. It is here where the initial health and other checks are completed prior to moving into the community.

Offshore health assessments

Once a person's refugee claim has been verified the individual may be eligible for third-country resettlement. Prior to arrival in Australia or Aotearoa New Zealand, refugees must undertake the immigration medical examination (IME) arranged by the respective governments and performed by offshore medical panels (Department of Home Affairs, 2024a). It is important to understand the health assessments that are undertaken before arrival in the new country so that tests and assessments are not duplicated unnecessarily.

In addition to a medical examination, refugees are specifically tested for TB, syphilis, HIV and hepatitis B and C. A chest X-ray is undertaken to investigate for TB in all people over the age of 11 years, and antibody testing is undertaken for those aged 2–10 years. If a person is found to have TB, a treatment regime is commenced for 3–6 months and the person must be cleared of TB before they can travel. Additionally, for those with TB, a health undertaking is organised whereby these people are linked to a local chest clinic for assessment, free treatment, and follow-up for 2 to 5 years (Department of Home Affairs, 2023).

In addition, vaccinations are routinely given at a pre-departure screening (three to five days before departure to Australia or Aotearoa New Zealand) and include measles, mumps and rubella (MMR) and polio. Since 2020, an individual's COVID-19 vaccination status is also noted. Childhood immunisations are recorded, and any other issues of concern are noted (Mahimbo, Seale & Heywood, 2017).

The health records generated by the IME are made available to the host countries' health personnel and are vital to refugee health systems. Some refugees may also have a copy of their medical records; otherwise, they can be sourced by contacting refugee health services.

Settlement and health

Refugees are granted permanent residency from the day of arrival in Australia (Department of Home Affairs, 2023) and Aotearoa New Zealand (New Zealand Immigration, 2024). This is an important facet of resettlement as it entitles the person to services available to other permanent residents, in particular, access to health care systems. In most instances, refugees in Australia are granted temporary access to a health care card which also entitles them to access various publicly funded health schemes like dental services (Services Australia, 2023). The Australian and Aotearoa New Zealand Humanitarian Settlement Programs include case management, on-arrival health assessments and short-term support with accommodation, language classes, employment training and community participation. These programs are recognised internationally as a best-practice model that provide refugees timely support at the start of the resettlement journey (Russell et al., 2013).

Despite the ongoing political rhetoric surrounding 'boat people' in the Australian political landscape, most asylum seekers arrive by plane with recognised travel documents, such as a student or tourist visa. Once on shore, they lodge a claim for protection to the government. The time taken by the government to grant asylum can be lengthy, and delays of five to six years in Australia are not uncommon (RCOA, 2024a). Unlike the situation in Aotearoa New Zealand, where people seeking asylum are entitled to access the Aotearoa New Zealand public health system at no charge, asylum seekers in Australia are not permanent residents and, therefore, have limited or no access to Medicare. This has a profound effect on their ability to access health care, as a lack of Medicare access generally precludes asylum seekers from using services such as general practices without a cash payment. Health care for the small number of people in administrative detention (254 at the end of December 2023) is provided by a private company contracted by the Australian government (RCOA, 2024b).

As Medicare is also linked to work rights, many asylum seekers are denied the right to work and/or seek social services support, for example, unemployment benefits. Some asylum seekers, therefore, rely on charities, church groups or family/friends for living expenses (Services Australia, 2023). Government and non-government services offer non-chargeable health care in all states and territories, such as the New South Wales (NSW) Refugee Health Service and the Asylum Seeker Resource Centre in Melbourne. Additionally, most states and territories have policies that direct their public health facilities to offer assessment and treatment to people seeking asylum at a non-chargeable rate. This is a sensible public health policy that enables, for example, an expectant mother to receive appropriate antenatal care or for the treatment of people with acute conditions such as heart attacks or surgical emergencies.

Regardless of visa status, many refugees and asylum seekers come from countries where doctors and nurses are health professionals they commonly encounter. Most refugees understand what doctors do and they are held in high esteem by the various communities. Less understood is the role of the nurse in sophisticated health systems such as Australia and Aotearoa New Zealand. Many nurses working in primary care practice at an advanced level may take the lead in chronic disease management, health education, wound management, women's health screening and immunisation programs. Nurses need to explain (and maybe defend) their scope of practice to a newly arrived refugee who may be unsure about their ability to undertake these activities independently of the doctor.

Refugee health assessment

All refugees are encouraged to undergo a comprehensive health assessment within 28 days of arrival in Australia (Foundation House, 2024). This health assessment is generally undertaken by a refugee health nurse or in a community setting, depending on location and service delivery model. Regardless of setting or health practitioner, there are common approaches to quality care.

The use of qualified **health care interpreter services** is imperative to ensure safe clinical care (Paradise et al., 2019). Although convenient, it is never appropriate to use family members, friends or settlement support staff due to the risks of misunderstandings,

Health care interpreter services – access to professional interpreters 24 hours a day to facilitate communication between health professionals and clients.

censorship of information and breaches of confidentiality. If on-site interpreters are not available, then phone interpreters should be used. In addition, some concepts that we take for granted in Australia, such as confidentiality, may be unknown to many new arrivals, and time must be taken to reassure people about their rights and responsibilities as health consumers.

Australia and Aotearoa New Zealand's health care systems are sophisticated, unfamiliar and difficult for newly arrived refugees to navigate. Access to health care is further complicated by limited finances, difficulties with transportation and inadequate use of interpreters (Langlois et al., 2016). Written information, handouts and pamphlets (in different languages) can be helpful for people to read and understand at a later time rather than trying to explain systems during the health assessment. However, many refugees have low health literacy and health beliefs and behaviours linked to their cultural backgrounds. This needs to be assessed when providing health education and health promotion (Fox et al., 2021).

The process of settling into a new country is daunting, with multiple obligations, conflicting priorities and appointments. Nurses must be prepared to negotiate with people about suitable days and times for ongoing appointments.

A comprehensive health assessment includes the following (Foundation House, 2024):

- migration history – country of birth, reason for displacement, transit locations and countries, length of displacement, time in immigration or other detention facilities either in Australia or overseas
- preferred language
- health literacy assessment
- past medical history, family history, medications and allergies
- infectious diseases screening – consider TB, malaria, parasitic infections such as strongyloidiasis and schistosomiasis, hepatitis B and C, HIV, sexually transmitted infections (STIs) based on country of origin, and medical history
- review of respiratory and cardiac systems, including measurement of blood pressure, smoking history or other substances (shisha or water pipe smoking), indoor smoke exposure
- other common diseases, including thyroid disorders and diabetes (both with history, clinical assessment and pathology)
- gastrointestinal system, including nutritional screening (height, weight, head circumference, length, body mass index (BMI))
- sexual/reproductive health history, including gravidity, parity, sexual violence, contraception, sexual dysfunction, and sexual orientation and identity
- immunisation history, including calculation of catch-up schedules
- hearing and vision
- women's health, including preventative health screening (cervical screening and breast screening), female genital mutilation (FGM)/cutting
- mental and psychological health screening, including evidence of torture or other injuries
- oral health examination.

A translated appointment letter is available to assist people in understanding what appointments they have. This is an online translation tool available in addition to reminder apps on smartphones and text services. It is available to anyone worldwide at www.mhcs.health .nsw.gov.au/publications/appointment-reminder-translation-tool/create_an_appointment (Multicultural Health Communication Service, 2019).

A comprehensive health assessment is usually complemented by pathology screening and tests already performed during the offshore medical examination. Screening usually includes, but is not limited to, full blood count, vitamin D levels, hepatitis B surface antibodies, surface antigen and core antibodies, strongyloidiasis serology and vitamin B12 (Foundation House, 2024).

Individual risk assessments based on a comprehensive health assessment should guide the clinician to order additional tests. Like other populations, refugees can present with a range of health conditions, including disabilities, chronic diseases, gender-based violence and developmental issues, so referral to specialist services may be necessary.

Mental health

The mental health of refugees, like all of us, is affected by a myriad of life events. The experience of grief, loss, persecution and powerlessness all impact the lives of refugees, and hence their mental well-being (Chen et al., 2017). Approximately 25 per cent of refugees have been physically tortured or subjected to severe psychological abuse prior to their arrival in Australia (Forum of Australian Services for Survivors of Torture and Trauma (FASSTT), 2018). In many other cultures mental health is still steeped in myth, religion and discrimination. So, there can be understandable reluctance and fear to disclose symptoms of mental health distress and dysfunction (Slobodin, Ghane & De Jong, 2018).

As such, nurses should be aware of the phenomenon of somatisation, whereby mental health distress may be expressed as physical symptoms, commonly headaches, stomach upsets and other vague non-malignant complaints. These 'socially acceptable' symptoms legitimise mental health symptoms and allow individuals to express their feelings without being labelled as 'mentally ill' (Satinsky et al., 2019).

Low rates of health literacy about mental health may also impact on health-seeking behaviours and individuals may rely on traditional customs, such as consulting spiritual or community leaders and the use of traditional medicines rather than seeking assistance from a health professional (Satinsky et al. 2019).

PTSD is well documented with classic symptoms described as hyperarousal, a low threshold to certain stimuli such as noise, sleep disruption, nightmares and intrusive memories (Armour, Mullerova & Elhai, 2016). PTSD can be debilitating and frequently associated with comorbid health conditions including poor functioning and increased health care utilisation (Greene, Neria & Gross, 2016).

In addition to PTSD, anxiety and depression contribute significantly to the burden of mental health in refugees (Lechner-Meichsner, Comtesse & Olk, 2024; Nickerson et al., 2019). Post-migration stressors such as language barriers, family being left behind, finance and unemployment, housing and the lack of understanding about life in a new country contribute significantly to mental health anguish and symptoms.

REFLECTION

The mental health of newly arrived refugees can be dependent on the attitudes of the host country. What are the prevailing attitudes in your community towards refugees and asylum seekers?

In primary health care (PHC) and community settings, the opportunities to recognise and assist those with mental health symptoms are endless. Understanding the background of the person and what supports are available, along with curiosity, underpin cultural competency and trauma-informed care. Understanding the mental health symptoms commonly seen in refugee populations is fundamental to PHC nursing practice among refugee populations. Additionally, the use of psychometric assessment tools such as Kessler's Psychological Distress Scale (K10) and the Refugee Health Screener (RHS-15) can assist in formal assessment (Hocking, Mancuso & Sundram, 2018; Hollifield et al., 2013; Shawyer et al., 2017).

Effective management and treatment for those with serious mental health issues may be challenging in the busy general practice environment. In Australia and Aotearoa New Zealand, specialised services are available to assist refugees with psychological issues resulting from their experiences of torture and trauma. Nurses should also investigate protective factors and incorporate these strategies into the holistic care they provide. Some protective factors that could arise from their community and community groups include spiritual support.

CASE STUDY 22.1

Ali is a 24-year-old man from Iran who identifies as homosexual. He was betrayed by an uncle who accused him of bringing shame upon the family. He was arrested, threatened with castration and subjected to severe beatings, which left him with a facial nerve palsy. He fled Iran and was granted refugee status by the UNHCR. He arrived in Australia under the Refugee and Humanitarian Program and has resettled in your community.

You have organised an assessment and briefed the health care interpreter about the situation. When you greet Ali, you note that he looks exhausted and has a flat affect.

You gently advise Ali that he is in a safe space in your clinic, the assessment is confidential, and findings will only be shared if he consents to releasing information.

You also reassure him that it is not against the law to be homosexual in Australia and that same-sex marriage is legal. At this point, Ali begins to softly weep.

After a short break, you continue your assessment. The physical examination is unremarkable except for a heavy smoking burden of 25 cigarettes a day and the obvious facial nerve palsy. Ali discloses he is not sleeping well, experiencing nightmares and flashbacks about his imprisonment and torture. He is frightened by sudden loud noises. Ali has no friends in Australia and is unsure about his future. You complete the RHS-15, and he scores highly for depression, anxiety and PTSD. You are aware of the services provided by the local FASSTT provider and discuss the potential referral with Ali. He expresses alarm at the suggestion, asking you. 'Am I insane?'

You explain to Ali that the symptoms he is experiencing are because of his imprisonment and torture, and they are, in fact, commonly seen in refugee populations. He is reassured by that information and once you confirm the confidentiality of the counselling services he agrees to a referral. You also offer him nicotine replacement therapy to assist him in reducing the number of cigarettes that he smokes per day and discuss some other strategies to manage his psychological distress, including regular exercise and deep breathing.

After giving Ali some translated health information, you make another appointment to see Ali in two weeks to check his psychological state. He thanks you profusely and promises to return for his follow-up.

REFLECTION

1. Is your work environment a 'safe space' for the LBGTQIA+ community? Why/why not?
2. At the next appointment, a health care interpreter refuses the assignment as he believes that homosexuality is an offence against God. How would you manage this situation?

CASE STUDY 22.2

Fatima is a 28-year-old woman from Somalia who arrived four months ago as a refugee. Fatima has completed her post-arrival health assessment, and the GP has referred her to you for a women's health check and education. Fatima has already been diagnosed with a urinary tract infection (UTI) and has been prescribed antibiotics. You have booked a female health care interpreter who speaks Somali, and the interpreter greets Fatima warmly when she arrives for her appointment.

Fatima tells you that she suffers from recurrent UTIs and tells you it is because of the 'cutting down below'. She was not comfortable disclosing this to the male GP and he did not enquire about her sexual health. She agrees to a physical examination, and you confirm that she has undergone FGM stage three – infibulation.

FGM is deeply rooted in the cultural mores and beliefs of the community (United Nations Population Fund (UNFPA), 2022). Most of the procedures are done by women (sometimes family members) with little knowledge of sanitation or pain relief. Deaths due to infections, haemorrhage and shock are not uncommon, with some estimates as high as 1 in 500 (Ivazzo, Sardi & Gkegkes, 2013).

The long-term health complications from FGM are well known and include chronic UTIs, incontinence, menstrual problems, anaemia and obstructed labour resulting in fistulae and maternal and infant deaths (UNFPA, 2022).

FGM is banned in many countries (including Australia and Aotearoa New Zealand) and it is a crime to procure or arrange the procedure, including sending young girls overseas for the procedure to be performed. It is also a crime to resuture an infibulated woman following childbirth (Australian Institute of Health and Welfare, 2019).

Following your assessment, you discuss possible ways to reduce the incidence of Fatima's UTIs (fluid intake, hygiene, etc.) plus information about self-collection for cervical screening and arrange for her to see a female GP for ongoing care.

REFLECTION

Fatima did have a question at the end of her assessment. She asks if it is possible to have her infibulation reversed.

1. What services are offered in your local health district?
2. What would be the benefits of a reversal procedure?

Conclusion

Refugee health is an evolving specialty in nursing. Australia and Aotearoa New Zealand have a long history in providing world-class health services to refugees on resettlement. Nurses play an important role in promoting and protecting the health of refugees, whether in the immediate post-arrival period or at the end of their lives in palliative and aged care settings. Importantly, nurses also play a key role in supporting refugees' access to health systems, case management and advocacy.

CRITICAL THINKING ACTIVITIES

1. A four-year-old girl arrives from Afghanistan with no immunisation records. Calculate a catch-up immunisation schedule for her using the *Australian Immunisation Handbook* (Department of Health and Aged Care, 2024).
2. A 15-year-old teenager discloses that she is about to be sent overseas to be married to a man she has never met. What are the laws in Australia and/or Aotearoa New Zealand in this situation? What is your advice to this young woman?
3. *Helicobacter pylori* (*H. pylori*) is a common finding in refugee populations. Signs and symptoms can be subtle, so newly arrived refugees should be assessed for the disease. What are the signs and symptoms of *H. pylori* infection? How do you confirm the presence of the bacteria? What is the current recommended therapy?

FURTHER READING

Amarasena, L., Samir, N., Sealy, L., et al. (2023). Offshore detention: Cross-sectional analysis of the health of children and young people seeking asylum in Australia. *Archives of Disease in Childhood, 108*, 185–91. https://doi.org/10.1136/archdischild-2022-324442

Foundation House. (2024). *Australian Refugee Health Practice Guide 2024.* https://refugeehealthguide.org.au/refugee-health-assessment/

Guo, L., Li, L., Xu, K., et al. (2023). Characterization of premigration and postmigration multidomain factors and psychosocial health among refugee children and adolescents after resettlement in Australia. *JAMA Network Open, 6*(4), e235841. https://doi.org/10.1001/jamanetworkopen.2023.5841

Refugee Nurses of Australia. (2018). *Standards of Practice for Australian Refugee Health Nurses 2018.* http://refugeenursesaustralia.org/wp-content/uploads/2018/10/Standards-of-Practice-for-Australian-Refugee-Health-Nurses-2018_final.pdf

REFERENCES

Abbara, A., Almalla, M., AlMasri, I., et al. (2020). The challenges of tuberculosis control in protracted conflict: The case of Syria. *International Journal of Infectious Diseases, 90*, 53–9. https://doi.org/10.1016/j.ijid.2019.10.015

Armour, C., Mullerova, J. & Elhai, J. (2016). A systematic literature review of PTSD's latent structure in the Diagnostic and Statistical Manual of Mental Disorders: DSM-IV to DSM-5. *Clinical Psychological Review, 44*, 60–74. https://doi.org/10.1016/j.cpr.2015.12.003

Australian Institute of Health and Welfare. (2019). *Towards estimating the prevalence of female genital mutilation/cutting in Australia.* Australian Government. www.aihw.gov.au/reports/men-women/female-genital-mutilation-cutting-australia/contents/summary

Bausch, F.J., Beran, D., Hering, H. et al. (2021). Operational considerations for the management of non-communicable diseases in humanitarian emergencies. *Conflict and Health, 15*(9). https://doi.org/10.1186/s13031-021-00345-w

Chen, W., Hall, B., Ling, L. & Renzaho, A. (2017). Pre-migration and post-migration factors associated with mental health in humanitarian migrants in Australia and the moderation effect of post-migration stressor: Findings from the first wave data of the BNLA cohort study. *The Lancet Psychiatry, 4*(3), 218–29. https://doi.org/10.1016/S2215-0366(17)30032-9

Department of Health and Aged Care. (2024). *Australian Immunisation Handbook.* Commonwealth of Australia. https://immunisationhandbook.health.gov.au

Department of Home Affairs. (2023). *Refugee category visas: Subclass 200, 201, 203, and 204.* Australian Government. https://immi.homeaffairs.gov.au/visas/getting-a-visa/visa-listing/refugee-200

—— (2024a). *Australian Panel Member Instructions: Immigration Medical Examinations July 2024.* Australian Government. https://immi.homeaffairs.gov.au/support-subsite/files/panel-member-instructions.pdf

—— (2024b). *Refugee and Humanitarian Program.* Australian Government. https://immi.homeaffairs.gov.au/what-we-do/refugee-and-humanitarian-program/about-the-program/about-the-program

Forum of Australian Services for Survivors of Torture and Trauma (FASSTT). (2018). *Never Turning Away: Australia's World-Leading Program of Assistance to Survivors of Torture and Trauma (PASTT).* https://fasstt.org.au/wordpress/wp-content/uploads/2018/12/FASSTT_BOOKLET_2017_A4_FA_web.pdf

Foundation House. (2024). *Australian Refugee Health Practice Guide 2024.* https://refugeehealthguide.org.au/refugee-health-assessment/

Fox, S., Kramer, E., Agrawal, P. & Aniyizhai, A. (2021). Refugee and migrant health literacy interventions in high-income countries: A systematic review. *Journal of Immigrant and Minority Health, 24*, 207–36. https://doi.org/10.1007/s10903-021-01152-4

Garry, S. & Checchi, F. (2021). Erratum to Armed conflict and public health: Into the 21st century. *Journal of Public Health, 43*(1), e110. https://doi.org/10.1093/pubmed/fdaa036

Greene, T., Neria, Y. & Gross, R. (2016). Prevalence, detection and correlates of PTSD in the primary care setting: A systematic review. *Journal of Clinical Psychology in Medical Settings, 23*(2), 160–80. https://doi.org/10.1007/s10880-016-9449-8

Hocking, D.C., Mancuso, S.G. & Sundram, S. (2018). Development and validation of a mental health screening tool for asylum-seekers and refugees: The STAR-MH. *BMC Psychiatry, 18*(1), 69. https://doi.org/10.1186/s12888-018-1660-8

Hollifield, M., Verbillis-Kolp, S., Farmer, B., et al. (2013). The Refugee Health Screener-15 (RHS-15): Development and validation of an instrument for anxiety, depression, and PTSD in refugees. *General Hospital Psychiatry, 35*(2), 202–9. https://doi.org/10.1016/j.genhosppsych.2012.12.002

International Organisation for Migration (IOM). (2024). *Key migration terms.* www.iom.int/key-migration-terms

Ivazzo C., Sardi T.A. & Gkegkes I.D. (2013). Female genital mutilation and infections: A systematic review of the clinical evidence. *Archives of Gynecology and Obstetrics, 287*(6), 1137–49. https://doi.org/10.1007/s00404-012-2708-5

Jawad, M., Hone, T., Vamos, E.P. et al. (2020). Estimating indirect mortality impacts of armed conflict in civilian populations: panel regression analyses of 193 countries, 1990–2017. *BMC Medicine, 18*(266). https://doi.org/10.1186/s12916-020-01708-5

Kapp, C. (2022, November 1). The Devastating Use of Sexual Violence as a Weapon of War: Three new UN reports details atrocities in Ethiopia, Haiti, and Ukraine. *Think Global Health.* https://www.thinkglobalhealth.org/article/devastating-use-sexual-violence-weapon-war

Langlois, E.V., Haines, A., Tomson, G. & Ghaffar, A. (2016). Refugees: Towards better access to health-care services. *The Lancet*, *387*(10016), 319–21. https://doi.org/10.1016/S0140-6736(16)00101-X

Lechner-Meichsner, F., Comtesse, H. & Olk, M. (2024). Prevalence, comorbidities, and factors associated with prolonged grief disorder, posttraumatic stress disorder and complex posttraumatic stress disorder in refugees: A systematic review. *Conflict and Health*, *18*, 32. https://doi.org/10.1186/s13031-024-00586-5

Levy, B.S. & Sidel, V.W. (2016), Documenting the effects of armed conflict on population health. *Annual Review of Public Health*, *37*(1), 205–18. https://doi.org/10.1146/annurev-publhealth-032315-021913

Mahimbo, A., Seale, H. & Heywood, A.E. (2017). Immunisation for refugees in Australia: A policy review and analysis across all States and Territories. *Australian and New Zealand Journal of Public Health*, *41*, 635–40. https//doi.org/10.1111/1753-6405.12710

Multicultural Health Communication Service. (2019). *Appointment translation*. NSW Government. www.mhcs.health.nsw.gov.au/publications/appointment-reminder-translation-tool/create_an_appointment

New Zealand Immigration. (2022). *New Zealand Refugee Resettlement Strategy*. New Zealand Government. https://www.immigration.govt.nz/documents/refugees/refugeeresettlementstrategy.pdf

————— (2024) *New Zealand Refugee Quota Programme*. New Zealand Government. www.immigration.govt.nz/about-us/what-we-do/our-strategies-and-projects/supporting-refugees-and-asylum-seekers/refugee-and-protection-unit/new-zealand-refugee-quota-programme

Ngo C.C., Maidment C., Atkins L., Eagar S. & Smith M.M. (2018). Blood screen findings in a 2-year cohort of newly arrived refugees to Sydney, Australia. *Public Health Research & Practice*, *28*(1), e2811804. https://doi.org/10.17061/phrp2811804

Nickerson, A., Hadzi-Pavlovic, D., Edwards, B., et al. (2019). Identifying distinctive psychological symptom profiles among a nationally representative sample of refugees resettled in Australia. *Australian and New Zealand Journal of Psychiatry*, *53*(9), 908–19. https://doi.org/10.1177/0004867419846403

Paradise, R., Hatch, M., Quessa, A., et al. (2019). Reducing the use of ad hoc interpreters at a Safety-Net Health Care system. *The Joint Commission Journal on Quality and Patient Safety*, *45*(6), 397–405. https://doi.org/10.1016/j.jcjq.2019.01.004

Philips, J. (2017). *Australia's Humanitarian Program: A quick guide to the statistics since 1947* (Research Paper Series 2016–17.) Parliament of Australia, Department of Parliamentary Services. https://parlinfo.aph.gov.au/parlInfo/download/library/prspub/3599552/upload_binary/3599552.pdf

Refugee Council of Australia (RCOA). (2023). *Statistics of refugees settling in Australia over the past 10 years*. www.refugeecouncil.org.au/settlement-statistics/2/

————— (2024a). *Refugee frequently asked questions: Get the facts*. www.refugeecouncil.org.au/rcoa-refugee-get-the-facts/

————— (2024b). *Statistics on people in detention in Australia*. www.refugeecouncil.org.au/detention-australia-statistics/3/

Refugee Nurses of Australia. (2017). Resources. https://refugeenursesaustralia.org./resources

Rehr, M., Shoaib, M., Ellithy, S., et al. (2018). Prevalence of non-communicable diseases and access to care among non-camp Syrian refugees in northern Jordan. *Conflict and Health*, *12*(33). https://doi.org/10.1186/s13031-018-0168-7

Rozanov, V., Frančišković, T., Marinić, I, et al. (2019). Mental health consequences of war conflicts. In A. Javed & K.N. Fountoulakis (eds), *Advances in Psychiatry* (pp. 281–304). Springer. https://doi.org/10.1007/978-3-319-70554-5_17

Russell, G., Harris, M., Cheng, I.-H., et al. (2013). *Coordinated Primary Health Care for Refugees: A Best Practice Framework for Australia*. Australian Primary Health Care Research Institute.

Satinsky, E., Fuhr, D. C., Woodward, A., Sondorp, E. & Roberts, B. (2019). Mental health care utilisation and access among refugees and asylum seekers in Europe: A systematic review. *Health Policy, 123*(9), 851–63. https://doi.org/10.1016/j.healthpol.2019.02.007

Services Australia. (2023). *Payments*. Australian Government. www.servicesaustralia.gov.au/payment-for-refugees-and-asylum-seekers?context=60041

Shawyer, F., Enticott, J.C., Block, A.A., et al. (2017). The mental health status of refugees and asylum seekers attending a refugee health clinic including comparisons with a matched sample of Australian-born residents. *BMC Psychiatry, 17*, 76. https://doi.org/10.1186/s12888-017-1239-9

Slobodin, O., Ghane, S. & De Jong, J. (2018). Developing a culturally sensitive mental health intervention for asylum seekers in the Netherlands: A pilot study. *Intervention, 16*(2), 86–94. https://doi.org/10.4103/INTV.INTV_2_18

United Nations (UN). (2022). *Ninety per cent of war-time casualties are civilians, speakers stress pressing Security Council to fulfil responsibility, protect innocent people in conflicts.* https://press.un.org/en/2022/sc14904.doc.htm

United Nations Development Fund for Women (UNIFEM). (2022). *Rape as a Tactic of War.* www.unwomen.org/sites/default/files/Headquarters/Media/Publications/UNIFEM/EVAWkit_06_Factsheet_ConflictAndPostConflict_en.pdf

United Nations High Commissioner for Refugees (UNHCR). (2010). *Convention and Protocol Relating to the Status of Refugees.* www.unhcr.org/en-au/3b66c2aa10

———— (2022). *Global trends: Forced displacement in 2021.* www.unhcr.org/publications/global-trends-2021

———— (2023a). *Global trends: Forced displacement in 2022.* www.unhcr.org/global-trends

———— (2023b). *UNHCR mid-year trends 2023.* www.unhcr.org/mid-year-trends-report-2023

———— (2024). *UNHCR global appeal 2024.* https://reporting.unhcr.org/global-appeal-2024

United Nations Population Fund (UNFPA). (2022). *Female genital mutilation frequently asked questions.* www.unfpa.org/resources/female-genital-mutilation-fgm-frequently-asked-questions

23 Occupational health nursing

Donna Burt, Fiona Groome, Sally Kane,
Fiona Landgren and Michelle Stirrup
With acknowledgement to Rhonda Brown

LEARNING OBJECTIVES

At the completion of this chapter, you should be able to:

- explain the importance and key components of occupational health and safety (OHS).
- identify how occupational health nurses (OHNs) support health, safety and well-being safe work policies and strategies.
- understand the role that OHNs have in the provision of safe and healthy workplaces.
- understand the diverse roles of nurses in health and safety.
- describe how OHNs contribute to health-promoting workplaces.

Introduction

The role of OHNs is to improve mental and physical health outcomes and the well-being of workers. These benefits can often extend to family and community.

The World Health Organization (WHO) (2023) defines occupational health as 'an area of work in public health to promote and maintain the highest degree of physical, mental and social well-being of workers in all occupations'.

Workers' health is impacted by several factors, including fatigue, gender, culture, age, language, living conditions, access to nutritious food, level of physical activity, sleep patterns, personal health practices and coping strategies, levels of social support and inclusion, personal safety and freedom from violence (discussed in Chapter 1).

An effective OHS program reduces injuries and illnesses, work absenteeism and staff turnover, and improves staff morale, operational efficiency, productivity, and worker's compensation insurance premiums. The strength of an organisation as a preferred employer often relates to its attention to OHS. The **OHN** plays an important role in ensuring safety and promoting healthy workplaces. The roles and major responsibilities of their OHN may vary depending on the size and nature of the employing organisation.

Occupational health nurse (OHN) – a nurse employed by a business or organisation to develop, provide and deliver occupational health programs under the broader health and safety umbrella. Occupational health programs aim to promote, maintain and restore health; prevent illness and injury; and protect workers from work-related hazards.

OHS

The WHO defines a healthy workplace as one where workers and managers collaborate around processes for continued improvement that protect and promote the health, safety and well-being of workers (WHO, 2010). These processes should be developed based on iden-tified health, safety and well-being concerns in the physical and psychosocial work environ-ment as well as workplace culture (WHO, 2010). There should also be an emphasis on making personal health resources available in the workplace and opportunities to participate in the community to improve the health of workers, their families and other community members (WHO, 2010).

Under Work Health and Safety Regulations (Australian Government, 2011b), workers have a right to stop work if they feel it is unhealthy or unsafe. **Employers** have a legal obliga-tion to provide a safe and healthy work environment.

Employers – people who engage the services of employees for financial payments or other compensation.

There has been a significant shift in occupational health in Australia and Aotearoa New Zealand towards the promotion of workers' health and well-being, not only to prevent work-related injury and health problems, but also to address broader health issues. The pro-vision of health and safety programs has the potential to not only improve worker safety but also to prevent and improve health outcomes of a range of health conditions such as cardio-vascular disease and mental health (Wolf et al., 2018). However, the development and imple-mentation of appropriate strategies to promote and improve workers' health is a significant task for any organisation. The enormity of this task requires a collaborative approach between employers, **employees** and health professionals to achieve common goals and develop steps, not only to prevent work-related injury and ill health, but also to promote workers' health and well-being.

Employees – people who are engaged to work for a business or organisation and are paid in wages, a fee or other form of payment.

Legislative framework

In Australia and Aotearoa New Zealand, all persons conducting a **business** or undertak-ing must ensure the health and safety of their workers (Australian Government, 2011b; Parliamentary Counsel Office, 2023). Workers have the right to a safe and healthy work-place and working environment, fair treatment, freedom from discrimination and equal opportunity.

Business – a legal term for an enterprise conducted by a person or organisation with a view to making a profit.

Workplace health and safety is governed by legislation in Australia under the *Work Health and Safety Act 2011* (Australian Government, 2011a) and in Aotearoa New Zealand under the Health and Safety at Work Act 2015 (Parliamentary Counsel Office, 2023). These laws and regulations provide a systematic risk-based approach to OHS. Employers are required to involve their workers in all aspects of OHS including the development, implementation, monitoring and evaluation of health and safety management systems, with a focus on risk management. Codes of practices and standards can assist in the management of workplace risks specific to an industry.

In Australia, each state and territory has the responsibility for formulating its own occupational health laws, standards and enforcement. Given their role in the promotion of workplace health and safety and supporting injured workers, OHNs must be familiar with the relevant statutory requirements of the country, state or territory in which they practise.

Occupational health aims to maintain and promote worker's health and working capacity, to improve working conditions, working environments, work organisation and workplace culture. Occupational health professionals include those in various disciplines such as occupational physicians, OHNs, occupational hygienists, physiotherapists, psychologists and occupational therapists.

Occupational health risks, such as chronic back pain, hearing loss, chronic obstructive pulmonary disease and asthma, account for a significant proportion of the burden of chronic disease. Further, workplace health risks such as physical, chemical, ergonomic, psychosocial and biological risks can aggravate pre-existing health conditions, for example, cardiovascular disease, diabetes and respiratory disease. (WHO, 2017; World Health Organization and International Labour Organization (WHO & ILO,) 2021).

OHNs, occupational physicians, occupational hygienists and the broader health and safety team look to reduce risk to the health and safety of workers by liasing with management, engineers and workers. Examples of this in practice may include:

- substituting or replacing a more powerful carcinogenic chemical with a less toxic equivalent
- implementing engineering controls, for example installing noise buffers to reduce noise levels
- rotating workers to ensure manual handling risks are reduced as an administrative control
- recommending the use of personal protective equipment such as masks and gloves for health care workers (Schulte et al., 2012).

The role of the nurse in OHS

The WHO (2010, p. 6) defines a healthy workplace as 'one in which workers and managers collaborate to use a continual improvement process to protect and promote the health, safety and well-being of all workers and the sustainability of the workplace by considering the following, based on identified needs:

- health and safety concerns in the physical work environment;
- health, safety and well-being concerns in the psychosocial work environment, including organisation of work and workplace culture;
- personal health resources in the workplace; and
- ways of participating in the community to improve the health of workers, their families and other members of the community'.

This definition reflects the key role OHNs have in the workplace. The workplace is increasingly being used as a setting for health promotion and preventive health activities – not only to prevent occupational injury, but to assess and improve people's overall health (Koinig & Diehl, 2021). OHNs are registered nurses (RNs) who have specialised in leading and working in a range of working environments and businesses. OHNs work to enhance the health, safety and well-being of workers in workplaces and beyond (Gok Metin & Yildiz, 2023). As a distinct group of primary health care nurses, the OHN's role is to prevent work-related ill health and disease (La Torre et al., 2020). They do this by collaboratively creating healthy workplaces that are safe, efficient and inclusive. OHNs champion workplace health and well-being strategies that recognise the impact of health on work and the value of work to health.

OHNs maintain continual practice to remain at the forefront of the health system and emerging health trends to influence at strategic and industry levels, creating a healthy workforce for the present and the future (Gok Metin & Yildiz, 2023). Thinking strategically, but acting locally, OHNs use business acumen along with knowledge of health and safety to provide operational services to enable a healthy, safe, and productive environment for workforces within businesses, organisations and sectors.

OHN practice focuses on:

- health promotion and well-being: improving the quality of health and long-term health outcomes in a working population by preventing diseases, controlling risk, improving well-being and enhancing the fitness of workers to work and function in society
- health protection: protecting the worker from work related health risks and ensuring prompt intervention if adverse health trends are identified in an individual or employee population
- disease prevention: primary prevention (the prevention of disease), secondary prevention (through periodic health surveillance) and tertiary prevention (through rehabilitation services after an injury and illness) (Guidotti, 2011; Oliver & Cameron, 2020) (Figure 23.1).

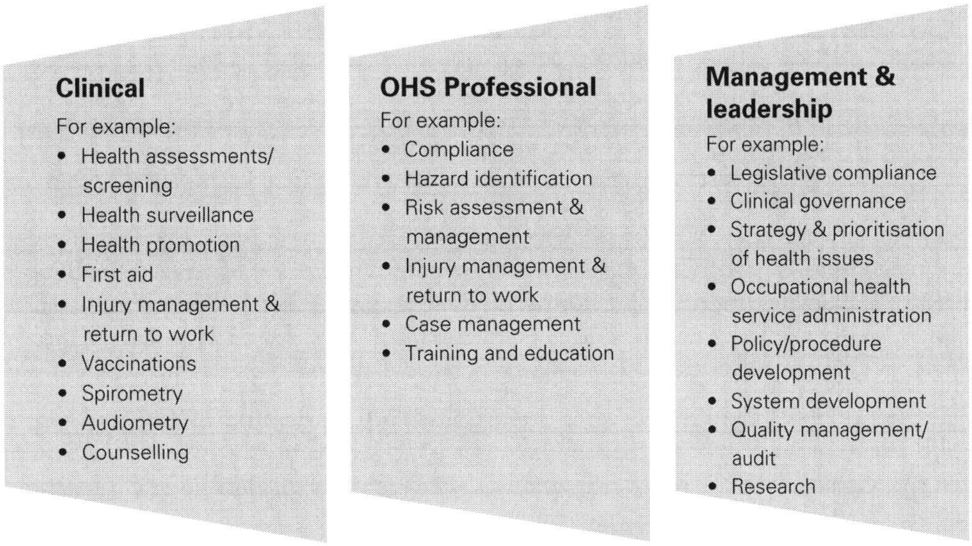

Figure 23.1 Scope of OHN practice
Source: Australian and New Zealand Society of Occupational Medicine (2023).

The OHN plays a major role in the protection and promotion of workers' health through risk assessment, risk management and proactive strategies that promote the health of workers, addressing a wide range of needs of employers and employees (Gok Metin & Yildiz, 2023; La Torre et al., 2020). Through good working relationships with managers, operations and the safety teams, OHNs make a significant contribution to improving workplace health and safety. OHNs are key contributors to site safety teams and operations projects and promote the proactive role of the organisation's health services.

OHNs play a key role in coordinating a holistic, multidisciplinary approach to the delivery of safe, quality and comprehensive occupational and environmental health programs and services (Australian and New Zealand Society of Occupational Medicine (ANZSOM), 2023). These programs serve to protect and manage the health and well-being of people at work. OHNs work with employers and employees to ensure where work is undertaken and how work is undertaken have considered steps to mitigate negative impact on workers' health (ANZSOM, 2023). For example, they may provide expertise and advice in risk assessment in relation to manual handling and ergonomics. As OHNs are also often the first point of contact for workers who are injured or have other health issues, they need to be approachable, accessible and responsive to the needs of employees and employers with regard to health risks, injuries, workplace hazards and the prevention of health problems. OHNs should include human resource advisors and managers as part of a broader multidisciplinary team when a worker's health is impacting an individual's ability to perform their full contractual role, or is being impacted by the workplace (ANZSOM, 2023). Working in occupational health draws on clinical knowledge, understanding of the impacts of work on health and health on work, and the legislative obligations for work health and safety (ANZSOM, 2023).

REFLECTION

How well prepared do you believe the graduate nurse is to work in OHS?

Health promotion and disease prevention

Medical health screening identifies workers who may be at increased risk of developing an occupational health-related illness where exposure to the risk cannot be eliminated. For example, a candidate with pre-existing health conditions could be aggravated by the proposed role. Current best practice requires baseline testing, or health screening, as part of a pre-employment medical assessment. These medical screens become the reference point for all further **health monitoring** throughout a worker's employment (Schulte et al., 2012).

Health monitoring throughout a worker's employment enables the detection of adverse health effects at an early stage so that steps can be taken to protect workers from further injury. Further, health surveillance is useful in assessing whether measures for controlling hazards are effective, provides an opportunity to reinforce preventive measures and safe work practices, and helps to identify any changes that need to be made to the work environment or work practices (WorkSafe Victoria, 2022).

Health surveillance is important to ensure the health of workers exposed to hazardous substances and other risks (Gok Metin & Yildiz, 2023). **Exposure monitoring** and health monitoring may be required by law for workers exposed to substances and situations that are hazardous to health. Such substances and situations include ionising radiation, solvents, biological agents, vibration and working with compressed air (New Zealand Occupational Health Nurses Association (NZOHNA), 2021).

Examples of necessary health screening and monitoring include:

- audiometry testing for those exposed to noise
- blood tests and medical examinations for those exposed to lead (**biological monitoring**)
- respiratory function tests and X-rays for those exposed to respirable dusts such as coal and silica.

Health monitoring – 'looks at whether a worker's health is being harmed because of what they are being exposed to while they are at work' (Worksafe Mahi Haumaru Aotearoa, 2024).

Exposure monitoring – measures and evaluates what your workers are being exposed to while they are at work. Usually undertaken by a qualified occupational hygienist (Worksafe Mahi Haumaru Aotearoa, 2024).

Biological exposure monitoring – 'involves taking blood or urine samples to test for a substance (or a metabolite of a substance) workers are working with' (Worksafe Mahi Haumaru Aotearoa, 2024).

REFLECTION

The role of the OHN involves a wide range of activities including health and risk assessment, emergency response, clinical care and health promotion. What level of knowledge and skill mix is required by OHNs to respond to the wide variety of incidents and presentations in the workplace?

Workers' compensation and rehabilitation

Workers' compensation is an insurance scheme that provides compensation including wage replacement, medical benefits and rehabilitation for employees injured in the course of employment (The Behaviour Change Collaborative, 2022). The scheme is funded by employers through payment of insurance premiums. The purpose of workers' compensation is to provide early intervention when a worker is injured in the workplace, and to maximise the opportunity for the worker to return to work (Perry et al., 2019).

OHNs have a key role in retaining workers in their employment through comprehensive holistic return-to-work support. OHNs are involved in many aspects of an injured worker's recovery from injury or surgery and return to work programs (Harriss, 2019; Perry et al., 2019). This can include multidisciplinary support and employee assistance programs.

OHNs aim to enhance optimal rehabilitation outcomes for the employee while balancing the needs of the business. This is achieved by engaging the key stakeholders in the process, that is, the injured person, line manager, claims manager, company-appointed doctor and other health care providers. In some states in Australia, it is a legislated requirement to employ a return-to-work coordinator within a business. This role may be undertaken by an OHN working in the business. The return-to-work coordinator is the main point of contact for injured workers and assists in ensuring that return-to-work obligations are met by the business by assisting injured workers to remain at work or return to work as soon as is safely possible after injury. The development of appropriate procedures helps to ensure a comprehensive rehabilitation process. This can include management of non-work-related injury and illness and the provision of appropriate duties if available.

Health-promoting workplaces

Employers bear many of the indirect costs associated with a range of non-work-related health conditions and illnesses through absenteeism and presenteeism (not fully functioning at work due to a medical condition or attending when sick). Workplaces provide an ideal opportunity for health promotion given the high proportion of the adult population employed and the considerable time spent at work (Harriss, 2020). This has been increasingly recognised with a significant shift in occupational health from primarily focusing on minimising the risk of physical hazards in the workplace to the inclusion of broader psychosocial, personal and lifestyle factors that affect health.

Providing health promotion in the workplace is conducive to creating a healthy working environment and can also positively influence workers' health and well-being through healthier lifestyle choices (Vargas-Martínez, Romero-Saldaña & De Diego-Cordero, 2021). There is an opportunity to optimise the health of the workforce to reduce the effects of chronic disease and ill health. Some common workplace-based health-promoting programs initiated and implemented by OHNs include health risk assessments, smoking cessation programs, providing vaccinations, advice on healthy food options in staff cafeterias, exercise and stress management programs, counselling, and support for drug and alcohol use and abuse. These health-promoting and well-being strategies, developed and implemented by OHNs, need to be meaningful, measurable, cost-effective and of benefit to employees and employers.

However, there are other factors within the workplace that the OHN needs to consider in order to maintain and promote the health of workers and their capacity to remain in work. The Royal Australasian College of Physicians' (RACP) Australasian Faculty of Occupational and Environmental Medicine (AFOEM) has set out an evidence-based consensus statement – the Health Benefits of Good Work (HBGW). The statement outlines the key determinants of an employee's health, well-being, engagement and productivity in the workplace, and the fundamental principles of the health benefits of accessing and engaging in good work. Individuals should be supported to access the benefits of good work when recovering at work following illness or injury or commencing new employment (RACP, 2024).

REFLECTION

What factors do you think contribute to a healthy workplace?

CASE STUDY 23.1

Mandy is an OHN working for a mining company in a remote location. Mandy describes her role as wide and varied. She is not only a nurse but is also sometimes a counsellor, safety coordinator, physiotherapist, occupational therapist or dietitian. She is responsible for the health and medical care of 310 onsite miners, administration workers and managers. Mandy not only has to be available during working hours, but she must also be on call 24 hours to respond to accidents or if someone becomes ill overnight.

On a typical day, Mandy has consultations for workers at the medical centre. She might see up to 10–12 workers who present with coughs, colds, rashes, gastrointestinal upsets, wounds to be redressed, or workers needing a review of other treatments. This is followed by checking, restocking and reordering medical supplies and equipment. Usually, Mandy will then attend meetings to report to management about workers requiring sick leave or lighter or modified duties and to report and identify problems, risks and hazards. Mandy will usually be involved in planning and/or conducting screening, prevention, health promotion and worker education programs. Recently, she worked closely with the head chef and kitchen staff to address concerns about the high volume of fried food being served. They have now reduced the fried food options and added more fruit, vegetable-based dishes, salads, whole grain bread and pasta. Mandy is also running a back-injury prevention program for workers and is responsible for first aid training for workers who can provide an important support role.

Mandy is called out on an emergency. A mining worker has become short of breath and has collapsed in one of the tunnels. After liaising with the first aider, who was first on the scene, she retrieves her emergency kit and drives the four-wheel-drive ambulance down into the mine to assess the worker's condition further. After an initial assessment, and with the assistance of the first aider, she transfers the worker to the medical centre where she continues to administer oxygen, monitors his vital signs and conducts an electrocardiogram (ECG). Mandy's assessment suggests that he may need to be transferred out for further treatment at a regional hospital, which is 300 km away. She contacts the Royal Flying Doctor Service (RFDS), which says there will be a delay as their crew is responding to another emergency. Mandy is able to speak with a doctor at the RFDS to discuss the worker's condition and get advice on further treatment while waiting for the transfer.

REFLECTION
Consider the ethical and legal implications of providing nursing services to 310 workers in a remote location.

1. What are the possible benefits and challenges of working in such an environment?
2. Can you think of any factors that might impact Mandy?

Occupational health nursing practice

OHNs fulfil many roles including that of clinician, manager, leader, educator, researcher, consultant and case manager (Gok Metin & Yildiz, 2023). They may be working independently or within a multidisciplinary health care team. They also work in collaboration with employees, employers and other health practitioners, including doctors, occupational and physical therapists, and counsellors.

Occupational health nursing incorporates illness and injury prevention, health promotion and restoring health and rehabilitation (Gok Metin & Yildiz, 2023). OHNs also have an integral role in facilitating and promoting onsite occupational health programs and prevention of work-related risks and hazards. They require competency in clinical governance and quality improvement, teaching and educational supervision, and management (Gok Metin & Yildiz, 2023). Their scope of practice spans several areas of health and well-being including health and risk assessment, education, counselling and crisis intervention, disease management, environmental health, legal and regulatory compliance, return to work programs for injured workers and response to emergencies (Harriss, 2020). OHNs are well placed to work towards addressing inequalities through their practice, and influencing relevant policies (NZOHNA, 2021). OHNs require a high level of training, postgraduate qualifications and clinical expertise across a wide range of health conditions and emergency presentations (Gok Metin & Yildiz, 2023).

CASE STUDY 23.2

The Robinsons Floor Sanding and Polishing Company employs 250 workers. They provide floor services in private homes and businesses across the inner and outer metropolitan areas. The work involves driving, lifting heavy portable sanding machines, handling sharp hand tools for floor preparation – including knives and chisels – bending and kneeling for extended periods, removing old floor finishes – including carpet – painting and varnishing, sanding and applying a range of finishes. Workers often work alone. Sanding and polishing floors exposes workers to dust, noise, lead in old paint and fumes from varnishes and other finishes.

REFLECTION

1. What are the potential risks for worker health and safety in this organisation?
2. What are the implications of these risks from the organisation's perspective?
3. What responsibilities does the organisation have for its employees?
4. What are the roles the OHN has in promoting the health, safety and well-being of these workers?

Conclusion

OHNs have an important role in the management of workplace health risks and the prevention of work-related illness and injury. They offer a range of beneficial, cost-effective occupational health services to assist businesses in meeting their legislative requirements to ensure a safe and healthy workplace and assist workers in managing and improving their health and well-being. The role of OHNs continues to evolve in health and safety management as legislation and regulations change. There is an increasing focus on emerging risks, especially psychosocial risks in the workplace, and general health promotion to manage risks in chronic conditions.

This chapter has discussed the implications of legislative requirements for OHS and the issues relevant to occupational health nursing. Occupational health and safety is achieved through collaboration between employers, employees and health care providers. Its strategies are designed to protect and promote the health, safety and well-being of all workers and these are a shared responsibility between employers, managers, employees and heath care professionals. In addition, workplace health-promoting strategies assist employees in making informed, healthy choices. The OHN has a significant and varied role in prevention, health promotion, provision of primary care services and development of strategies that ensure the health and safety of workers.

CRITICAL THINKING ACTIVITIES

1. What difference to worker health and safety can an OHN make in a workplace?
2. How can an OHN influence worker health?
3. What challenges might an OHN face in the workplace?
4. What guides the practice of the OHN in identifying unsafe work practices or concerns that affect the health and well-being of workers?

FURTHER READING

Harber, P., Alongi, G. & Su, J. (2014). Professional activities of experienced occupational health nurses. *Workplace Health & Safety, 62*(6), 233–42. https://doi.org/10.1177/216507991406200603

Royal Australian College of Physicians (RACP). (2024) *It pays to care*. https://www.racp.edu.au/policy-and-advocacy/division-faculty-and-chapter-priorities/faculty-of-occupational-environmental-medicine/it-pays-to-care

Wolf, J., Prüss-Ustün, A., Ivanov, I., et al. (2018). *Preventing Disease Through a Healthier and Safer Workplace*. World Health Organization (WHO). https://apps.who.int/iris/bitstream/handle/10665/272980/9789241513777-eng.pdf

REFERENCES

Australian and New Zealand Society of Occupational Medicine (ANZSOM). (2023). *Competency Standards for Occupational Health Nurses*. ANZSOM.

Australian Government. (2011a). *Work Health and Safety Act 2011*. Australian Government. www.legislation.gov.au/Details/C2016C00887

—— (2011b). *Work Health and Safety Regulations 2011*. Australian Government. www.legislation.gov.au/Details/F2011L02664

Gok Metin, Z. & Yildiz, A. N. (2023). Update on occupational health nursing through 21st century requirements: A three-round Delphi study. *Nurse Education Today, 120*, 105657. https://doi.org/10.1016/j.nedt.2022.105657

Guidotti, T.L. (ed) (2011). *Global Occupational Health*. Oxford University Press.

Harriss, A. (2019). A place at the table for OH nurses? *Occupational Health & Wellbeing, 71*(10), 24–28.

—— (2020). Name of the game–is it time for OH to change its name? Occupational *Health & Wellbeing, 72*(4), 26–30.

Koinig, I. & Diehl, S. (2021). Healthy leadership and workplace health promotion as a pre-requisite for organizational health. *International Journal of Environmental Research and Public Health, 18*(17), 9260. https://doi.org/10.3390/ijerph18179260

La Torre, G., D'Andreano, F., Lecce, G., et al. (2020). The occupational health nurse and his/her role in the prevention of work-related diseases: Results of an observational study. *Annali di Igiene, 32*(1), 3–15. https://doi.org/10.7416/ai.2020.2325

New Zealand Occupational Health Nurses Association (NZOHNA). (2021). *Proposed Framework for OHN Standards of Nursing Practice for Registered Nurses in Aotearoa New Zealand*. NZOHNA. www.nzohna.org.nz/assets/Uploads/Education-Project/OHN-FRAMEWORK-DOCUMENT-2.pdf

Oliver, K. & Cameron, B. (2020). Occupational health nursing. In N. J. Wilson, P. Lewis, L. Hunt and L. Whitehead (eds), *Nursing in Australia* (pp. 261-67). Routledge.

Parliamentary Counsel Office. (2023). *Health and Safety at Work Act 2015*. New Zealand Government. www.legislation.govt.nz/act/public/2015/0070/latest/DLM5976660.html

Perry, T., Cheung, A., Asumbrado, A. & McBee, K. (2019). Current concepts in occupational health: Managing an acute injury that limits work participation. *The Journal of Orthopaedic & Sports Physical Therapy & Practice, 31*(2), 101–05.

Royal Australasian College of Physicians (RACP). (2024). *Health benefits of good work*. www.racp.edu.au/advocacy/division-faculty-and-chapter-priorities/faculty-of-occupational-environmental-medicine/health-benefits-of-good-work

Schulte, P., Pandalai, S.D., Wulsin, V. & Chun, H. (2012). Interaction of occupational and personal risk factors in workforce health and safety. Framing health matters. *American Journal of Public Health, 102*(3), 434–48. https://doi.org/10.2105/AJPH.2011.300249

The Behaviour Change Collaborative. (2022). *Australian Workers' Understanding of Workers' Compensation Systems and their Communication Preferences [Final Report]*. Safe Work Australia. www.safeworkaustralia.gov.au/doc/australian-workers-understanding-workers-compensation-systems

Vargas-Martínez, A. M., Romero-Saldaña, M. & De Diego-Cordero, R. (2021). Economic evaluation of workplace health promotion interventions focused on Lifestyle: Systematic review and meta-analysis. *Journal of Advanced Nursing*, *77*(9), 3657–91. https://doi.org/10.1111/jan.14857

Wolf, J., Prüss-Ustün, A., Ivanov, I., et al. (2018). *Preventing Disease Through a Healthier and Safer Workplace*. World Health Organization. https://apps.who.int/iris/bitstream/handle/10665/272980/9789241513777-eng.pdf

WorkSafe Mahi Haumaru Aotearoa. (2024). *Exposure monitoring and health monitoring – guidance for businesses*. New Zealand Government. www.worksafe.govt.nz/topic-and-industry/monitoring/guidance-for-businesses/

WorkSafe Victoria. (2022). *Occupational health and safety – your legal duties*. Victoria State Government. www.worksafe.vic.gov.au/occupational-health-and-safety-your-legal-duties

World Health Organization (WHO). (2010). *WHO Health Workplace Framework and Model: Background and Supporting Literature and Practices*. www.who.int/publications/i/item/who-healthy-workplace-framework-and-model

——— (2017). *Protecting workers' health*. www.who.int/news-room/fact-sheets/detail/protecting-workers'-health

——— (2023). *Occupational health*. www.who.int/health-topics/occupational-health

World Health Organization (WHO) and International Labour Organization (ILO). (2021). *WHO/ILO Joint Estimates of the Work-Related Burden of Disease and Injury, 2000-2016: Global Monitoring Report*. www.who.int/publications/i/item/9789240034945

Nursing in general practice

Elizabeth Halcomb and Cristina Thompson
With acknowledgement to Eileen McKinlay

24

LEARNING OBJECTIVES

At the completion of this chapter, you should be able to:

- describe the context of general practice and understand how it fits in the broader health system.
- describe the role of general practice nurses (GPNs).
- identify workforce issues for nurses employed in general practice.
- recognise the standards that describe the nursing role in general practice.

Introduction

A GPN is a registered or enrolled nurse employed in a **primary care** (general practice) setting. Approximately 82 000 nurses are working outside of hospital settings in Australia, and two-thirds (68%) of these work in general practice (Australian Institute of Health and Welfare (AIHW), 2020). It is estimated that over 90 per cent of general practices employ nurses (The Royal Australian College of General Practitioners (RACGP), 2023). Aotearoa New Zealand workforce data reveals that in 2018–19, 5.5 per cent of the total nursing workforce worked in general practice, accounting for some 3018 nurses (Nursing Council of New Zealand (NCNZ), 2019). This places general practice as one of the ten largest practice areas within the Aotearoa New Zealand nursing workforce (NCNZ, 2019). In countries like Aotearoa New Zealand and the United Kingdom, general practice nursing has been established over many years. However, in Australia it is a more recent development, and the size of the Australian general practice nursing workforce has expanded greatly since the early 2000s (Australian Medicare Local Alliance, 2012; Heywood & Laurence, 2018b). This has come about in response to positive government policy and financial incentives to enhance the provision of nursing services in primary care to address the growing problem of chronic and complex conditions associated with an aging population (Halcomb et al., 2017; Halcomb et al., 2021). Nurses enter general practice employment either directly following graduation (McInnes et al., 2019; Thomas et al., 2018) or as the result of a career change from other clinical areas (Ashley et al., 2017).

Primary care –
a person's first point of contact with the health system and the focal point for all ongoing health care needs (Department of Health, 2022). For most people in Australia and Aotearoa New Zealand, this refers to the general practice setting.

The general practice setting

Australian general practices are predominantly run as small businesses comprising self-employed doctors who are funded via fee-for-service payments (Department of Health, 2022). Many practices are owned by GP 'principals' who have the joint role of the nurses' employer and their clinical colleague (McInnes et al., 2017b).

The Australian health system is complex, as the federal government sets a scheduled fee for services under the Medicare payment scheme and then reimburses up to 85 per cent of the scheduled fee for the service (Australian Government, 2022). Individual practices then decide whether the client will be charged an additional 'gap' fee. The nature of general practice operating as a business creates a significantly different clinical practice environment to government-funded acute care services. While in the small business setting there is an emphasis on recouping costs for equipment and staff time, in the acute sector these resources are funded more broadly. The GPN needs to understand the nature of the general practice business model and the impact that this has on service delivery to appreciate the impact of their role and service delivery on the business.

General practice funding has previously been demonstrated to significantly impact the role of the GPN (Halcomb et al., 2008). Historically, Australian GPNs were funded for specific items of service provided for and on behalf of the GP. In 2012, the Practice Nurse Incentive Program introduced a new block funding model to support general practice nursing (Department of Health and Aged Care, 2012). In February 2020, this was replaced by the Workforce Incentive Program, which has since been revised in response to feedback (Department of Health and Aged Care, 2023). These models provide funding for nursing services based on factors such as the practice location, size and nature of the practice population, and the hours worked by nurses (Department of Health and Aged Care, 2012). While block funding is an attempt to expand the range of services provided by GPNs, its impact on the nurses' role, service delivery and patient outcomes has yet to be fully evaluated.

In Australia, there have been significant changes to the organisation of general practice service delivery. This includes the changing mix of health professionals in practice teams, the corporatisation of practice and advances in technology (Department of Health, 2022; RACGP, 2023). Currently, across Australia, 31 primary health networks (PHNs) are funded to improve the efficiency and effectiveness of health services and primary care service coordination within particular geographical areas (Lane et al., 2017). In addition to their role in overseeing service delivery, PHNs also support the general practice workforce, providing professional support and education for GPs, GPNs and other health professionals in their region (Lane et al., 2017).

In 2022, the Australian government's Department of Health (2022) released *Australia's Primary Health Care 10 Year Plan 2022–2032* which outlines three key reform streams. This plan identified priorities of future-focused health care, person-centred primary health care (PHC), and locally delivered integrated care. A major change being introduced as a part of this plan is voluntary patient registration with general practices, known as MyMedicare. Having people voluntarily register with a single practice for their health care will facilitate some level of formalisation of the relationship between general practices and patients to promote a level of care continuity that can enhance health outcomes.

In 2001, within Aotearoa New Zealand, The Primary Health Care Strategy (Ministry of Health, 2001) initially set the framework for the current delivery of PHC services across

Aotearoa New Zealand. This strategy led to district health boards (DHBs) funding primary health organisations (PHOs) as not-for-profit services. The Health and Disability System Review in 2020 followed the Waitangi Tribunal Wai 2575 inquiry of 2017–19 and both found much more was needed to improve the health of Māori (Ministry of Health, 2020; 2021). These resulted in the Pae Ora (Healthy Futures) Act 2022 (Parliamentary Counsel Office, 2022), which focuses on equity by aiming to ensure that everyone can access quality health care, no matter who or where they are. A single entity called Te Whatu Ora Health New Zealand has replaced the former DHBs and a parallel entity Te Aka Whai Ora Māori Health Authority now focuses on implementing services to improve health outcomes for Māori following a growing focus on the importance of Te Tiriti o Waitangi (Health New Zealand, 2024). The PHOs still exist but vary in size and structure and continue to function to oversee the provision of essential PHC services to those residing within their geographical boundaries (McMurray & Clendon, 2015; Ministry of Health, 2019). Several subsidised schemes serve low-income and/or high-needs clients in general practice. There has been considerable growth in the number of nurse practitioners (NPs), a scope established in 2004, and many NPs work in PHC settings, including general practice (Adams & Carryer, 2021). Similarly, there has been a growth in interprofessional collaborative practice in primary health care. This has included new health coach, health improvement practitioner and kaiawhina roles, with nurse and pharmacy prescribers as well as other pharmacy roles, such as practice pharmacists, being embedded in general practice (Morris et al., 2024).

The general practice workforce

The general practice workforce has changed dramatically in recent decades in Australia, Aotearoa New Zealand and internationally (Department of Health, 2022; Department of Health, 2009; Heywood & Laurence, 2018a). The shift to a multidisciplinary team-based approach has stemmed from a need to strengthen primary care services to meet the growing burdens of an aging population and its associated increase in chronic and complex conditions. Strengthening primary care nursing has been a key strategy to facilitate lifestyle modifications such as quitting smoking, reducing body weight and increasing physical activity, as well as improving chronic disease management. GPNs can contribute significantly to improving the implementation of adherence to best practice clinical guidelines, as well as enhancing health literacy and promoting self-management (Halcomb et al., 2017; Halcomb et al., 2019).

The growth in the general practice nursing workforce has necessitated revisiting how services are delivered in general practice and which health professional is best placed to provide them. Advances in the delivery and organisation of primary care favour team-based models of care and facilitation of GPNs to work to the full extent of their practice scope (Department of Health, 2022; Flinter et al., 2017). In Australia, the aftermath of the COVID-19 pandemic has resulted in greater reliance on telehealth, changes to primary medical care funding arrangements and enhanced multidisciplinary practice (Duckett, 2020). These trends have implications for the GPN role and strategies, such as skill mix change, where tasks usually undertaken by the GP are transferred to other practitioners including GPNs (Spooner et al., 2022). A key to optimising outcomes, however, is teamwork and collaboration between multidisciplinary health professionals. Indeed, collaborative relationships between GPs and GPNs have been shown to improve primary care delivery (Lukewich et al., 2022). Despite the benefits of collaboration, the frequent status of the GP as the employer of GPNs, the previously medically driven model of general practice and a lack of focus on the integration of the nursing workforce has created challenges in achieving good teamwork (McInnes et al., 2017a; McInnes et al., 2017b).

REFLECTION

1. What have you observed about the delivery of health care in general practice when you or your family/friends have received health care?
2. What have you noticed about nurses working in general practice?

The role of the GPN

Scope of practice – 'the full spectrum of roles, functions, responsibilities, activities and decision-making capacity that individuals within that profession are educated, competent and authorised to perform' (NMBA, 2013).

Various levels of nurses may be employed within general practice including enrolled nurses, registered nurses (RNs) and NPs. Each of these individuals is educated and skilled to provide nursing care within a specific **scope of practice**. The various regulatory frameworks that define the standards and competence expected of nurses in their professional practice articulate these specific scopes of practice (Nursing and Midwifery Board of Australia (NMBA), 2019; NCNZ, n.d.). Additionally, the education, clinical experience and demonstrated competency of the individual nurse in the specific practice environment will further define their practice scope (Halcomb et al., 2016; Halcomb et al., 2017). To guide nurses in making decisions about whether a particular activity is within their individual scope of practice, the NMBA (2013) provides a decision-making framework. Given the relative isolation from other nurses in which many nurses work in general practice, every nurse must ensure that the care they provide is within their scope of practice.

Common clinical activities for nurses working in general practice include health assessment, care planning, immunisation, patient education/self-management support, chronic condition management, recall and reminders for screening, and support for lifestyle risk factor modification (Halcomb et al., 2017; Halcomb & Ashley, 2019). Some GPNs may collect samples for pathology testing and, if appropriately educated, may perform specialised assessments such as pap tests, spirometry and exercise testing. Experienced GPNs are increasingly providing nurse-led clinics for a range of conditions such as cardiovascular disease, sexual health, diabetes, wound care, antenatal care or arthritis management (Halcomb & Ashley, 2019). Additionally, NPs provide clinics with a greater level of autonomy and ability to order tests, implement treatment, prescribe and refer within their scope of practice. There is growing evidence that these kinds of interventions have a positive impact on health outcomes (Halcomb et al., 2017; Halcomb & Ashley, 2019; Lukewich et al., 2022; Stephen et al., 2022).

The specific tasks undertaken by nurses working in general practice are shaped by various factors including:

- the nurse's professional experience and skill
- the individual practice population
- the practice's business orientation
- community resources and health system issues.

Each nurse comes into general practice with a different educational and clinical background (Ashley et al., 2017). The nature of this previous experience will impact the individual's scope of practice and thus the role the nurse plays within the general practice. The practice population and business orientation of the practice will also influence the activities required of the GPN. For example, a practice with a proportionately young population and a high birth rate may employ a GPN to provide antenatal, postnatal and family-focused services. In contrast, a practice with a largely aging practice community may engage a GPN to improve chronic disease management, reduce lifestyle risk factors and reduce avoidable hospitalisations. As employers of GPNs, GPs have a significant input into the services that they provide (McInnes et al., 2017a). The increasing sizes of general practices, the employment of more dedicated staff specifically to perform administrative functions and changes in the funding of GPN services have all contributed to alterations in GPN roles, enabling an increased focus on treatment and preventative health functions (Halcomb et al., 2017).

REFLECTION

1. How might a nurse in general practice help keep a person living with a chronic condition out of hospital care?
2. How could a GPN incorporate health promotion into their daily practice?

CASE STUDY 24.1

Steve is a 60-year-old plumber who recently divorced his wife and lives alone. He is overweight and is taking medication for his hypertension. Steve stops at the local hotel on his way home from work, having a few drinks and a counter meal most nights as he hates cooking. He visits the practice for a routine blood pressure check-up and is seen by the GPN.

Upon checking Steve's blood pressure, Sally (a RN) notices that although it is similar to his previous readings, it is still above best practice guidelines—even though he has been prescribed antihypertensive medication. The nurse asks Steve conversationally about his lifestyle to assess his cardiovascular risk. As they talk, Sally acknowledges Steve's difficulty in incorporating physical activity into his daily routine. However, she reinforces the importance of exercise to general physical well-being and identifies how exercise can also improve emotional well-being. Sally then asks Steve about his visits to the hotel for dinner and a few drinks after work. Following some gentle probing, Steve admits he goes to the pub after work each night because he does not want to go home to an empty house. He acknowledges that he is drinking more alcohol than ever before. Steve justifies this by saying that he keeps drinking to stay at the pub without being out of place and that he enjoys the company. Steve then becomes visibly upset and states that his life is 'pathetic'.

Sally observes that Steve does not appear to be content with his current habits and suggests that they could explore some strategies for healthier and more satisfying outcomes for him. Steve agrees and apologises for becoming upset. Sally reassures Steve that it is quite

CASE STUDY 24.1 Continued

natural for him to be upset, as it is likely that he is still grieving over the end of his marriage and his previous life. Sally asks Steve if he has spoken to anyone about the end of his marriage and divorce. Steve reflects that, apart from the divorce lawyers and a few friends and family, he has not really talked about it. He says that most of his friends and family tell him that he is better off without his ex-wife and suggest he should start dating again. Steve says that he does not feel ready for another relationship after 30 years of marriage. However, he does acknowledge that he has to make some changes in his life, or he will 'end up a sad old drunk who sits at the pub all day watching the horse races'.

Steve and Sally discuss possibilities for lifestyle change. By the end of the consultation, Steve agrees to consider counselling to work through issues related to his divorce. Steve also decides to go to the animal shelter and adopt a dog. He says that he would have a reason to go straight home after work to take it for a walk each evening and it would provide him with company in the evenings and on the weekends. Steve also plans to investigate having prepared meals delivered – as he still is not interested in having to make his own. He thinks this would be convenient and would give him more time to walk his dog.

REFLECTION

1. What differences did Sally make to Steve's perspectives on his health (and potentially health outcomes) through monitoring his blood pressure and undertaking a lifestyle assessment?
2. What kinds of additional services and support might help Steve?
3. What activities could Sally, in conjunction with the GP, do to support Steve?

Professional practice standards

In 2014, the Australian Nursing and Midwifery Federation released revised professional practice standards for nurses working in Australian general practice (Australian Nursing and Midwifery Federation (ANMF), 2014; Halcomb et al., 2017). These standards articulate the parts of the registered and enrolled nursing role that are unique to the general practice context and unlike those expected of nurses practising in other clinical contexts. As such, these build on the national nursing standards (NMBA, 2019) to provide additional standards relevant to this specific area of practice. The standards divide the work of the GPN into four domains:

1. Professional practice
2. Nursing care
3. General practice environment
4. Collaborative practice (ANMF, 2014).

Key performance indicators within the standards document allow nurses to evaluate their current clinical performance and plan appropriate professional development to consolidate skills in the various domains of practice.

In Aotearoa New Zealand, like in the United Kingdom, primary care nursing competency standards are embedded within a career framework (Stillwell & New Zealand College of Primary Health Care Nurses, 2019). In 2019, standards of practice specifically for Aotearoa New Zealand PHC nurses were developed (Stillwell & New Zealand College of Primary Health Care Nurses, 2019). These four standards are:

1. Promoting health
2. Building capacity
3. Improving access and equity
4. Working together, better and smarter.

CASE STUDY 24.2

Regentville Medical Practice has just employed Michael as a GPN. Michael graduated last year and has only worked in an aged care facility for a few months since becoming an RN. Michael was pleased to find that Regentville Medical Practice employs an experienced RN so he can be supported. However, as the other RN has a day off today, Michael is working alone. This means that Michael is seeing all the patients booked with the nurse for dressings, immunisations and health assessments, as well as providing support for the four GPs on duty.

While in the middle of a health assessment, Dr Blight comes in and asks Michael to cut Mrs Brown's toenails as they are rubbing on her shoes. He also asks Michael to do an electrocardiogram (ECG) on Mr Smith as he has been feeling a bit short of breath today. Before Michael can respond, Dr Blight tells him that the patients are waiting outside and walks out. Michael finishes the assessment but is very worried about what to do next. He has never done an ECG with the old-style machine that the practice has and has never been shown or taught about trimming toenails.

REFLECTION

1. How do you decide whether a specific clinical task is within your scope of practice?
2. Where can you find information or support to help you make decisions about your scope of practice?
3. What should Michael do now?
4. What could Michael do differently in the future?

Conclusion

Nursing in general practice is an exciting opportunity to contribute to the health care of individuals, their families and communities. Our contemporary context sees an increasing emphasis being placed on the delivery of health care within the community. In this context, there is great potential for nurses to work to the extent of their scope of practice in collaboration with GPs, allied health and specialist services to reduce avoidable hospital presentations/admissions and improve health outcomes, well-being and quality of life.

CRITICAL THINKING ACTIVITIES

1. What are some of the challenges that you might face being a nurse employed by a GP to work in general practice?
2. How might the small business model of general practice impact your role?
3. What factors might enable and hinder you from being able to collaborate with GPs in the practice?

FURTHER READING

Australian Nursing and Midwifery Federation. (2014). *National Practice Standards for Nurses in General Practice*. Australian Nursing and Midwifery Federation.

Calma, K., Stephens, M. & Halcomb, E.J. (2019). The impact of curriculum on nursing students' attitudes, perceptions and preparedness to work in primary health care: An integrative review. *Nurse Education in Practice*, *39*, 1–10. https://doi.org/10.1016/j.nepr.2019.07.006

Department of Health. (2022). *Future Focused Primary Health Care: Australia's Primary Health Care 10 Year Plan 2022–2032*. Commonwealth of Australia.

McInnes, S., Halcomb, E., Huckel, K. & Ashley, C. (2019). The experiences of new graduate registered nurses in a general practice based graduate program: A qualitative study. *Australian Journal of Primary Health*, *25*(4), 366–73. https://doi.org/10.1071/PY19089

Stillwell, Y. & New Zealand College of Primary Health Care Nurses. (2019). *Aotearoa New Zealand Primary Health Care Nursing Standards of Practice*. New Zealand.

REFERENCES

Adams, S. & Carryer, J. (2021). How the institutional and policy context shapes the establishment of nurse practitioner roles and practice in New Zealand's primary health care sector. *Policy, Politics, & Nursing Practice*, *22*(1), 17–27. https://doi.org/10.1177/1527154420965534

Ashley, C., Halcomb, E., Brown, A. & Peters, K. (2017). Exploring why nurses transition from acute care to primary health care: A mixed methods study. *Applied Nursing Research, 38*, 83–7. https://doi.org/10.1016/j.apnr.2017.09.002

Australian Government. (2022). *Strengthening Medicare Taskforce Report*. Australian Government. www.health.gov.au/resources/publications/strengthening-medicare-taskforce-report?language=en

Australian Institute of Health and Welfare (AIHW). (2020). *A profile of primary health care nurses*. Australian Government. www.aihw.gov.au/reports/primary-health-care/a-profile-of-primary-care-nurses/data

Australian Medicare Local Alliance. (2012). *General Practice Nurse National Survey Report*. Australian Medicare Local Alliance.

Australian Nursing and Midwifery Federation (ANMF). (2014). *National Practice Standards for Nurses in General Practice*. www.anmf.org.au/media/ouzgnqft/anmf_national_practice_standards_for_nurses_in_general_practice.pdf

Department of Health. (2009). *Primary Health Care Reform in Australia: Report to Support Australia's First National Primary Health Care Strategy*. Commonwealth of Australia.

——— (2022). *Australia's Primary Health Care 10 Year Plan 2022–2032*. www.health.gov.au/resources/publications/australias-primary-health-care-10-year-plan-2022-2032

Department of Health and Aged Care. (2012). *The Practice Nurse Incentive Program*. Commonwealth of Australia.

——— (2023). *Workforce Incentive Program Practice Stream Guidelines*. Commonwealth of Australia.

Duckett, S. (2020). What should primary care look like after the COVID-19 pandemic? *Australian Journal of Primary Health, 26*(3), 207–11. https://doi.org/10.1071/PY20095

Flinter, M., Hsu, C., Cromp, D., Ladden, M.D. & Wagner, E.H. (2017). Registered nurses in primary care: Emerging new roles and contributions to team-based care in high-performing practices. *Journal of Ambulatory Care Management, 40*(4), 287–96. https://doi.org/10.1097/jac.0000000000000193

Halcomb, E. & Ashley, C. (2019). Are Australian general practice nurses underutilised? An examination of current roles and task satisfaction. *Collegian, 26*(5), 522–7. https://doi.org/10.1016/j.colegn.2019.02.005

Halcomb, E., Ashley, C., Middleton, R., et al. (2021). Understanding perceptions of health, lifestyle risks and chronic disease in middle age. *Journal of Clinical Nursing, 30*(15–16), 2279–86. https://doi.org/10.1111/jocn.15711

Halcomb, E.J., Davidson, P.M., Salamonson, Y. & Ollerton, R. (2008). Nurses in Australian general practice: Implications for chronic disease management. *Journal of Clinical Nursing, 17*(5A), 6–15. https://doi.org/10.1111/j.1365-2702.2007.02141.x

Halcomb, E.J., McInnes, S., Moxham, L. & Patterson, C. (2019). Nurse-delivered interventions for mental health in primary care: A systematic review of randomised controlled trials. *Family Practice, 36*(1), 64–71. https://doi.org/10.1093/fampra/cmy101

Halcomb, E.J., Stephens, M., Ashley, C., Foley, E. & Bryce, J. (2016). Nursing competency standards in the primary health care setting: An integrative review. *Journal of Clinical Nursing, 25*(9), 1193–205. https://doi.org/10.1111/jocn.13224

Halcomb, E.J., Stephens, M., Bryce, J., Foley, E. & Ashley, C. (2017). The development of national professional practice standards for nurses working in Australian general practice. *Journal of Advanced Nursing, 73*(8), 1958–69. https://doi.org/10.1111/jan.13274

Health New Zealand. (2024). *Māori Health*. New Zealand Government. https://www.tewhatuora.govt.nz/health-services-and-programmes/maori-health

Heywood, T. & Laurence, C. (2018a). An overview of the general practice nurse workforce in Australia, 2012–15. *Australian Journal of Primary Health, 24*(3), 227–32. https://doi.org/10.1071/PY17048

—— (2018b). The general practice nurse workforce: 'Estimating future supply'. *Australian Journal of General Practice, 47*(11), 788. https://doi.org/10.31128/AJGP-01-18-4461

Lane, R., Halcomb, E., McKenna, L., et al. (2017). Advancing general practice nursing in Australia: Roles and responsibilities of primary health care organisations. *Australian Health Review, 41*(2), 127–32. https://doi.org/10.1071/AH15239

Lukewich, J., Martin-Misener, R., Norful, A.A., et al. (2022). Effectiveness of registered nurses on patient outcomes in primary care: A systematic review. *BMC Health Services Research, 22*(1), 740. https://doi.org/10.1186/s12913-022-07866-x

McInnes, S., Halcomb, E., Huckel, K. & Ashley, C. (2019). Experiences of new graduate registered nurses in a general practice based graduate program: A qualitative study. *Australian Journal of Primary Health, 25*(4), 366–73. https://doi.org/10.1071/PY19089

McInnes, S., Peters, K., Bonney, A. & Halcomb, E. (2017a). A qualitative study of collaboration in general practice: Understanding the general practice nurse's role. *Journal of Clinical Nursing, 26*(13–14), 1960–8. https://doi.org/10.1111/jocn.13598

—— (2017b). The influence of funding models on collaboration in Australian general practice. *Australian Journal of Primary Health, 23*(1), 31–6. https://doi.org/10.1071/PY16017

McMurray, A. & Clendon, J. (2015). *Community Health and Wellness: Primary Health Care in Practice*. Elsevier Health Sciences.

Ministry of Health. (2001). *The Primary Health Care Strategy*. New Zealand Government. www.health.govt.nz/system/files/documents/publications/phcstrat_0.pdf

—— (2019). *About primary health organisations*. New Zealand Government. www.health.govt.nz/strategies-initiatives/programmes-and-initiatives/primary-and-community-health-care

———— (2020). *Health and Disability System Review. 2020. Health and Disability System Review – Final Report – Pūrongo Whakamutunga*. New Zealand Government.

———— (2021). *Wai 2575 Health Services and Outcomes Inquiry*. New Zealand Government. www.health.govt.nz/maori-health/wai-2575-health-services-and-outcomes-inquiry

Morris, C., McDonald, J., Officer, T.N., et al. (2024). A realist evaluation of the development of extended pharmacist roles and services in community pharmacies. *Research in Social and Administrative Pharmacy, 20*(3), 321–34. https://doi.org/10.1016/j.sapharm.2023.11.006

Nursing and Midwifery Board of Australia (NMBA). (2013). *National Framework for the Development of Decision-Making Tools for Nursing and Midwifery Practice – September 2007*. www.nursingmidwiferyboard.gov.au/codes-guidelines-statements/frameworks.aspx

———— (2019). *Professional standards*. www.nursingmidwiferyboard.gov.au/Codes-Guidelines-Statements/Professional-standards.aspx

Nursing Council of New Zealand (NCNZ). (2019). *The New Zealand Nursing Workforce: A profile of Nurse Practitioners, Registered Nurses and Enrolled Nurses 2018–2019*. NCNZ.

———— (n.d.). *Registered nurse: Scope of practice*. https://nursingcouncil.org.nz/Public/ncnz/nursing-section/registered_nurse.aspx

Parliamentary Counsel Office. (2022). *Pae Ora (Healthy Futures) Act 2022*. New Zealand Government. www.legislation.govt.nz/act/public/2022/0030/latest/LMS575405.html

Spooner, S., McDermott, I., Goff, M., Hodgson, D., McBride, A. & Checkland, K. (2022). Processes supporting effective skill-mix implementation in general practice: A qualitative study. *Journal of Health Services Research & Policy, 27*(4), 269–77. https://doi.org/10.1177/135581962210913

Stephen, C., Halcomb, E., Fernandez, R., et al. (2022). Nurse-led interventions to manage hypertension in general practice: A systematic review and meta analysis. *Journal of Advanced Nursing, 78*(5), 1281–93. https://doi.org/10.1111/jan.15159

Stillwell, Y. & New Zealand College of Primary Health Care Nurses. (2019). *Aotearoa New Zealand Primary Health Care Nursing Standards of Practice*. New Zealand Nurses Organisation.

The Royal Australian College of General Practitioners (RACGP). (2023). *General Practice: Health of the Nation 2023*. RACGP. https://www.racgp.org.au/general-practice-health-of-the-nation/executive-summary

Thomas, T.H.T., Bloomfield, J.G., Gordon, C.J. & Aggar, C. (2018). Australia's first transition to Professional Practice in Primary Care Program: Qualitative findings from a mixed-method evaluation. *Collegian, 25*(2), 201–8. https://doi.org/10.1016/j.colegn.2017.03.009

Correctional nursing

Grant Kinghorn, Rebecca Bosworth and Elizabeth Halcomb

25

LEARNING OBJECTIVES

At the completion of this chapter, you should be able to:

- outline the purpose of the correctional health systems.
- describe the role of nurses in correctional settings.
- identify the opportunities of nursing in correctional settings.

Introduction

Globally, people in prison often come from the most deprived sections of society due to adverse political, economic, environmental, social and lifestyle factors (Ismail et al., 2021). This group experiences chronic and complex mental and physical health conditions at higher rates than the general population (Australian Institute of Health and Welfare (AIHW), 2023a), including mental health conditions, chronic non-communicable and communicable conditions and acquired brain injury (AIHW, 2023a; McLeod et al., 2020). They also have higher rates of tobacco smoking, high-risk alcohol consumption, illicit drug use and injecting drug use (AIHW, 2023a; McLeod et al., 2020). As many as 90 per cent of people in custody have a diagnosis of either a mental health condition or addiction (Bell, Hopkin & Forrester, 2019; Trimmer et al., 2019). Often, people in prison have under-utilised health care in the community and, for many, the first interaction with health services occurs during incarceration (Borschmann et al., 2020). Therefore, incarceration may provide an opportunity to access treatment to improve health and for appropriate health care to be initiated (Besney et al., 2018; Bouchaud, Brooks & Swan, 2018; Lafferty et al., 2018).

Fundamental national and international standards govern the provision of health care in correctional settings (United Nations Office on Drugs and Crime (UNODC), 2015). Globally, the declaration of 'prison health is part of public health' released by the (World Health Organization (WHO), 2003), is the underpinning principle of health care in correctional facilities today. Internationally, the United Nations Basic Principles for the Treatment of Prisoners, Principle 9 highlights that 'Prisoners shall have access to the health services available to those in the country without discrimination on the grounds of their legal situation' (United Nations Human Rights Office of the High Commissioner (OHCHR), 1990). In some countries, people in prison may not receive community-equivalent care (Winkelman et al., 2022); however, in Australian and Aotearoa New Zealand prisons, health is high on the agenda (Corrective Services Administrators' Council (CSAC), 2018; Justice Health NSW, 2023a). Successful health interventions implemented during incarceration can mean that individuals return to the community with a more positive attitude to health and improved health compared to when they entered custody (Justice Health NSW, 2023a; Ramaswamy & Freudenberg, 2022; Trimmer et al., 2019). Improving the health and well-being of people in custody improves the health of the entire community (AIHW, 2023a).

Nurses play a key role in the delivery of health care in correctional environments. **Correctional nursing** involves the assessment, planning and implementation of health care within all kinds of correctional environments (Shelton, Maruca & Wright, 2020). Given the unique environment and patient needs, correctional nurses are required to have specific skill sets, knowledge and personal attributes beyond those of nurses in other settings (Caro, 2021; Goddard et al., 2019). Correctional nurses need practical and theoretical knowledge of the criminal justice system, the function of the courts and health legislation (American Nurses Association, 2021).

This chapter provides an overview of the correctional health system, highlighting the complex needs of this population and the important role of nurses. It also identifies some of the challenges of correctional nursing and the skills needed by nurses to work effectively in this environment.

Correctional nursing –
'Correctional nursing is the protection, promotion and optimization of health and abilities, prevention of illness and injury, alleviation of suffering through the diagnosis and treatment of human response, advocacy, and delivery of health care to individuals, families, communities, and populations under the jurisdiction of the criminal justice system' (American Nurses Association, 2021).

Correctional health systems

Traditionally, health care staff in correctional environments were employed as part of the correctional services workforce (Burton, Chiarella & Waters, 2022; Shelton et al., 2020). With the expansion of public health systems in recent decades, correctional health care services have either become more closely affiliated with public health services or outsourced to private health care providers (McLeod et al., 2020; Sasso et al., 2018; Trimmer et al., 2019). Across Australia, each state and territory provides health care services to most correctional settings. The local health department provides correctional health services in some jurisdictions, while the justice or corrections department takes responsibility in others (AIHW, 2023a). Similarly, in Aotearoa New Zealand, correctional health care services are the responsibility of the local district health board. However, health care services need to work closely with corrective services staff to organise care delivery (Brooke, 2020; Burton et al., 2022; Gorman et al., 2018).

While an increasingly multidisciplinary approach has been integrated to ensure holistic care is provided, the first level of contact a person staying in prison has with correctional health services is predominantly with nurses (Caro, 2021; Shelton et al., 2020). Correctional nurses deliver care in a range of settings including minimum-, medium- or high-security custodial settings, courts, police cell complexes and community-based settings (American Nurses Association, 2021; Gould & Brent, 2020). The role and skills/knowledge required by the nurse vary across settings. For example, nurses in custody services, courts and community teams provide assessments, recommendations and specialist advice to correctional staff and courts (Caro, 2021). They may also assist in averting or managing alcohol and other drug withdrawal and mental health conditions (Shelton et al., 2020). Nurses who work in correctional centres and hospitals deliver direct care either in a specialist service (for example, forensic mental health) or with a more general primary health care (PHC) focus.

The profile of people in prison

In Australia, approximately 65 000 people cycle through correctional settings each year (AIHW, 2022). Between June 2021 and 2022, some 40 591 adults were in the Australian **prison** system (Australian Bureau of Statistics (ABS), 2024), representing around 0.15 per cent of the population (25.9 million). There are far fewer individuals incarcerated in Aotearoa New Zealand, with 8376 people reported to be incarcerated during 2023 across the country's 19 correctional facilities (Ara Poutama Aotearoa Department of Corrections, 2023). This represents some 0.17 per cent of the Aotearoa New Zealand population (4.9 million).

> **Prison** – an institution managed by correctional services that holds individuals who have been sentenced to a period of imprisonment by a court after being convicted of undertaking offences against the law.

Similar to the international profile of people incarcerated (Sasso et al., 2018), the Australian prison population is overwhelmingly male (92%), with an average age of 36 years (ABS, 2024; AIHW, 2024). In Aotearoa New Zealand, 94 per cent of the incarcerated population is male, with 35 per cent aged between 30 and 39 years (Ara Poutama Aotearoa Department of Corrections, 2023). Despite the lower numbers of incarcerated females, this group has recently increased in greater numbers than male offenders (ABS, 2024; Besney et al., 2018). Additionally, incarcerated females have a very high incidence of physical, sexual and emotional abuse as well as substance use disorders (Besney et al., 2018; Bright, Higgins & Grealish, 2023).

People in contact with the justice system and those housed in correctional environments represent some of the most at-risk and priority populations (AIHW, 2024; Lafferty et al., 2018). Priority populations are disproportionately represented in correctional environments internationally (Besney et al., 2018; WHO, 2022). In Australia, while Aboriginal and Torres Strait Islander people comprise 3 per cent of the general community, they remain overrepresented in the prison system, accounting for some 32 per cent of the total prison population (12 902) (ABS, 2024). In Aotearoa New Zealand, 52.8 per cent of those incarcerated in 2023 were Māori (Ara Poutama Aotearoa Department of Corrections, 2023).

In Australia, 31 per cent of those entering custodial environments have completed a school level at Year 9 or below and 43 per cent were homeless in the four weeks before entering custody (AIHW, 2023a). People in correctional environments have been shown to have a high level of physical health concerns including blood-borne viruses and various chronic conditions such as cardiovascular disease, diabetes and asthma (Besney et al., 2018; Bouchaud et al., 2018; Wong et al., 2018). Almost two in five (39%) of those entering custody report a long-term health condition or disability that limits their daily activities and affects their participation in education or employment (AIHW, 2023a). Longer incarceration periods and increased aging of patients within custodial services mean that the complexity of chronic health issues is also placing additional pressure on health care services and the responsibilities of nursing staff.

Young offenders are managed by juvenile justice services until they are 18 years old. These are often separate facilities or discrete units within adult correctional services. In Australia, an average of around 800 young people are in detention each night (AIHW, 2023b). Like the adult population, most of these are male (91%), however, in the juvenile offender population half (50%) are Aboriginal or Torres Strait Islander (AIHW, 2023b). The majority are aged between 10 and 17 years (83%) and unsentenced (72%) (AIHW, 2023b). In Aotearoa New Zealand, there is a strong emphasis on addressing the family and social issues that contribute to offending. Youth who have committed minor offences can be sent to youth justice centres that provide rehabilitative and social support to improve outcomes and reduce recidivism (Oranga Tamariki Ministry for Children, 2023). Intervening to address the health and socio-economic disadvantages being experienced by young offenders presents an opportunity to change outcomes for young people.

REFLECTION

Given what you have read about people in prison, what opportunities and challenges do you think exist for a registered nurse in providing care for this priority population?

The correctional nursing role

The core role of correctional nurses is to engage with and provide assessment, planning, treatment and follow-up. Nurses' responsibilities include conducting reception screenings for all incoming patients, undertaking comprehensive health screenings for patients staying long-term, and participating in the assessment, planning, implementation, and evaluation of nursing care (American Nurses Association, 2021; Goddard et al., 2019). Nurses are also responsible for providing for the day-to-day health care requirements for people in correctional environments (AIHW, 2023a). This involves counselling, health promotion, advocacy, clinical teaching, supervising, mentoring and research (Gould & Brent, 2020). Responsibilities may also include assessment of psychiatric health needs, management of medical and psychiatric emergencies, suicide prevention, infection control, emergency care, health education and pathology collection (WHO, 2022).

While the role of correctional nurses may be similar to other community nursing roles, the practice environment is very different. Correctional nurses are often the first level of contact with the health care system as opposed to the general community where general practitioners (GPs) provide most of the primary care (Justice Health NSW, n.d.). Correctional nurses work in mostly autonomous positions with a large patient profile for whom they provide direct care and treatment, daily triage, emergency care, and health promotion while empowering self-care and promoting health literacy (Peternelj-Taylor & Woods, 2019; Trimmer et al., 2019).

There are several correctional nursing specialties including primary health, population health, women's health, Indigenous health, adolescent health, drug and alcohol, forensic mental health as well as specific chronic disease management (Ara Poutama Aotearoa Department of Corrections, 2014; Burton et al., 2022; Peternelj-Taylor & Woods, 2019; Wong et al., 2018). The workforce profile also includes generalist nurses, specialist nurses and nurse practitioners. Nursing staff work closely with the multidisciplinary team to address risk and support patients to improve their health (Burton, 2023).

The guiding principles that underpin the correctional health nurse role intertwine closely with those of drugs and alcohol and mental health nurses. These principles have been discussed further in Chapter 21. In brief, they include the alignment of all care with the United Nations' Sustainable Development Goals (Fields et al., 2021; United Nations Department of Economic and Social Affairs (UN DESA), 2023) to uphold the principle above all to 'do no harm', to use person-centred language to reduce stigma and discrimination (Alcohol and Drug Foundation, 2023), and deliver trauma-informed holistic care by treating the person and not the illness (Marel et al., 2022).

Health screening

Health screening is a key role of correctional nurses, particularly given the nature of the population and the frequent previous lack of access to and engagement with health services (Brooke, 2020). Time spent within the correctional system can provide an opportunity to engage people with individualised plans of health care to improve their health and risk factor profile (Besney et al., 2018).

Screening initially occurs upon arrival to the facility by reception nurses through interviewing, observation and physical assessment (Shelton et al., 2020). This initial screening facilitates the triage of individuals' needs across the domains of health, identification of required referrals and development of a care plan. The nature of the correctional environment necessitates that these assessments also include evaluation of mental health and potential risks to the people staying in prison themselves and/or others (Dickens et al., 2020).

Many people housed in correctional environments have lower health literacy than the general population and limited previous health service use (AIHW, 2023a; Mehay, Meek & Ogden, 2021). Additionally, the circumstances that led the individual to enter incarceration may either be a sequela of mental health issues or may result in a degree of confusion, disorientation, depression or anxiety. The correctional nurse needs to understand this context when undertaking initial assessments and use appropriate communication techniques to promote comfort and safety (Bright et al., 2023). Given the high frequency of transfers and movement of individuals across correctional environments, all health assessments must be well documented to avoid duplication and promote continuity of care.

Correctional nurses may also perform ongoing health screening related to changes in health status – such as mental health, and alcohol and other drug use disorders – or for specific purposes such as segregation or 'safe cell' assessment and clearance for work programs. With the rise in female incarceration, there is a growing need for gender-specific assessment services (Solell & Smith, 2019). Correctional nurses must become familiar with the requirements and purpose of each type of screening, and how each is best communicated to other members of the health care and correctional services team (Peternelj-Taylor & Woods, 2019).

PHC

PHC services within correctional settings are similar to those within the community (Bouchaud et al., 2018) and include the range of prevention, health promotion and disease management services delivered in mainstream general practice, as well as acute condition management (Justice Health NSW, n.d.). An 'application system' enables patients to access health services including those offered by doctors, dentists, psychiatrists, podiatrists and opticians (Brooke, 2020; Caro, 2021). However, unlike in the community where a person can directly refer to these health providers, in correctional settings much of the initial triage is undertaken by nurses (Gould & Brett, 2020). Correctional nurses must be able to think quickly and respond to a wide variety of health-related scenarios (Hancock, 2020). As GPs may only have limited clinic days, the correctional nurse has significant autonomy in triaging presentations and planning referrals or treatment (Brooke, 2020).

A key consideration in the delivery of PHC in correctional environments is the need for patient education and support to develop sustainable self-management, particularly for chronic and ongoing conditions. Providing such resources within the correctional environment has the potential to improve the health of patients on their return to the community (McLeod et al., 2020).

Alcohol and other drugs

An important specialisation within correctional health services is drug and alcohol nursing. The main roles include supporting individuals to reduce their risk from substance-related harm by risk assessment and management of intoxication and withdrawal from alcohol and other drugs (AOD) for all clients upon entry to the custodial system, and the provision of opioid treatment programs (OTPs) (for example, methadone, naltrexone and buprenorphine). After a person is released, it is essential to establish and maintain care arrangements for those on an OTP to guarantee seamless care continuation and referral to AOD services offered by the Corrective Services. This includes organising care arrangements and facilitating access to individual and group counselling as well as lifestyle education (Justice Health NSW, n.d.).

Forensic mental health

Within correctional environments, the forensic mental health nurse has various specialist roles including providing assessment and advice to courts. This nurse also needs a sound knowledge base of criminogenic factors and offending behaviour to assist in analysing previous and current behaviour and to guide an understanding of factors that may impact ongoing management and treatment (Marshall, Adams & Stuckey, 2019; Oates et al., 2020). In some jurisdictions, forensic mental health hospitals provide a combination of acute and ongoing care for people with significant mental health care needs that cannot be met within the mainstream correctional system. Appropriately addressing mental health issues while a person is in custody is important in reducing the risk of reoffending or harming themselves or others.

Emergency care

All correctional nurses are expected to have the skills and abilities to respond to a range of medical emergencies. The safety concerns within the correctional environment create challenges to ensure the security of staff and others during emergencies. As correctional nurses are most likely to be the first health professionals to respond, and at many times are the only health professionals on-site, they are expected to identify immediate care priorities and provide overall emergency response management (Woods & Peternelj-Taylor, 2022). The nurse needs to stabilise the patient and prepare for transport to an appropriate medical facility (Spycher et al., 2021). Nurses must work closely with correctional officers who can assist in securing and clearing the area, carrying equipment and facilitating off-site transport (Woods & Peternelj-Taylor, 2022).

CASE STUDY 25.1

Jane, a 36-year-old Caucasian woman, has been seeing the clinic nurse for the past two weeks for an infected cyst that requires cleaning and dressing. On the most recent visit, the nurse observed Jane to be more withdrawn and distracted than usual. The nurse asks Jane how she is feeling, and she states that it's been hard over the last week as her partner has broken up with her and she is scared that she will lose custody of her children, especially since she will be in prison for another four years. The nurse asks Jane if she has spoken to anyone about this but, instead of answering, Jane states: 'It's useless in talking … everything is useless when you're stuck in here with no real hope of anything … life is just pointless.'

REFLECTION

1. What is your initial impression of Jane and what are your initial concerns for her?
2. What essential information would you like to gain from Jane and what would be your approach to ensure that she feels safe talking to you?
3. Who else may you engage with to ensure Jane's immediate safety and well-being?

Correctional nursing challenges

> When I first started I was a bit confronted by the walls and the locked gates you have to negotiate, the razor wire and correctional officers in the towers but it is amazing how quickly that disappears into the background. While I am always aware that this is a very secure environment, I also find that my work is so challenging that I don't really think about those things anymore. (Quote from a nurse working in a Correctional Centre (Justice Health NSW, 2023b))

Correctional nursing can be rewarding and challenging particularly when working with patients living with complex health issues in largely autonomous roles. Service delivery is not always straightforward and can often be impacted by the prison environment, communication delays, and uncertainty regarding discharge dates which may impact the continuity of care following release into the community (AIHW, 2023a). However, the most common issue identified by correctional nurses is related to working within a security model, as this fundamentally conflicts with providing person-centred health services (Bouchaud et al., 2018; Gorman et al., 2018; Sasso et al., 2018). Those transitioning from working in a traditional health care setting to a correctional environment may find that their concept of care does not sit comfortably with the custodial ethos of such settings (Gorman et al., 2018; Lazzari et al., 2020; Sasso et al., 2018). This can lead to frustration and negatively impact on job satisfaction. For various reasons, people in prison may be suddenly moved between custodial settings and this can interrupt the continuity of health services. Conversely, 'lockdowns' and security concerns can limit the movement of individuals thus impacting their capacity to attend booked appointments or clinics (Bell et al., 2019; Dennard et al., 2021).

Another challenge relates to perceptions of the individuals within the correctional population. All nurses are expected to demonstrate respect for patients regardless of their background, criminal history and health diagnoses. A correctional nurse's ability to convey a non-judgemental attitude, while ensuring that the principles of equality, fairness and confidentiality are maintained, is often tested (Sasso et al., 2018; Solell & Smith, 2019). This is particularly the case where nurses have concerns about their safety (Bell et al., 2019; Dennard et al., 2021; Hancock, 2020). Correctional nurses must recognise that their feelings and attitudes about an individual may impact their behaviour and subsequent therapeutic relationships (Solell & Smith, 2019). As correctional nurses work with many priority populations, they must be continuously aware of their professional boundaries and ensure that their relationship with their patients is positive and beneficial to both parties (Hancock, 2020; Lazzari et al., 2020; Solell & Smith, 2019). In recognition of the continued over-representation of Indigenous people in prison, health care must be underpinned by cultural safety and creating an environment that is respectful and values the identity, culture and experience of consumers (Minister for Corrections, 2023). Multicultural treatment considerations must also be embedded for people from culturally and linguistically diverse backgrounds (Rose et al., 2019).

The stress and burnout created by providing nursing care to priority populations within a complex environment is an issue (Bell et al., 2019). Dealing with complex mental health issues such as episodes of self-harm, suicide and assaults, combined with adverse working conditions, can potentially impact the health of nurses. Correctional nurses must practise good self-care strategies and engage in workplace support to optimise their well-being (NSW Health, 2021).

REFLECTION

Consider what the professional opportunities and challenges would be for a registered nurse adapting to work in a correctional environment. Think about how these nurses would develop their confidence and competence in providing autonomous and holistic care to a complex patient group. Reflect on your own feelings about working with people who have come into contact with the criminal justice system.

1. What would your immediate feelings be?
2. How would you ensure that you treated these patients with respect?
3. How would you balance your security and personal boundaries with that of providing adequate and person-centred care?

CASE STUDY 25.2

Peter, a 22-year-old man, arrives at a reception centre after being arrested for armed robbery. It is his sixth arrest and induction into a correctional environment in the last three years. Peter comments that he is happy to be in custody as he has been homeless for the last three months and has nowhere else to go. According to his file, Peter has a history of intravenous drug and alcohol use but has refused to see either a drug and alcohol or population health nurse on his previous admissions. Once again, he refuses to be referred to any specialist while in custody and declines to have baseline physical health observations undertaken. The nurse observes that Peter appears malnourished and is unsteady on his feet. Before finishing the assessment, Peter asks if the nurse can prescribe an antipsychotic for him, stating: 'I'm not crazy, I just find it is the only thing that helps me get off to sleep these days.'

REFLECTION

1. What do you think are the essential health concerns for Peter?
2. Considering that Peter has refused any referrals, what follow-up could the nurse put in place?
3. What strategies could the nurse use to help Peter engage with available services?
4. What would your attitude be towards Peter if you saw him for each admission? Would it be considered therapeutic?

Conclusion

Correctional nursing provides an essential service to people in prison whose needs may not have been met by the current health care system. The complexities of the role transcend the various physical environments and backgrounds of patients by providing therapeutic care within a security model. Nurses working in correctional environments require a comprehensive level of skills and knowledge to be able to undertake assessment and ongoing and emergency care for a variety of health care concerns. Often working in small teams and autonomous positions, correctional nurses provide an essential link with the patients and other health team members.

CRITICAL THINKING ACTIVITIES

You have just commenced work in a high-security correctional environment.

1. How would you balance the needs of your patients while addressing the security needs of the environment?
2. How would you ensure that you had the appropriate and up-to-date knowledge and skills set to be able to work in an autonomous role?
3. What would you do to continue your own reflective and professional development in such a working environment?

FURTHER READING

Ara Poutama Aotearoa Department of Corrections. (2023). *Prison facts and statistics – March 2023.* New Zealand Government. www.corrections.govt.nz/resources/statistics/quarterly_prison_statistics/prison_stats_march_2023

Australian Institute of Health and Welfare (AIHW). (2023a). *The Health of People in Australia's Prisons 2022.* (Cat. no. PHE 334.) Australian Government. www.aihw.gov.au/getmedia/e2245d01-07d1-4b8d-81b3-60d14fbf007f/aihw-phe-33-health-of-people-in-australias-prisons-2022.pdf?v=20231108163318&inline=true

Burton, J., Chiarella, M. & Waters, D. (2022). Historical context of custodial health nursing in New South Wales, Australia. *Journal of Forensic Nursing, 18*(4), 221–8. https://doi.org/10.1097/JFN.0000000000000357

Dean, K., Browne, C. & Dean, N. (2022). *Stigma and Discrimination Experiences Amongst Those with Mental Illness in Contact with the Criminal Justice System: A Rapid Review Report for the Australian National Mental Health Commission.* University of New South Wales.

REFERENCES

Alcohol and Drug Foundation. (2023). *The power of words: Having conversations about alcohol and other drugs: A quick guide*. http://anyflip.com/line/fqdv/

American Nurses Association. (2021). *Correctional Nursing: Scope and Standards of Practice* (3rd ed.). American Nurses Association.

Ara Poutama Aotearoa Department of Corrections. (2014). *Change Lives, Shape Futures – Reduce Re-offending Among Maori*. New Zealand Government. www.mcguinnessinstitute.org/wp-content/uploads/2021/04/3e.-Change-Lives-Shape-Futures-Reducing-Re-offending-among-Maori.pdf

——— (2023). *Prison facts and statistics – March 2023*. New Zealand Government. www.corrections.govt.nz/resources/statistics/quarterly_prison_statistics/prison_stats_march_2023

Australian Bureau of Statistics (ABS). (2024). *Prisoners in Australia*. Australian Government. www.abs.gov.au/statistics/people/crime-and-justice/prisoners-australia/latest-release

Australian Institute of Health and Welfare (AIHW). (2023a). *The health of people in Australia's prisons 2022*. Australian Government. www.aihw.gov.au/getmedia/e2245d01-07d1-4b8d-81b3-60d14fbf007f/aihw-phe-33-health-of-people-in-australias-prisons-2022.pdf?v=20231108163318&inline=true

——— (2023b). *Youth detention population in Australia 2021*. Australian Government. www.aihw.gov.au/reports/youth-justice/youth-detention-population-in-australia-2021/contents/summary

——— (2024). *Health of people in prison*. Australian Government. www.aihw.gov.au/reports/australias-health/health-of-prisoners

Bell, S., Hopkin, G. & Forrester, A. (2019). Exposure to traumatic events and the experience of burnout, compassion fatigue and compassion satisfaction among prison mental health staff: An exploratory survey. *Issues in Mental Health Nursing*, *40*(4), 304–9. https://doi.org/10.1080/01612840.2018.1534911

Besney, J.D., Angel, C., Pyne, D., et al. (2018). Addressing women's unmet health care needs in a Canadian remand center: Catalyst for improved health? *Journal of Correctional Health Care*, *24*(3), 276–94. https://doi.org/10.1177/1078345818780731

Borschmann, R., Janca, E., Carter, A., et al. (2020). The health of adolescents in detention: A global scoping review. *The Lancet Public Health*, *5*(2), e114–e126. https://doi.org/10.1016/S2468-2667(19)30217-8

Bouchaud, M.T., Brooks, M. & Swan, B.A. (2018). A retrospective analysis of nursing students' clinical experience in an all-male maximum security prison. *Nurse Educator*, *43*(4), 210–14. https://doi.org/10.1097/NNE.0000000000000467

Bright, A.-M., Higgins, A. & Grealish, A. (2023). Women's experiences of prison-based mental healthcare: A systematic review of qualitative literature. *International Journal of Prisoner Health*, *19*(2), 181–98. https://doi.org/10.1108/IJPH-09-2021-0091

Brooke, J. (2020). Healthcare provision in prison. In J. Brooke (ed.), *Dementia in Prison: An Ethical Framework to Support Research, Practice and Prisoners* (pp. 21–43). Routledge. https://doi.org/10.4324/9780429291043

Burton, J. (2023). The emergence of custodial health nursing as a specialty whose time has come: An Australian experience. *International Nursing Review*, *70*(3), 273–8. https://doi.org/10.1111/inr.12815

Burton, J., Chiarella, M. & Waters, D. (2022). Historical context of custodial health nursing in New South Wales, Australia. *Journal of Forensic Nursing*, *18*(4), 221–8. https://doi.org/10.1097/JFN.0000000000000357

Caro, A.I. (2021). The role of prison nursing: An integrative review. *Revista Espanola de Sanidad Penitenciaria*, *23*(2), 76–85. https://doi.org/10.18176/resp.00034

Corrective Services Administrators' Council (CSAC). (2018). *Guiding principles for Corrections in Australia*. CSAC. www.corrections.vic.gov.au/guiding-principles-for-corrections-in-australia

Dennard, S., Tracy, D.K., Beeney, A., et al. (2021). Working in a prison: Challenges, rewards, and the impact on mental health and well-being. *Journal of Forensic Practice*, *23*(2), 132–49. https://doi.org/10.1108/JFP-12-2020-0055

Dickens, G.L., O'Shea, L.E. & Christensen, M. (2020). Structured assessments for imminent aggression in mental health and correctional settings: Systematic review and meta-analysis. *International Journal of Nursing Studies*, *104*, 103526. https://doi.org/10.1016/j.ijnurstu.2020.103526

Fields, L., Perkiss, S., Dean, B.A. & Moroney, T. (2021). Nursing and the sustainable development goals: A scoping review. *Journal of Nursing Scholarship*, *53*(5), 568–77. https://doi.org/10.1111/jnu.12675

Goddard, D., De Vries, K., McIntosh, T. & Theodosius, C. (2019). Prison nurses' professional identity. *Journal of Forensic Nursing*, *15*(3), 163–71. https://doi.org/10.1097/JFN.0000000000000239

Gorman, G., Singer, R.M., Christmas, E., et al. (2018). In a spirit of restoration: A phenomenology of nursing practice and the criminal justice system. *Advances in Nursing Science*, *41*(2), 105–17. https://doi.org/10.1097/ANS.0000000000000210

Gould, L.A. & Brent, J.J. (2020). *Routledge Handbook on American Prisons*. Routledge.

Hancock, S.L. (2020). The emotional burden of the correctional health care advanced practice nurse. *Journal of Correctional Health Care*, *26*(4), 315–26. https://doi.org/10.1177/1078345820953219

Ismail, N., Lazaris, A., O'Moore, É., Plugge, E. & Stürup-Toft, S. (2021). Leaving no one behind in prison: improving the health of people in prison as a key contributor to meeting the Sustainable Development Goals 2030. *BMJ Global Health*, *6*(3), e004252. https://doi.org/10.1136/bmjgh-2020-004252

Justice Health NSW. (n.d.). *Our Health Services*. NSW Government. https://www.nsw.gov.au/health/justicehealth/patients-families-carers/our-health-services

——— (2023a). *10 Year Strategic Plan 2023–32*. NSW Government. www.nsw.gov.au/sites/default/files/2023-07/224410-justice-health-strategic-plan_con8-signed.pdf

——— (2023b). *Our careers*. NSW Government. www.nsw.gov.au/health/justicehealth/work-with-us

Lafferty, L., Chambers, G.M., Guthrie, J., Butler, T. & Treloar, C. (2018). Measuring social capital in the prison setting: Lessons learned from the Inmate Social Capital Questionnaire. *Journal of Correctional Health Care*, *24*(4), 407–17. https://doi.org/10.1177/1078345818793141

Lazzari, T., Terzoni, S., Destrebecq, A., et al. (2020). Moral distress in correctional nurses: A national survey. *Nursing Ethics*, *27*(1), 40–52. https://doi.org/10.1177/0969733019834976

Marel, C., Siedlecka, E., Fisher, A., et al. (2022). *Guidelines on the Management of Co-occurring Alcohol and Other Drug and Mental Health Conditions in Alcohol and Other Drug Treatment Settings* (3rd ed.). The Matilda Centre for Research in Mental Health and Substance Use, The University of Sydney. https://comorbidityguidelines.org.au/pdf/comorbidity-guideline.pdf

Marshall, L.A., Adams, E.A. & Stuckey, M.I. (2019). Relationships, experience, and support: Staff perception of safety in a forensic mental health facility. *Journal of Forensic Psychiatry & Psychology*, *30*(5), 824–35. https://doi.org/10.1080/14789949.2019.1642368

McLeod, K.E., Butler, A., Young, J.T., et al. (2020). Global prison health care governance and health equity: A critical lack of evidence. *American Journal of Public Health*, *110*(3), 303–8. https://doi.org/10.2105/AJPH.2019.305465

Mehay, A., Meek, R. & Ogden, J. (2021). Understanding and supporting the health literacy of young men in prison: A mixed-methods study. *Health Education*, *121*(1), 93–110. https://doi.org/10.1108/HE-08-2020-0076

Minister for Corrections. (2023). *Cultural Review of the Adult Custodial Corrections System, Aboriginal participants and cultural safety*. Government of Victoria. https://www.vic.gov.au/sites/default/files/2023-03/Victorian-Government-response-to-the-Cultural-Review-of-the-Adult-Custodial-Corrections-System_.pdf

New South Wales (NSW) Health. (2021). *Handbook for Nurses and Midwives: Responding Effectively to People Who Use Alcohol and Other Drugs*. NSW Government. www.health.nsw.gov.au/aod/professionals/Publications/handbook-nurses-aod.pdf

Oates, J., Topping, A., Ezhova, I., Wadey, E. & Marie Rafferty, A. (2020). An integrative review of nursing staff experiences in high secure forensic mental health settings: Implications for recruitment and retention strategies. *Journal of Advanced Nursing, 76*(11), 2897–908. https://doi.org/10.1111/jan.14521

Oranga Tamariki Ministry for Children. (2023). *Youth justice residences*. New Zealand Government. www.orangatamariki.govt.nz/youth-justice/youth-justice-residences/

Peternelj-Taylor, C. & Woods, P. (2019). Saskatchewan provincial correctional nurses: Roles, responsibilities, and learning needs. *Journal of Correctional Health Care, 25*(2), 1078345819833661. https://doi.org/10.1177/1078345819833661

Ramaswamy, M. & Freudenberg, N. (2022). Health promotion in jails and prisons: An alternative paradigm for correctional health services. In R.B. Greifinger (ed.), *Public Health Behind Bars: From Prisons to Communities* (pp. 219–38). Springer. https://doi.org/10.1007/978-0-387-71695-4_13

Rose, A., Trounson, J., Skues, J., et al. (2019). Psychological wellbeing, distress and coping in Australian Indigenous and multicultural prisoners: A mixed methods analysis. *Psychiatry, Psychology and Law, 26*(6), 886–903. https://doi.org/10.1080/13218719.2019.1642259

Sasso, L., Delogu, B., Carrozzino, R., Aleo, G. & Bagnasco, A. (2018). Ethical issues of prison nursing: A qualitative study in Northern Italy. *Nursing Ethics, 25*(3), 393–409. https://doi.org/10.1177/0969733016639760

Shelton, D., Maruca, A.T. & Wright, R. (2020). Nursing in the American justice system. *Archives of Psychiatric Nursing, 34*(5), 304–9. https://doi.org/10.1016/j.apnu.2020.07.019

Solell, P. & Smith, K. (2019). If we truly cared: Understanding barriers to person-centred nursing in correctional facilities. *International Practice Development Journal, 9*(2), 7. https://doi.org/10.19043/ipdj.92.007

Spycher, J., Dusheiko, M., Beaupère, P., Gravier, B. & Moschetti, K. (2021). Healthcare in a pure gatekeeping system: Utilization of primary, mental and emergency care in the prison population over time. *Health & Justice, 9*(1), 1–16. https://doi.org/10.1186/s40352-021-00136-8

Trimmer, W., Fuller, C., Kake, C. & Asbury, E. (2019). Collaborative primary mental health education for correctional nurses. *Journal of Correctional Health Care, 25*(1), 55–64. https://doi.org/10.1177/1078345818819885

United Nations Department of Economic and Social Affairs (UN DESA). (2023). *The 17 Goals*. https://sdgs.un.org/goals

United Nations Office on Drugs and Crime (UNODC). (2015). *The United Nations Standard Minimum Rules for the Treatment of Prisoners (the Nelson Mandela Rules)*. www.unodc.org/documents/justice-and-prison-reform/Nelson_Mandela_Rules-E-ebook.pdf

United Nations Human Rights Office of the High Commissioner (OHCHR). (1990). *Basic Principles for the Treatment of Prisoners*. United Nations. https://www.ohchr.org/en/instruments-mechanisms/instruments/basic-principles-treatment-prisoners

Winkelman, T.N., Dasrath, K.C., Young, J.T. & Kinner, S.A. (2022). Universal health coverage and incarceration. *The Lancet Public Health, 7*(6), e569–e572. https://doi.org/10.1016/S2468-2667(22)00113-X

Wong, I., Wright, E., Santomauro, D., et al. (2018). Implementing two nurse practitioner models of service at an Australian male prison: A quality assurance study. *Journal of Clinical Nursing 27*(1–2), e287–e300. https://doi.org/10.1111/jocn.13935

Woods, P. & Peternelj-Taylor, C. (2022). Correctional nursing in Canada's Prairie provinces: Roles, responsibilities, and learning needs. *Canadian Journal of Nursing Research, 54*(1), 59–71. https://doi.org/10.1177/0844562121999282

World Health Organization (WHO). (2003). *Declaration on prison health as part of public health: adopted in Moscow on 24 October 2003*. https://apps.who.int/iris/handle/10665/352130

——— (2022). *Health in prisons: addressing the public health gap to ensure that no one is left behind*. www.who.int/europe/multi-media/item/health-in-prisons-addressing-the-public-health-gap-to-ensure-that-no-one-is-left-behind

Nurse practitioners

Kathleen Tori

26

LEARNING OBJECTIVES

At the completion of this chapter, you should be able to:

- discuss the key attributes that contribute to the nurse practitioner's (NP's) role.
- discuss the scope of practice of primary health care (PHC) NPs.
- compare the NP scope of practice with other community nursing roles.
- explore the career progression for nurses considering the NP role in the Australian and Aotearoa New Zealand contexts.

Introduction

Nurse practitioners (NPs) are a valued addition to the PHC team and are well-placed to increase accessibility to quality health care services while offering consumer choice (Kelly et al., 2017). NPs have undertaken advanced education and clinical training. In addition, they have demonstrated their competency, capacity and capability to provide high-quality, effective and efficient clinically focused health care delivery (Nursing and Midwifery Board of Australia (NMBA), 2023). Although many NPs practise in rural or underserviced communities, NPs practise across a diverse range of health care settings, delivering either specialist or generalist health services. Recognised as advanced practice nurses (APNs) internationally and nationally, the NP role has emerged as a response to meet the challenges of rising health care demand and is proving effective in promoting transformational changes within the PHC sector (Grant et al., 2017; Jennings, Lowe & Tori, 2021). The NP's role is a blended model of health care in which the nurse seamlessly combines advanced diagnostic and therapeutic interventional nursing care in clinical practice when assessing, treating and caring for patients (Tori, 2017). In PHC, the role of the NP is to augment health care provision, either in collaboration with medical professionals or independently, to enable greater access to health services for all patients, particularly in socio-economically disadvantaged communities, Indigenous and priority populations (Ortiz et al., 2018; Poghosyan et al., 2018; Wilson et al., 2021).

Combining their advanced nursing knowledge and skills with diagnostic reasoning and therapeutic knowledge, NPs have the legal authority to practise beyond the level of a registered nurse (RN) and can effectively provide health care for a range of common and complex

Nurse practitioners (NPs) – nurse practitioners are registered nurses who have undertaken the relevant approved programs of study and are endorsed to practise within their scope under the legislatively protected title 'nurse practitioner' (NMBA, 2023, pp. 3–4), in Australia or have the legal authority to practise beyond the level of a registered nurse in Aotearoa New Zealand (Ministry of Health, 2024).

conditions (Ministry of Health, 2024). As such NPs can augment current health care provision, offering increased accessibility to affordable and high-quality health care (Barraclough, Longman & Barclay, 2016; Jennings et al., 2021). However, with barriers to enabling full implementation of the NP role, in the Australian and Aotearoa New Zealand contexts, the uptake and envisaged benefits of NPs in primary health care environments have yet to be realised (Rossiter et al., 2023).

NPs are well-established within the nursing profession internationally, having been in existence in varying contexts since the 1960s in the United States and the 1980s in the United Kingdom (Currie, Chiarella & Buckley, 2015). Most international NPs are employed within PHC settings, particularly in the United States, where as many as 90 per cent of NPs practise within the community (Poghosyan et al., 2018). While noting the argument that NPs can be viewed as general practitioner (GP) 'replacements' (Carryer & Adams, 2022, p. e36), the NP role should be seen as one that extends the traditional biomedicine model while remaining underpinned by the nursing paradigm, an extended and advanced nursing role which remains true to the philosophy of nursing (Carryer & Adams, 2022).

NPs were introduced into the Australian health care system over 23 years ago (Rossiter et al., 2023). In Aotearoa New Zealand, the NP role was first mooted following a Ministerial Taskforce in 1998, where the NP role was viewed as a way to improve access to health services (Carryer & Adams, 2022, p. e36; Scanlon et al., 2018) and was formally introduced in 2001 (Adams et al., 2022). Although the development of the NP role and increase in numbers of NPs in Australia and Aotearoa New Zealand has been relatively slow over the past two decades (Adams et al., 2022; Currie et al., 2015; Whitehead et al., 2022), the NP role represents a growing workforce in both countries. In Australia, there are now over 2656 endorsed NPs (NMBA, 2024), while in Aotearoa New Zealand some 60 per cent of the approximately 300 NPs practise in PHC settings (Adams et al., 2022; Ministry of Health, 2024). The role of the NP in both countries is regulated by the relevant health professional regulatory boards and accredited postgraduate master's degree courses must be undertaken prior to applying for endorsement as an NP. The Australian NP role has been recognised with a legislatively protected title that only endorsed or authorised NPs can use (NMBA, 2023), whereas the Aotearoa New Zealand NP role has a separate legislated scope of practice to that of the RN, but the 'title' is not protected (Ministry of Health, 2024).

Scope of practice

Globally, NPs have an integral role within their respective health care systems (Scanlon et al., 2018). Contemporary NPs are defined by their specialty practice area (for example, primary care, palliative care, emergency care) and their designated scope of practice (Scanlon et al., 2015). The scope of practice enables NPs to manage episodes of care as a primary provider and/or as part of a collaborative care team. It is influenced by the context in which NPs practise, the policy requirements of the service provider and their level of education, confidence and competence. In Australia, it is also determined by permissions under national and state legislative and regulatory requirements governing the NP role (NMBA, 2023; Scanlon et al., 2015). The NP's scope of practice is further bounded by legislative amendments and jurisdictional regulatory decisions that are implemented and contextually different depending on the country and state or territory the NP practices in (Scanlon et al., 2015).

Consider your current scope of practice and reflect upon the following:

1. What legislation, regulations, standards of practice and/or organisational policies govern and influence your professional practice?
2. Reflecting on your most recent clinical placement, what information did you have to take into consideration to ensure you were practising within your scope of practice?

Career progression to nurse practitioner

NPs are RNs who are educated to practise in a range of clinical contexts collaboratively and /or independently (Rossiter et al., 2023). The legislated scope of the NP, in Australian and Aotearoa New Zealand contexts, builds upon that of the RN and is the highest clinical designation within the nursing profession (Victorian Department of Health, 2017). Once endorsed, NPs can manage episodes of care as the primary provider of care, including wellness-focused care, autonomously or as part of collaborative health care teams. The NP role enables experienced nurses to extend their scope of practice to include advanced assessment, initiating and interpreting diagnostic investigations, referrals to other health care practitioners, and prescribing (or deprescribing if necessary) medications (Wilson et al., 2021). In effect, NPs are able to provide care for their clients for the full episode of care – from presentation through to disposition, depending on the context in which they practise – and, as such, they have proven integral to the provision of high-quality, safe, efficient and effective PHC (Halcomb et al., 2016).

The practice of the NP is differentiated from other levels of nursing as it integrates education, leadership, research, management, consultation, service evaluation and clinical decision-making that are inherent in advanced and extended nursing positions (Woods & Murfet, 2015). It enables the career path for clinical RNs to be extended, while at the same time acknowledging that the NP role remains embedded within 'the nursing profession's values, knowledge, theories and practices and provides innovative, flexible health care delivery that embraces the true philosophy of nursing' (Carryer & Adams, 2022).

For endorsement as an NP in Australia, RNs must complete either an Australian Nursing and Midwifery Accreditation Council (ANMAC) accredited master's level degree course (referred to as 'Pathway 1') or apply for equivalency under the 'Pathway 2' avenue (NMBA, 2016). For an educational provider (university) to be accredited by the ANMAC to provide an NP master's program, it must ensure 'that graduate[s] have the common and transferable skills, knowledge, behaviours, and attributes required to practice' (ANMAC, 2015, p. 9). Core components of a typical accredited NP master's program include academic and administrative governance and clinically focused subjects, such as advanced physical assessment, differential diagnoses, radiology, pathology and pharmacology subjects, that prepare the NP for advanced practice (ANMAC, 2015). Prerequisites for entry into most Australian NP programs are relatively consistent and include three years of full-time (or equivalent part-time) advanced clinical practice and postgraduate clinical specialty education in which the NP intends to apply for endorsement.

The endorsement pathway for NP roles under Aotearoa New Zealand legislation is similar the Australian pathway. In Aotearoa New Zealand, RNs must demonstrate a minimum of four years in a specific specialty area and the successful completion of a master's degree, including advanced practice nursing and prescribing competencies incorporating theoretical and concurrent clinical practice components (Ministry of Health, 2024). Additionally, the RN seeking approval to practise as an NP must pass a panel assessment that focuses on NP competencies and must have completed 300 hours of supervised clinical practice (Ministry of Health, 2024).

PHC NPs

It should be noted that PHC NPs are not only located within the rural or remote regions; they are also actively employed within the more populated areas and augment general practice teams (Helms, Crookes & Bailey, 2015). With increasing emphasis on health education, health promotion, illness prevention and effective management of chronic conditions, PHC refers to the types of care rather than the geographical location of the service delivery (see Chapter 1). Primarily, the PHC NP works with a variety of health care services to ensure that optimal care is provided. This includes liaising with local hospital networks, planning and coordinating care, integrating health care delivery with other health care practitioners, problem-solving with colleagues, and arranging or providing ongoing monitoring and evaluation of interventions.

The PHC NP role was designed to improve access to appropriate health care at a reduced cost to the consumer and the health care system, and also target at-risk populations (Jennings et al., 2021; Rossiter et al., 2023), effectively addressing health service 'gaps' (Clifford et al., 2020). The introduction of PHC NPs offered an alternate health provider, effectively allowing nurses to formally undertake primary care clinical activities previously considered only the domain of the GP, both augmenting current services and offering nurse-led care options. With the majority of GPs located in 'urban, affluent areas and lower numbers and poorer doctor/patient ratios in rural and poor areas' (Carter, Owen-Williams & Della, 2015, p. 647), the introduction of the PHC NP was:

- seen as a way to meet the challenge of providing the increased need for PHC in geographically diverse communities
- a method of empowering local communities, being driven by the search for cost-effective, quality health services targeting at-risk populations
- a way of delivering equivalent health care outcomes for a wide range of complex, acute or chronic conditions (Carryer & Adams, 2022).

The presence of the PHC NP has realised many benefits in the provision of health care and offers a committed approach to improving patient health outcomes (Halcomb et al., 2016). The PHC NP can enhance service delivery in several ways, including client-focused benefits such as improved access, longer consults, improved continuity, decreased fragmentation of care and increased patient satisfaction. The introduction of the PHC NP role addresses the needs of the community by significantly reducing avoidable admissions to urgent care or emergency departments for presentations within their scope of practice, effectively reducing associated admissions and ambulance transports to larger health facilities outside the community catchment area (Department of Health, 2019). Figure 26.1 explores the flexibility, breadth and overview of the scope of practice of a PHC NP. Carter and colleagues (2015) note: 'Australian NPs are well positioned to meet the emerging increased demand for primary care' (p. 650), a view that is mooted by other contemporary authors of NP research (Jenning et al., 2021; Rossiter et al., 2023) and particularly for rural health facilities (Mills, Giles & Hooker, 2023). Contemporary research indicates that the PHC NP contributes effectively to addressing the increased demands for primary care in Australia (Currie et al., 2020) and Aotearoa, New Zealand (Adams & Carryer, 2021).

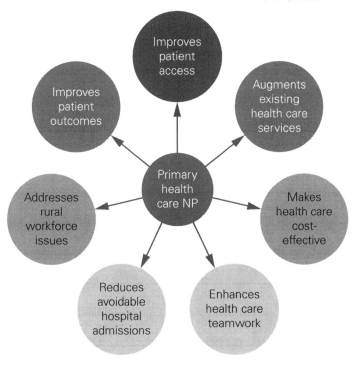

Figure 26.1   The PHC NP
Source: Adapted from Adams & Carryer (2021); Jennings et al. (2021); Rossiter et al. (2023).

REFLECTION

1. What types of conditions do you think the PHC NP would be able to see and treat within community settings?
2. With whom do you think the PHC NP collaborates in the coordination of health care?

CASE STUDY 26.1

Mr Rogers is an 83-year-old man who has been recently referred to the NP from the community clinic for opinion and treatment following a short stay in the local health facility for general deterioration in health status.

He had been undergoing treatment for a right heel ulcer for 18 months. During this time, Mr Rogers was often non-compliant with attending the clinic at designated dates

CASE STUDY 26.1 Continued

and times to have review assessments and dressings organised for him, often only making every third scheduled visit which coincided with when he came into town for other supplies, or when one of his daughters was able to bring him. Home visits by the Home Nursing Service were not initially an option as Mr Rogers, being a very independent and private person, had previously refused access on numerous occasions.

With a history of multiple medical, mental health, social and chronic pain issues, Mr Rogers has had extensive and frequent inpatient stays at the local hospital, particularly over the past six months. During his last admission, he was referred to the NP, who could meet and assess him the next day while he was still in hospital. The NP was also included in the discharge planning meeting with Mr Rogers and his immediate family. At this meeting, Mr Rogers, urged by his daughters, agreed to allow follow-up and care at his home scheduled for a few days post-discharge.

Under the NP's care, the planned dressing schedule by the Home Nursing Service has been re-established. The NP has enabled several referral and health care linkages with other services and supports to be implemented, such as the aged care mental health service, social worker referrals and aged care assessment services. All of these have been accepted by Mr Rogers with encouragement from his daughters. Specialist referrals included a dermatologist and the commencement of peripheral vascular disease investigations in collaboration with the GP clinic. Seeing the benefits of having the NP supporting his care, Mr Rogers remains compliant with his suggested health care arrangements and now understands the need for additional health care team services.

REFLECTION

1. Why do you think Mr Rogers was agreeable with the health care plan that the NP arranged?
2. What may have been the consequences for Mr Rogers' overall health if he had not agreed to accept the suggested multidisciplinary health care plan?

CASE STUDY 26.2

Mrs Jones, a 64-year-old female with advanced cancer, has recently been admitted to the palliative care ward of a large regional hospital. She is a retired nurse and a farmer's wife and for most of her life, has resided in a small rural community, marrying locally and raising her children on the outskirts of town. Her family has difficulty visiting her, as her elderly husband does not drive, there is very limited local transport and her sons live interstate. Mrs Jones does not want to be in the large regional facility and has expressed the preference to 'die at home'.

Mrs Jones is experiencing uncontrolled pain, nausea and vomiting from prescribed medications. She has also been diagnosed with severe depression due to being away from home, feeling isolated and her poor prognosis. At the request of the family, the NP organised a visit to Mrs Jones at the hospital which resulted in a case management meeting with the palliative care consultant. Following this initial meeting, Mrs Jones is transferred to the local rural hospital, with support put in place for a holistic assessment and care review.

During her stay, the NP checks that her medications can be prescribed and administered at home and arranges for home support visits to be set up by the palliative care and NP so that Mrs Jones can be transferred directly to her home. This is welcomed by Mrs Jones and her family, and all feel well supported by the collaborative approach to her care.

Mrs Jones passes away a few days after she was transferred home, comfortable at home and surrounded by her family and friends.

REFLECTION

1. Why do you think it was important for Mrs Jones to pass away in her home community, in particular, her home environment?
2. What may have been the consequences for Mrs Jones' family if the NP had not been able to organise the transfer?

Conclusion

The NP movement has gathered momentum in the Australian and Aotearoa New Zealand health care systems. NPs in both countries increase health care accessibility, safely and efficiently, by providing care to existing services. Research demonstrates that the NP role can contribute to the growing primary care health demands within the community and is pivotal in improving access to care and to patient outcomes.

CRITICAL THINKING ACTIVITIES

1. Consider the likely benefits for communities that have NPs.
2. Consider the considerations that the NP would need to take into account when arranging health care plans for patients.
3. In your words, how would you describe the role of the NP? How is this role different to that of the registered nurse?

FURTHER READING

Australian College of Nurse Practitioners (ACNP). (2024). *Home page.* www.acnp.org.au

Ministry of Health. (2024) *Nurse practitioners in New Zealand.* New Zealand Government. https://www.health.govt.nz/strategies-initiatives/programmes-and-initiatives/nursing/nurses-in-new-zealand/nurse-practitioners

Nursing and Midwifery Board of Australia (NMBA). (2016). *Registration Standard: Endorsement as a Nurse Practitioner.* www.nursingmidwiferyboard.gov.au/Registration-Standards/Endorsement-as-a-nurse-practitioner.aspx

REFERENCES

Adams, S. & Carryer, J. (2021). How the institutional and policy context shapes the establishment of nurse practitioner roles and practice in New Zealand's primary health care sector. *Policy, Politics, & Nursing Practice 22*(1), 17–27.

Adams, S., Mustafa, M., Bareham, C., et al. (2022). The organizational climate for Nurse Practitioners working in primary health care in New Zealand: A national study. *The Journal for Nurse Practitioners, 18*(7), 736–40. https://doi.org/10.1016/j.nurpra.2022.04.024

Australian Nursing and Midwifery Accreditation Council (ANMAC). (2015). *Nurse Practitioner Accreditation Standards.* ANMAC.

Barraclough, F., Longman, J. & Barclay, L. (2016). Integration in nurse practitioner-led mental health service in rural Australia. *Australian Journal of Rural Health, 24*, 144–50.

Carryer, J. & Adams, S. (2022) Valuing the paradigm of nursing: Can nurse practitioners resist medicalization to transform healthcare? *Journal of Advanced Nursing, 78*(2), e36–e38. https://doi.org/10.1111/jan.15082

Carter, M.A., Owen-Williams, E. & Della, P. (2015). Meeting Australia's emerging primary care needs by nurse practitioners. *The Journal for Nurse Practitioners, 11*(6), 647–52.

Clifford, S., Lutze, M., Maw, M. & Jennings, N. (2020). Establishing value from contemporary nurse practitioners' perceptions of the role: A preliminary study into purpose, support and priorities. *Collegian, 27*(1), 95–101. https://doi.org/10.1016/j.colegn.2019.05.006

Currie, J., Carter, M., Lutze, M. & Edwards, L. (2020) Preparing Australian Nurse Practitioners to meet health care demand. *The Journal for Nurse Practitioners, 16*(8), 629–33. https://doi.org/10.1016/j.nurpra.2020.06.023

Currie, J., Chiarella, M. & Buckley, T. (2015). Preparing a realist evaluation to investigate the impact of privately practicing nurse practitioners on patient access to care in Australia. *International Journal of Nursing, 2*(2), 1–10.

Department of Health. (2019). *Cost Benefit Analysis of Nurse Practitioner Models of Care.* KPMG. www.health.gov.au/resources/publications/cost-benefit-analysis-of-nurse-practitioner-models-of-care?language=en

Grant, J., Lines, L., Darbyshire, P. & Parry, Y. (2017). How do nurse practitioners work in primary health care settings? A scoping review. *International Journal of Nursing Studies, 75*, 51–7.

Halcomb, E., Stephens, M., Bryce, J., Foley, E. & Ashley, C. (2016). Nursing competency standards in primary health care: An integrated review. *Journal of Clinical Nursing, 25*(9–10), 1193–205. https://doi.org/10.1111/jocn.13224

Helms, C., Crookes, J. & Bailey, D. (2015). Financial viability, benefits and challenges of employing a nurse practitioner in general practice. *Australian Health Review, 39*, 205–10.

Jennings, N., Lowe, G. & Tori, K. (2021) Nurse practitioner locums: A plausible solution for improving sub-regional healthcare access. *Australian Journal of Primary Health. 27*, 1–5. https://doi.org/10.1071/PY20103

Kelly, J., Garvey, D., Biro, M. & Lee, S. (2017). Managing medical service delivery gaps in a socially disadvantaged rural community: A nurse practitioner-led clinic. *Australian Journal of Advanced Nursing, 34*(4), 42–9.

Mills, J., Giles, F. & Hooker, L. (2023, February 6). With training to diagnose, test, prescribe and discharge, nurse practitioners could help rescue rural health. *The Conversation.* https://theconversation.com/with-the-training-to-diagnose-test-prescribe-and-discharge-nurse-practitioners-could-help-rescue-rural-health-199287

Ministry of Health. (2024). *Nurse practitioners in New Zealand.* New Zealand Government. www.health.govt.nz/strategies-initiatives/programmes-and-initiatives/nursing/nurses-in-new-zealand/nurse-practitioners

Nursing and Midwifery Board of Australia (NMBA). (2016). *Registration Standard: Endorsement as a Nurse Practitioner*. www.nursingmidwiferyboard.gov.au/Registration-Standards/Endorsement-as-a-nurse-practitioner.aspx

———— (2023). *Nurse Practitioner Standards for Practice*. www.nursingmidwiferyboard.gov.au/Codes-Guidelines-Statements/FAQ/Nurse-practitioner-standards-for-practice.aspx

———— (2024). *Nurse and Midwife Registration Data Table – 30 June 2023*. www.nursingmidwiferyboard.gov.au/About/Statistics.aspx

Ortiz, J., Hofler, R., Bushy, A., et al. (2018). Impact of nurse practitioner practice regulation on rural population outcomes. *Healthcare, 6*(2), 65. https://doi.org/10.3390/healthcare6020065

Poghosyan, L., Norful, A.A., Liu, J. & Friedberg, M.W. (2018). Nurse practitioner practice environments in primary care and quality of care for chronic diseases. *Medical Care, 56*(9), 791–7.

Rossiter, R., Phillips, R., Blanchard, D., Wissen, K. & Robinson, T. (2023). Exploring nurse practitioner practice in Australian rural primary health care settings: A scoping review. *Australian Journal of Rural Health, 31*(4), 617–30. https://doi.org/10.1111/ajr.13010

Scanlon, A., Cashin, A., Bryce, J., Kelly, J.G. & Buckley, T. (2016). The complexities of defining nurse practitioner scope of practice in the Australian context. *Collegian, 23*(1), 129–42.

Scanlon, A., Murphy, M., Tori, K. & Poghosyan, L. (2018). A national study of Australian nurse practitioners' organizational practice environment. *Journal for Nurse Practitioners, 14*(5), 414–18.

Scanlon, A., Smolowitz, J., Honig, J. & Barnes, K. (2015). Building the next generation of advanced practice nurses through clinical education and faculty practice: Three international perspectives. *Clinical Scholars Review, 8*(2), 249–57.

Tori, K.E. (2017). *The role of the emergency nurse practitioner: An ethnographic study [Unpublished doctoral thesis]*. La Trobe University.

Victorian Department of Health. (2017). *Urgent Care Centres: Models of Care Toolkit Rural Health Urgent Care Centres*. TDC3 Richmond. Victorian Government.

Wilson, E., Hanson, L.C., Tori, K.E. & Perrin, B.M. (2021). Nurse practitioner led model of after-hours emergency care in a rural urgent care centre: Health service staff and stakeholder perceptions. *BMC Health Services Research, 21*(1), 1–11. https://doi.org/10.1186/s12913-021-06864-9

Whitehead, L., Twigg, D.E., Carman, R., et al. (2022) Factors influencing the development and implementation of nurse practitioner candidacy programs: A scoping review. *International Journal of Nursing Studies, 125*, 104133. https://doi.org/10.1016/j.ijnurstu.2021.104133

Woods, M. & Murfet, G. (2015). Australian nurse practitioner practice: Value adding through clinical reflexivity. *Nursing Research and Practice*, 1–14. https://doi.org/10.1155/2015/829593

Postface

The world we live in is constantly changing. However, in recent years, these changes have been especially rapid and have had a significant impact on the way that people live. The COVID-19 pandemic highlighted the impact of the social determinants of health, transforming how many view and experience health and well-being. COVID-19 has also negatively impacted a range of social and economic factors within our communities. As many countries face economic downturn, issues such as food insecurity and housing affordability are rising in prominence. At the same time, the world is facing increasing impacts of climate change and more frequent natural hazard events such as bushfires, floods, and earthquakes (Inglis et al., 2023). All of these changes impact the physical and mental health of our community (Halcomb et al., 2023; Thompson et al., 2024). In whatever setting they work, nurses play a key role in supporting individuals, families and communities to adapt to these new conditions and maintain health and well-being.

In Australia and Aotearoa New Zealand, government policy is placing an increasing emphasis on primary health care and community-based health services to meet the needs of aging populations and emerging health needs (Australian Government, 2022; Department of Health and Aged Care, 2022; Health New Zealand, 2024; Ministry of Justice, 2021). Broadly, such policy seeks to strengthen the role of nurses within the multidisciplinary primary health care team and develop advanced practice roles for nurses to work to an extended scope of practice. These changes create a range of opportunities for nurses to seek and forge diverse and exciting new career pathways outside of the hospital. Capitalising on such an opportunity requires the nursing profession and individual nurses to continue contributing to, and advocating for, socially-just health and health care underpinned by primary health care principles. Nurses need to be at the table as new services are being co-designed and planned. Nurses need to highlight the full extent of their practice scope and the contribution that they can make as health professionals to team-based care. Finally, nurses need to be creative and innovative in applying their skills to the health system and care needs of the community. It is an exciting time to be entering the nursing profession or looking to enter the community and primary health care sector. Now, more than ever, the community's health and well-being are dependent on a strong health workforce. As the contexts of practice are shifting in the community, nurses need to embrace the growth that this provides for the profession and the opportunity this provides for their career and professional development.

REFERENCES

Australian Government. (2022). *Strengthening Medicare Taskforce Report.* Australian Government. www.health.gov.au/sites/default/files/2023-02/strengthening-medicare-taskforce-report_0.pdf

Department of Health and Aged Care. (2022). *Future Focused Primary Health Care: Australia's Primary Health Care 10 Year Plan 2022–2032.* Commonwealth of Australia. www.health.gov.au/resources/publications/australias-primary-health-care-10-year-plan-2022-2032

Halcomb, E., Thompson, C., Morris, D., et al. (2023). Impacts of the 2019/20 bushfires and COVID-19 pandemic on the physical and mental health of older Australians: a cross-sectional survey [Primary care]. *Family Practice, 40*(3), 449–57. https://doi.org/10.1093/fampra/cmac138

Health New Zealand. (2024). *Te Aka Whai Ora: Maori Health Authority.* New Zealand Government. www.teakawhaiora.nz/

Inglis, S., Ferguson, C., Eddington, R., et al. (2023). Cardiovascular nursing and climate change: A call to action from the CSANZ Cardiovascular Nursing Council. *Heart, Lung and Circulation, 32*, 16–25. https://doi.org/10.1016/j.hlc.2022.10.007

Ministry of Justice. (2021). *Health Services and Outcomes Inquiry (Wai 2575).* New Zealand Government. www.health.govt.nz/maori-health/wai-2575-health-services-and-outcomes-inquiry

Thompson, C., Dilworth, T., James, S., et al. (2024). The self-care of older Australians during bushfires and COVID-19: A qualitative study. *Disaster Medicine and Public Health Preparedness, 18*, e219. https://doi.org/10.1017/dmp.2024.96

Index

Printed in the United States
by Baker & Taylor Publisher Services